My Best Regards for
Your Health & Happiness
Howard T. Knoblock

An American Pediatrician's Odyssey

My Life and Memoirs
Composed at Nine Decades

Howard Thomas Knobloch, M.D.

Associate Clinical Professor of Pediatrics,
Michigan State University of Medicine, Emeritus

WingSpan Press

Printed in the United States of America

Published by WingSpan Press, Livermore, CA
www.wingspanpress.com

ISBN 978-1-59594-155-8

First edition 2007

Library of Congress Control Number 2007925487

Dedication

I hereby dedicate my book as a legacy to my children in their order of birth:

1. Susan Caroline, including thanks for her indefatigable typing of the first part of the book. "Suzy" in fact was the prime instigator and motivator for my writing this book. She was my constant guiding light and inspiration. She got the ball rolling.

2. John Howard Thomas, including thanks for his part in securing, along with Susan and Melissa, typing of the rest of the book. They also were mighty inspirational and motivating in the book's writing.

3. Gregory Haines, including thanks for his preparation of the book photographs and cover. Greg is a professional photographer extraordinaire in his own right, and quite passionate and innovative in his work.

4. Melissa Mary, the caboose, including thanks for her efforts as producer of this book. She was also indispensable as chief cook, organizer, and editor. "Lissa" is also very enthusiastic, a tireless worker, full of great ideas, and has a very sweet disposition to boot.

I am grateful to my progeny for all of their indispensable contributions in the formulation of my book.

I dedicate my book to my parents, Margaret Reamer and Howard Harrer Knobloch, who supported and encouraged me through medical school; to both of my wives – Doris Mathilde, to whom I was married 24 years and was the mother of all of my children, and Mildred Stephie, with whom I've been these past 42 years; and finally, last but not least, to my three dearest grandchildren, Jon Prengel, Lisa Heidan, and Sara Prengel.

I would also like to thank Joan Cummings and Dr. Farrel LeVasseur for their assistance with the cover photograph for the book.

Contents

Foreword

This book has been a long time in the making, almost 96 years of eventful living by my Father as of the book's publishing date. I am so grateful that he has taken the time to recount his remarkable life in writing and share it with all of us. I wrote the following poem for him to commemorate his 90th birthday, now way back then. I believe this poem fairly evokes his essence:

My Dad

How does he age with such grace?
He ignores it and quickens his pace.

It's medical journals, lectures, dinners and such.
It's the Tigers, the Dead Sea Scrolls - nothing's too much.
Marathon cribbage games, skunks left and right,
Out playing pinochle to wee hours of the night.

Today it's a day trip with family around.
Today we laugh, family stories abound.
We hear about Greg and his shot giving days,
We hear about Tom and his upchucking ways,
How Melissa kept crying til scotch was prescribed,
And Susan was silenced, a pail of water applied.

Who can forget the famed Snow Bowl affair?
Dad's sprint for the train and leap into air.
He caught the caboose and got pulled on in time,
And got to the game to freeze his behind.

What age is his goal? Right now it's 100,
But next time 110, and then add another,
For Dad never ceases to do things anew,
For him time doesn't matter, he'll never be through!

By Melissa Mary Knobloch Meder

Introduction

I feel I was extremely lucky to have lived during the "golden years" era for doctors (1930 to 2000 AD). Physicians were really in control of their destiny and were subservient to no one. Lawyers, HMO plans, industry or insurance companies did not shackle us. Money was secondary, and we truly represented the patients' best interests and health problems. I have never turned one patient away and never closed my practice at any time. I was never away for more than a few days, and then only a few times a year. We did not have all the amazing diagnostic X-ray and lab tools at our disposal. We were fine-tuned in diagnostic judgment; and analysis of diseases was imperative. Cookbook or Armed Service medicine was not in vogue for most of my years. Like firemen, we were "on call" 24 hours a day and ready for all medical demands at a moment's notice at all times. As long as we had the bare necessities of life, we were content and did not strive to build up an empire of wealth. Honesty, loyalty, kindness, and faith in human nature were our prime values. However, times change constantly. As the saying goes, 'mutable semper'.

Medicine has shown an almost cataclysmic change in the past century. It's been a change almost like day and night, much like the change from medieval to modern times. The genetic code or human genome is being dissected in minute detail to eventual completion and this will revolutionize medical practice. Antibiotics are being discovered literally by the dozens to combat bacteria, viruses, mycoses, rickets, parasites, and worms, aerobic and anaerobic mental and emotional disturbances. Medical diagnosis and treatment have advanced immeasurably with new medicines and methods, just like advancing from the dark ages to present times. All body systems and tracts have come under extensive scrutiny with diagnosis, treatment, and prognosis making insurmountable advances in every field. Allergy has exhibited marked forward strides in diagnosis and treatment. There have been remarkable strides made in the life saving measures available for the treatment of accidents and emergencies. We have benefited greatly with the advances during the World Wars in wound care, both medically and surgically. Special problems in the fetus and neonate have been mastered to a remarkable degree. Special problems in adolescence have also had excellent solutions. The treatment of psychiatric illness has catapulted by leaps and bounds since the time Freud reigned supreme. Curative miracle medications have and are being discovered. However, medicine still has many mountains to climb including those solving issues relating to tobacco, alcohol, psychedelic drugs, teen pregnancy, and premature newborn problems.

I remember vividly, when elementary grade classmates would suddenly succumb to diphtheria, typhoid fever, meningitis, shiga infection, pneumonia, grade-A hemolytic strep, erysipelas and brucellosis. I hated to see summer come before the advent of polio immunization because of numerous episodes of paralysis of extremities and especially the bulbar paralytic type. My Professor of Pediatrics at the University of Maryland Medical School died from poliomyelitis at the beginning of my freshman year. I was a pallbearer at my classmate and cousin Amy Mae's funeral, a second grader who died due to complications of scarlet fever. I remember clearly my buddy and neighbor, Carl Foster, who died a victim of salmonellosis at 7 years of age. A paternal aunt died of puerperal sepsis and Irene, my father's sister, died from malignant hyper-thyroidism. It is almost inconceivable to realize the tremendous advances that medicine has made in the field of oncology with diagnosis and treatment. It is like the aphorism "baby you've come a long way". But, pragmatically speaking, we have just opened Pandora's Box and medicine has a long way to go. Man has been on the planet some 75,000 years, but medicine has only actually advanced beyond the basics in the 20th century. Lucky me! Onward, and forward, and upward march!

Please excuse a few vital, mandatory repeat passages in my book due to the necessity for emphasis and logical continuity of the thread of each event. In most instances I am tying up loose ends of the octopus of stories.

Chapter 1

Birth to Two Years Old – Trafford, PA.

My Mother, Margaret Reamer Haines Knobloch, at age 18 years, gave birth to me on a Saturday, June 3, 1911. I was born at 11:30 p.m. in Trafford City, Pennsylvania, just 10 miles east of Pittsburgh, in a second floor apartment above a pharmacy. A general family doctor, J. R. Tilbrook, M.D, attended my Mother. My Mother at age 17 years, had "run off" by train to Cumberland, Maryland, (the Las Vegas marriage capital) to marry my Father, Howard Harrer Knobloch, age 24 years, on 30th June, 1910 A.D.

This was the first marriage for both my parents. Her Father, John Thomas Haines, had debated seriously at 2 a.m. on June 30th about canceling the marriage plans. But, he came to a succinct, favorable decision thinking, "Howard's a good man and Margaret's made up her mind. So she's made her bed, let her lie in it!"

My Mother and Father had a whirlwind courtship of a few months before they decided to elope by train to Cumberland. Prior to their meeting, Mother had been romancing a young man by the name of Ike Tinsley from Canada. They had become quite serious in their relationship until Ike lost his cool over an argument one night and bit my Mother's lower lip very cruelly. That finished their friendship. Mother often related to me that Ike had the most gorgeous green eyes and she was hoping strongly that I would have green eyes, and I did! She had ebony black eyes.

Mentally and temperamentally I favor my Mother more so and physically and emotionally I favor my Father; but really I am an impartial combination of both parents.

My Grandfather, J. T., had a stringent unbreakable rule that his daughters could not, under any circumstances, form romantic friendships with any young man whose religion was Catholicism. He would meet all male contenders who vied for the favor of his female children at the door and check their religious credentials. If they were not the correct ones (for him), expulsion ruled. Knowing J. T. as I did, I'm pretty sure this dictum was true and obeyed to the letter.

My Father, Howard, when an early adolescent, was withdrawn from the 8th grade when his father, a renowned newspaper printer, died suddenly of a cataclysmic stroke at age 43 years. Shockingly, at 13 years of age Howard went to work at Kelly and Jones, a manufacturing plant in south Greensburg, Pennsylvania, to help support a single mother and seven children. It was really a cruel quirk of fate, because my Dad was a brilliant student and showed flashes of unlimited intellectual possibilities. Anyhow, back to reality, he accepted his cruel destiny and complied with the best of his ability. In Trafford he learned the trade of wood pattern making, which came naturally to him, and he excelled to the highest degree. He was manually very adept and skillful instinctively.

On the first floor of the apartment building at Cavitt and Fifth streets where my parents lived, there was Haupt's Pharmacy. They had a daughter, Christine, exactly my age and she was a formidable playmate. I caught a lashing for pulling her ears.

From my Mother's tales, I was the worst hellion imaginable. I was an ungodly scourge and had continuous Cole Porter "Night and Day" colic for one year. It was impossible to find any formula, which would agree in the least with this recalcitrant baby. In the end, the doctor, driven to distraction, finally prescribed condensed milk, which is unheard of today, but it worked! Dr. Tilbrook told my parents emphatically <u>not</u> to have any more children because of a congenital abnormality of my Mother's uterus. Before delivery he also warned Margaret Reamer Haines Knobloch that I would either be born dead on arrival or would be the worst, cantankerous child (brat) that God had ever created. Poor Mother claims she walked me at least 24 hours a day for the first nine months. Fortunately, a middle-aged Danish couple, the Danvers, resided on the third floor and they really came to her rescue. Mr. and Mrs. Danvers put in a daily presence and contributed a great relief from a constantly screaming infant by rocking, talking, walking, swinging, and swaying in shifts. My recollection of them is vivid sucking and squashing of orange halves against my mouth while grunting and growling.

Mother also had some tangible support from her sister, Verna, who was single and a year younger than my Mother. Verna came to live with us that first year in Trafford. Verna was at the romantic crossroads of life and highly valued male relationships.

I remember going to church with my parents and creating a turbid atmosphere, which resulted in the removal of my presence. This was somewhere about 3 to 12 months of age. Also, it crosses my mind that I attended a carnival with a lot of music, lights, candy, and pop at about 1 year of age.

We three used to go to Greensburg, thirty miles easterly, on weekends by train from Trafford on the Pennsylvania Railroad, which originated from Pittsburgh some 10 miles westerly, for there was no highway then. These trips were begun after my intense colic was ameliorating. I remember the trips, especially in the winter with snow on the ground and me on a sled. All I saw was red from sun reflections while being hauled to the station by sled.

I remember explicitly many summer evenings circa 1 year when Mother and Dad would take me to the crest of a hill near our home. They would sit on a bench and romance each other while I played on the hill in front of them. Sometimes my Aunt Verna would entertain a Swiss suitor who would bring me a striped bag (poke) of penny candy and he would yodel when I begged him vigorously.

At another time I recall distinctly playing with at least 5 dogs in the middle of the streetcar tracks in front of our apartment. We stopped the streetcar, fortunately! The conductor got out of the city streetcar, dispersed the canines, and then took me to find Mother.

Another time, while at play in front of the building, I remember a photographer coming by and taking my picture at age 21 months. I was reluctant, but gave in when he conned me with a candy bar. I still have the picture.

Another incident occurred when I sustained a very painful, second plus degree right forearm burn from a red hot register. I did not cry following the burn, my Mother said, but just gritted my teeth, groaned, and hissed.

The Danvers were really wonderful friends of my parents and were frequent visitors to our apartment. They were childless, lived a floor above us, and were quite happy and mirthful middle-aged people. They were always laughing, joking, and telling stories. In fact, Mrs. Danver was instrumental in inducing me to take my first steps alone at 9 months of age by offering me one of her delicious cookies. They got a huge kick out of the way I would sleep invariably with my arms extended fully over my head and would tease me about my high buttoned shoes. Actually, to this very day my sleeping posture still embodies my upper extremities at full extension superior to my cranium. They really died laughing at my antics when I crushed oranges and bananas to my mouth.

I remember one particular event that occurred when I was about 16+ months old. It jarred my psyche a bit. I knew my Father worked in a plant across a small river about 3 blocks from the apartment building. I had the brilliant idea of going to see him by crossing a vacant area full of bull rushes, which were almost as tall as I. I hadn't advanced very far when I became totally lost and a pang of fear of the unknown crossed my mind. After about an hour of wandering and searching, my guardian angel in the form of Aunt Verna, came to my rescue. My poor tortured Mother gave me a bit of dressing down to be sure.

I will relate two episodes narrated by my Mother, but not remembered by myself. Number one episode happened at age one plus year of age when my dear second Mother, Verna, took me for a buggy ride (literally and figuratively). We stopped by the Pennsylvania Railroad in Trafford for Verna to converse with an unknown male suitor. I must have become bored and crawled out of the buggy, unseen by Verna, to investigate the train station. I finally ended up on the train tracks. In 5 minutes a crack fast train from Pittsburgh was due to pass through on the track I was on. This time, my guardian angel was a postal clerk, who came out to hang up the mailbag for this train, which was passing through Trafford. The train was a through P.R.R. train on its way easterly to Greensburg, Johnstown, Altoona, and the far destination of Harrisburg. The postman was a bit surprised when he spied me but he managed to quickly grab me from the jaws of death and deliver me to my surprised and amazed Aunt.

The second episode concerns our friend Mrs. Danver, who inhabited the 3rd story apartment. I must have been getting near the 2-year stage in growth and development and was reaching for the age of independence. While at play outside the building after escaping a sleeping and harrowed Mother, I discovered the fire escape at the side of the building. I decided to climb up the escape to see where it led. It had no side rails and was open between steps. Carefully, I gradually ascended to the third floor and fortunately my guardian angel, Mrs. Danver plus providence this time, coaxed me into her third story apartment window, again with a plate of homemade cookies. After recovering from the shock, my neighbor and benefactress, Mrs. Danver, carried me nervously to my home and presented me to a bewildered, unbelieving, and thankful Mother.

Finally, when I reached the "terrible" age of two, going on three, Father got a good job at Elliott Company in Jeanette, Pennsylvania, situated five miles from Greensburg. Greensburg was a small city 30 miles northeast of Pittsburgh, where the lion's share of our close relatives resided. We rented an apartment in the basement of the residence of my maternal grandparents, Emma and J.T. Haines, who lived at 515 Sidney Street. I grieved to leave my roots at Trafford, especially my buddy, Christine Haupt, with whom I had many interesting battles. However, I believe it was the fear of unknown changes that really alarmed me.

Chapter 2

The Move to Greensburg, Pennsylvania

Greensburg, Pennsylvania was founded circa 1790. It has a population of 35,000 and is the County seat of Westmoreland County. Greensburg is in Southwestern Pennsylvania about 30 miles east of Pittsburgh. There was no highway between these two cities when I was born. Greensburg was named after the renowned General Nathaniel Greene, the "swamp rat", who was a Revolutionary War hero fighting his major battles in the Carolinas. Greensburg was primarily a small residential city in the middle of the bituminous coal country. Greensburg's climate was quite similar to the lower one third of Michigan's Lower Peninsula.

Greensburg was often compared to Rome, Italy, with its seven steep hills, and was situated in the foothills of the Allegheny Mountains, otherwise known as the Appalachian Mountains. In fact, the Greensburg hills had a 20 to 30% grade. With a good snowfall, I could travel over a mile on my trusty Flexible Flyer sled in winter, from the top of Alexander Street, then down Foster and Sidney Streets, and away out to Plough's Grocery Store, which was beyond Brandon Street. Fortunately, in the teens of the 20th Century, there were very few automobiles in existence to interfere with sledding. Automobiles compulsorily had to have wheel chains in the winter because of the heavy snow, hills and ice. Maneuvering over those hills was really hazardous. In fact the hill at the bottom of Foster Street, on which I lived, had a 35% grade.

Our new home in Greensburg at 520 Foster St. was quite cozy and comfortable. It was built by my father in 1920. Mother did extensive entertaining of friends and relatives. Actually there was never a dull moment.

My Grandfather (Mother's Father), John Thomas Haines, was a very virile person and possessed a very strong character physically, mentally, and morally. He ran a tight ship, but was quite fair and square. He was reputed to be the strongest man in Westmoreland County, and the only person able to lift a steel railroad tie. His wife, Emma, was an extremely loving and forgiving person. She was happy-go-lucky, a superb cook, and her trademark was always being calm, cool, and collected under stress.

John and Emma had 7 children. My Mother was the third born along with 6 siblings and the distribution was 5 girls and 2 boys. Alice was the second born and she had married Samuel Francis Hammer Senior, a civil engineer graduate of West Virginia University at Morgantown. He was a premier football linesman and a wizard in math who won a $50.00 gold award for receiving the highest mark in math. They had 2 children named Samuel Junior and Mary Frances. Mary was the first-born child in the Reymer-Haines family and she married William Andrews, a postal clerk. They had 2 children, Frances and John. Verna was number 4 and she married Austin Craven, a Vaudeville musician and magician. The Cravens had an adopted daughter, Betty, who was the daughter of Frank Haines. Frank was Verna's brother. Verna was unable to have children due to a uterine abnormality. Number 5 child was Robert Jamison, a pattern maker who served in World War I. He married Ethel Manos, who died with vascular and arthritic complications and was childless. Robert's second marriage was to Edna Kemp and they had one daughter, Sally Haines. Sally was one of my dearest friends ever. Number 6 was Frank, a prime coronetist, who married Ethel Price. They had 5 children: Frank Junior, who died with rheumatic fever at age 7 years, Dorothy, Judy, Betty, and John - in that order. Isabel, the baby of the Haines family, married Paul Sindorf, an electrician. They had 2 girls, Jane and Mary Lou. Thus, luckily, I had an even dozen first cousins on my Mother's side of the family but, unfortunately, I was an only and lonely child.

On my Father's side of the family, my grandparents Anna and John Knobloch begat 7 children only the genders were reversed. My Father had 4 brothers and 2 sisters. Edward, a Scout Leader primarily, was the eldest and he married Pearl Slonacher. Edward and Pearl had one child, Jay, who later became a chiropractor. My Dad was the number 2 in the family. John, an industrial worker, was the third child and he married Anna Armbruster. They had 2 children, namely Donald and Ruby. The fourth child was Arthur, a highly trained industrial mechanic, who married Alice Hahnemann. They had one son, Arthur Junior. The fifth was Irene, who married Walter Stockberger, a journey salesman. They had 2 children, Anna and Mabel. The sixth and last daughter of my Father's family was Mabel, a very gifted artist, who married Frank Snedden, an inventive person and a near genius. They had 3 children, Frank Junior, Mary, and Eileen. Frank, the seventh child, was the youngest brother of my Grandfather's family and he married my Aunt, Hazel Jennings. They had 2 daughters, Louise and Myrna.

Irene, Dad's sister, died in her early thirties with acute thyrotoxicosis following thyroid surgery at Harper Hospital in Detroit, Michigan, which in 1931 was the cradle and birthplace of the American Academy of Pediatrics. The year of her death was 1916 and her body was buried from my grandparent's home in Greensburg with the Reverend Lawrence E Bair officiating. (Reverend Bair was a rookie in his first year of service as pastor of the First Reformed Lutheran Church in Greensburg, which was attended by the Haines family. I would become a very close friend of Reverend Bair when I reached my early teens.)

My parents adopted Mabel Stockberger, Irene's daughter, for two years after her mother died, because their father Walter needed to establish a home as a single parent for his children. Mabel's sister, Anna, was farmed out to her Aunt Pearl and Uncle Ed Knobloch for a period of several years. All in all, being an only child, I was blessed with 10 paternal first cousins to keep me in playmates. Most of them lived close by in hometown Greensburg. Six cousins lived in Pittsburgh, two cousins lived in Mount Pleasant, which was twenty miles east, and two cousins lived in Jeanette, 5 miles west of Greensburg.

My family was very closely linked with the Hammers. Cousin Sam was only a year older than I, and Cousin Mary was just one year younger. They lived a block away. Their paternal grandparents lived on a farm between Johnstown and Jennerstown, Pennsylvania, and we would fairly often pay them a visit in my Uncle Sam's new Steven Salient Six automobile. We had to go over the Ligonier Mountains on our journey, and we would have to stop at least once midway to replace the water in the radiator, which had boiled over. The mountain scenery was superb and the narrow roads were awfully curvy and had steep grades, which made passing trucks very difficult. At the farm, we would go horseback riding, milk the cows, pick berries, feed the chickens, go to church and hike all over the countryside. Cousin Mary was a constant friend and playmate. Cousin Sam was feisty and aspired to become an M.D./surgeon in Pittsburgh.

My Uncle Samuel's Father, Matthew, was a devout Christian and always said a detailed blessing before all meals. He was an avid reader of the Bible and prayed twice daily. He never shaved and had a mighty, gray beard at least to his waist. His word was law and no one ever disputed his requests or "advise". His wife, Elsie, was a marvelous cook and had a docile, compliant, and pleasant temperament. His son, George, Uncle Sam's older brother, managed the farm efficiently and productively. George and his wife Bessie had two children, Elmer and Hortense, a bit older than we were, but quite friendly and sociable.

We were really intrigued by Grandfather, Matthew, who related many interesting stories about the infamous Johnstown flood, which occurred in

1888. The Cremahomian Dam burst after several inches of rain and the torrents of water rolled down a mountain like a tidal wave, causing great loss of life, billions of dollars in damage, and looting and pillaging followed in Johnstown.

Actually, the Hammers lived only a few houses from our residence on Sidney Street and later on Oakland Avenue in Greensburg. The entire Haines clan with all our nearby relatives would gather together on holidays and special occasions at the Hammers' or Haines' homes. We would go on picnics in or near Greensburg at Electric Park, Tollgate Park, Delmont Park, Oakford Park or Youngwood Park. All the relatives really were quite hospitable and friendly.

We lived with my Mother's parents on Sidney Street for three years in an apartment in the basement of their home and had lodging on the second floor with them and Mother's siblings (Uncles Robert, Frank, and Aunt Isabel). Robert Jamison (Bob) was in Greensburg in high school and a star guard on the 1916 football team, which won the State championship by beating Harrisburg Tech. Uncle Frank Haines was in Greensburg High School also. He was deeply engaged in studying the trumpet and was becoming a stellar musician. Isabel was in junior high school and was highly interested in cooking.

I remember one time while Frank was pursuing his daily practice on the trumpet; I came up unknowingly and devilishly from behind him and while standing on a chair pushed his back suddenly, forcing his teeth against the mouthpiece, but he sustained no dental injury. All Hades broke loose. Frank had a terrific temper and a low fuse. He was obsessed with almost a narcissistic perception of his body image. On another occasion, I somehow got hold of a knife and did a carving and sculpturing production on the bathroom framework. I had a head to head encounter with Grandpa Haines and, believe me, he instilled the fear of God in my mind. It was a huge lesson well learned. I didn't earn the sobriquet of "Peck's Bad Boy" for being angelic, for sure.

My Mother was an accomplished pianist and had aspirations for her superlative soprano voice. She had all the qualities and attributes to be an ideal nurse: She loved all people, especially children, was very empathetic, was an excellent conversationalist, very warm-hearted, intelligent, and had a wonderful sense of humor. My Father was a superb guitarist, very happy, understanding, extremely honest, sagacious, a workaholic, and endowed with the ability of hitting the nail on the head in a paucity of words.

My close friend, Robert Morris, lived across from us on Sydney Street. He was my age, had a very low fuse, and would bite his proximal knuckle of the right forefinger when angry, which was often as he was easily aroused. We played all kinds of games daily. Football, run sheepy run, horseshoes, skating, hopscotch, and tiddly winks were some of our exciting pursuits. We also played one which was a bit precarious - where a person would exhale all his air and the person facing him would rap his arms around the chest and squeeze him tightly, causing temporary unconsciousness. Fortunately, the Lord takes care of little children and drunks.

My other close playmates were Sam & Mary Hammer, my first cousins who lived five houses west of us. Once in awhile an older lad who lived five houses east of us, Rocky Booth, would join us but he was a bit of a prankster. He tried to steal my football and one time brought me a glass of "lemonade" to drink. Upon tasting it, I discovered it was urine and salty. Another friend, Harry McChesney, would visit me from time to time and we would play mumbly peg and shoot marbles.

"Maw" Craven, my Uncle Austin Craven's mother from Creekside, Pennsylvania, would visit me quite often and would read me biblical passages and relate many biblical stories. She gave me a book named Hurlburt's Story of the Bible to study. Austin Craven did a lot of Vaudeville featuring magic tricks, piano playing, and music played on a saw. He was a real expert magician and entertainer, who later became a barber and a master of the coiffure art. He cut my hair for many years.

One final episode is very prominent in my memory. It involves an injury incurred while I was running into the bathroom and bowled over a bucket of scalding hot water, intended for my bath. In those days, we did not have a water heater, although we did have a bathtub. The water flowed all over my entire right leg and it was exceedingly painful. A third degree burn of my lower leg occurred. It was a real emergency and Doctor Schneider came on the double. He instructed my poor, distraught Mother to soak my lower extremity in ice-cold water continuously for 24 hours, and this immediately relieved my painful weeping, wailing, and gnashing of teeth.

My cousin Mary Hammer, age 4 years, had a very serious encounter with a deep tissue infection of the left facial cheek, which all but claimed her life. She had picked a pimple on her left cheek two days prior to the symptoms. At that time we had no antibiotics or cultures. Our medical armory at that time was like a popgun and all her treatment was focused on hot, continuous normal saline packs. She remained at home and my dear, compassionate Mother was at her side day and night, changing her packs under Doctor McKelvey's able guidance. Mary was on the razor's edge of death, but with my Mother's excellent, continuous, expert care she managed to squeak by after 6 days. It was probably a hemophilus influenza or hemolytic A streptococcus rampant necrotizing cellulitis.

Mary's brother, Samuel Francis Hammer Junior, had many, many bouts of acute bilateral otitis media with purulent effusion. My Uncle Sam Hammer Senior had a brother physician, William; who did family practice in Johnstown, Pennsylvania, which was located about 10 miles from Brother George's farm that I discussed previously. Doctor William would come to Greensburg to the J. T. Haines residence to see Sam Junior when he had painful, pusy discharging ears. He would examine Sam and maybe do punctures of the eardrums on the dining room table. On one occasion he performed bilateral mastoid surgery to relieve the pus pressure in the mastoid bones under local anesthesia.

My cousin Sam and I were quite the adversaries. Sam was a year older, more corpulent, and muscular than I. One time we each received a pair of boxing gloves for Christmas. Grandpa Haines arranged a bout in front of the relatives. It was no contest and ended abruptly in the first round when I was getting pummeled unmercifully. Samuel, much larger physically, had more of the killer instinct and I, being softhearted, had inherited too much of my Father's genes. On another occasion, young Sam Junior also struck me on the forehead with a stone. We were both throwing rocks, but his aim was more accurate than mine - bull's eye. Afterwards he had the gall to pick off the scab and I carry the scar to this day.

The entire Haines clan was real closely knit and allied. We would all convene at each other's home (Hammer's or Haines's residence) on Christmas Eve for presents and on Christmas Day for a big turkey dinner. On the night before Christmas, either my Uncle Bob or Frank, Mother's brother, would get into a Santa Claus suit and have all the children recite a story, usually from Grimm's Fairy Tales or Aesop's Fables, and then pass out all the gifts. It was a gala affair and everyone was in a festive and congenial mood. Emma baked umpteen loaves of bread daily and lots of pot pies and cookies for her ravenous folks. Her culinary fare was simple, basic, and filling.

Austin Craven did a lot of Vaudeville featuring magic tricks, piano playing and music played on a saw. One time he extracted an egg from Grandpa Reamer's beard. He was a real expert magician and entertainer, who later became a barber and a master of the coiffure art. He cut my hair for many years.

One final episode is very prominent in my memory. It involves an injury incurred while I was running into the bathroom and bowled over a bucket of scalding hot water, intended for my bath. In those days, we did not have a water heater, although we did have a bathtub. The water flowed all over my entire right leg and it was exceedingly painful. A third degree burn of my lower leg occurred. It was a real emergency and Doctor Schneider came on the double. He instructed my poor, distraught Mother to soak my lower extremity in ice-cold water continuously for 24 hours, and this immediately relieved my painful weeping and wailing.

My Mother relates a "true" story about her Mother, Emma, after we moved into her home. She kneaded 5 loaves of bread almost daily for her rapacious family. One day, while in the middle of performing this household chore in the kitchen, the front doorbell rang. She left her dough to find her daughter, Mary, who was visiting from Mount Pleasant, PA. After their tête-à-tête and upon returning to her task of kneading and rolling the bread, she discovered to her consternation that her wedding ring was missing. She never removed her prized ring except for this household duty, but it was nowhere to be found. About a year later my Mother, who always had a deep, eternal interest in the supernatural side of life, was talking to a "medium". She asked the lady about the secret whereabouts of my Grandmother's wedding ring, it's loss being a major tragedy. The medium, while in deep concentration, came up with a logical solution. "The hallowed ring can be found behind the kitchen floor board to the right of where your Mother stood to prepare the bread." The explanation is as follows: while your Mother was entertaining her daughter in the living room, the mice came out to eat the uncooked bread dough and dragged the wedding ring to its final resting place. So! My Mother related this bit of information to Emma and, voila, after removing the designated floorboard, lo and behold there was the wedding ring in its pristine condition, dedoughed.

Incidentally, Emma was quite famous for her potpie dumplings and some kind of sugar pie, which I've never seen elsewhere. She was a truly superb chef of the old school and I'm positive that she never saw a cookbook. Likewise, my Mother who cooked with a pinch of this and a pinch of that followed in her footsteps. I, in my preschool years, would call her the "sandwich" Grandmother (not knowing her real name), for she almost daily made me "rat cheese" sandwiches to replenish my energy.

One very distinct incident is etched into my memory lanes and it occurred when I was 4 years of age. Mother sent me to Plough's grocery store for some needed victuals and offered some penny candy as my reward. Plough's store was about 3 blocks from our home on the corner of Sidney and Stanton Streets. After picking out my candy, Mr. Plough said he had something to show me. He had just been delivered a huge stalk of probably a hundred bananas. He laid the bananas on the wooden floor and opened up a large fruit jar about 10 feet away from the bananas. To my amazement a tremendous sized tarantula spider came out of the bananas and crept slowly into the fruit jar and Al Plough quickly, with dexterity, screwed the lid on the jar. I was standing behind Al and my eyes must have reached saucer size at least. This happening was quite an exciting revelation to me and I couldn't wait to get back to my domicile to tell my Mother. I was too young to be frightened and, not realizing the danger, was fearless.

Another tale concerning Mr. Plough revolves around the time, at about three years of age, when my Mother took me grocery shopping. While she was busily engaged in filling her grocery list, I was preoccupied with picking out some choice pieces of penny candies, unbeknownst to Mother and Al Plough. Voila! When we arrived home, to my Mom's embarrassment, I ecstatically exhibited to her my cache of sweets collected while she was busily engaged. After giving me a detailed lecture that my purloining of candy was exactly the antithesis of the commandment, "thou shalt not steal," she coerced me into returning, by myself, to Plough's store to return the merchandise. This I did sorrowfully. After giving back the candy to Mr. Plough, I apologized profusely, promising to never commit larceny in the future.

In another instance involving Margaret (my Mother), I was playing with my football, a third year birthday present, in the kitchen with Emma (Maternal Grandmother). After a while, I dropped the football at the beginning of a flight of steps leading from the kitchen to the lower floor level where we lived. I went into the dining room to play with my favorite toy, a battleship which had a target drawn in the middle. If someone hit the target with a cork from a popgun at 20 feet, the battleship would explode, hurtling its parts all over the room. This toy would occupy tons of my time. It so happened that my Mother had come upstairs to get one of Emma's favorite potpie recipes while I was busily engaged in exploding my battleship. After obtaining the famous recipe, my Mother started to descend the stairway leading to our basement. To her utter surprise and amazement, she stepped on the football at the stair top and miraculously rode the pigskin down from the kitchen to the basement including a wide turn, approximately 15 lucky steps. It wasn't the "Midnight Ride of Paul Revere", but one she never would put in the amnesia column.

The 1914 to 1918 World War I, "the war to end all wars" struck our household with penetrating vengeance. Mother's oldest brother, my Uncle Robert, enlisted in the U. S. Army Infantry in 1917 and was transported by ship to France where he fought under General Pershing in the battle of the Ardennes Forest. He unfortunately was exposed to noxious gas inhalations and sustained long lasting pulmonary damage, but otherwise survived the War intact. My Father's sister-in-law's brother was killed in a battle at the Maginot Line in France.

Mother was an accomplished piano player. She took lessons and taught lessons on the piano, and would sing war songs with her mellifluous soprano voice: "Over There.", "Til the Boys Come Home", and "In Flander's Fields".

My Haines relatives were mainly Republicans and did not relate as bosom buddies to President Woodrow Wilson's philosophy regarding the necessity of war. They blamed him mainly for our participation in World War I with the Allies and didn't approve of his "Alley Cat" morals. However, most presidents have been accused justly or unjustly of such animalistic behavior.

Prior to this war, my Father was a rabid sports person and was engaged in the pursuit and participation of baseball, a star second baseman in the shop league and a point guard of renown on the Trojan's basketball team in an amateur league. Football was his major "bleacher" sport. Our local high school football team was always high and foremost in the state rankings, and he would often take me at age 3 years to Saturday games at Offutt Field where Kiski Prep, Bellfonte Academy, University of Pittsburgh Panther Freshman, Slippery Rock, Johnstown and Harrisburg Tech played Greensburg High School. I really remember his taking me under the stands at halftime to empty my bladder. When I was older, about 10 years, I would walk over a mile to see games by crawling over fences. Many other children catapulted the fence uncontested to get a free pass to the end zone seats while the guards dozed.

My Dad was a real master of the guitar and we would visit with his brother (Uncle John) on Sundays after church at First Reformed Lutheran. He would play the guitar and Uncle John would play the mandolin. In duet they would play many symphonic pieces in concert fashion. Their renditions were really spellbinding for all of us. Dad also was an amateur horticulturist and had a true verdant thumb. He engaged in gardening every summer, and Mother would do a large amount of canning to consummate his labors. He was especially addicted to raising gladiolas, dahlias, and truly loved "beefsteak" tomatoes, the prodigious ones.

I distinctly remember a foolhardy incident that occurred when I was five years of age. My Mother's brother, Robert, was interested in cars and had an elderly Packard, vintage1905, in which he would take family members for rides. One time when he was driving into the garage on the east side of our residence, I asked him to run over my lower legs with the car. Fortunately, in those days the automobiles were much, much lighter in weight. The tires were smaller, and there were no windows. If it rained, we would have to snap on the "side curtains". Anyhow, Uncle Bob condescended to my request to run over my legs with the right front and back wheels. Well! Fortunately, no injuries were incurred except when I related this story to my Mother, Margaret. She berated her brother Robert to high heavens and also gave me a harangue I have never forgotten.

One of my most morbid and harrowing experiences happened in 1917 at age 6 years. There was a mighty awesome pandemic of Influenza A sweeping the globe. It was a world wide epidemic sweeping our planet with a vengeance rivaling the Bubonic Plague catastrophe of the sixteenth century. Over 500,000 humans succumbed. People in Greensburg, Pennsylvania, as well as in all parts of the United States, were dying by the thousands daily – literally just like flies, without any exaggeration. There were mass graves overrunning the demand for wooden caskets. People would show signs and symptoms of acute influenza overnight and then be a corpse 8 to 12 hours later, having succumbed to galloping pneumococus pneumonia. There was absolutely nothing in the medical armament which would make even a dent therapeutically to conquer this illness. Sink or swim was the order of the day. I remember that everyone was panic-stricken and "flu" was the all-permeating topic of the day and night. People were rushing to the YMCA for hot and cold "therapeutic" baths, which actually were about as useless as the orchids on the Marquis de Lafayette's horse.

To get back to my tale of woe, it involved my dear playmate, Robert Morris, who lived across the street from our habitation. Well, late one morning in September Robert appeared in our doorway and made a request that we go to his home and visit with his mother, Molly, who was confined to a sick bed with a light "cold". Molly was a ravishing, gorgeous, striking brunette. I can still explicitly visualize her beautiful Mona Lisa like face. Well, we did go upstairs to see Molly, and she was very exuberant and happy to see us. To tell the truth, she showed no ill symptoms. We made some cheese sandwiches and bean soup and shared our meal with her. We then went out to play, as though this were just a routine occurrence. Later in the afternoon, I returned home to relate the news about Molly's incarceration in bed to my Mom. Molly was considered a most lovely woman, physically and spiritually, almost heavenly, to those who knew her. On the following morning, deeply to our horrified surprise, Mother and I received the very sad news that Molly had met a shocking and unexpected demise. The night of the day after our visit to her bedside, I became sick with a similar bout of "The Flu", showing early signs of an acute cold episode. This illness was extremely contagious and highly transmissible.

Well, our family physician, Dr. Howard Hamman, M. D., came out to our home that same night to see me at Mother's emergent request. Doctor's house calls in that period were rationed and triaged to those who were absolutely the most severely ill. I have a clear vision of my Mother, Margaret, at my bedside with tears streaming down her cheeks, asking the physician bluntly the 64 dollar question, "Is he going to die, Doctor?" I can also visualize the doctor at that juncture staring into space somberly, expressionless, and studiously. After what seemed to me an interminable period of time, he said absolutely nothing. I was deeply impressed and thought I must be gravely ill, but really and truly I did not feel that bad or afraid. Well! Thanks to Divine Providence, God, Mother Nature, my Lord and Savior, or whomever, I dodged the fateful cannonball. It was a rank squeaker, but the end result was favorable. I had the "hard" measles two years before and had had acute juvenile tuberculosis one year after my escape from the flu experience. I remember being quite sick for 3 weeks with the hard measles and may have had a pneumonic complication.

However, I seemed to recuperate readily from the attack of a viral influenza without complications.

The tuberculosis (phthisis) was transmitted to me by Jack Muir, a dear family friend, and also from adult relatives on my paternal side of the family from known cases. In those "good old days", tuberculosis (TB) was extremely common and ranked very high as a cause of death. There was absolutely no cure or treatment. It was simply a matter of "kill or cure - sink or swim". There was no vaccine, no Health Department, and x-ray imaging was barely off the ground. Absolute bed rest and sanitariums were the prime treatment recourse. It was thought that the calcium in the form of milk could wall off the tubercule bacilli in the lungs and prevent cavitations (holes in the lungs). Other prominent dangers with TB were the septicemia (blood stream infection) with dissemination to the brain (tuberculoma or meningitis), kidney infection (nephritis), lymph node spread or cardiac involvement (percarditis). Body resistance or immune response was the key to recovery, and the younger the patient probably the less resistance present due to immaturity. My signs and symptoms of tuberculosis, or "galloping consumption" were uncontrollable cough, fever, night sweats, weight loss, malaise, loss of appetite, insomnia and increased irritability. Usually in children cavitation does not occur early but there is primarily infiltration of the lung hilar lymph nodes. The organisms are coughed up during sleep and can be recovered from the stomach contents early in the morning on awakening. I believe the tuberculin test was alive in 1918, but the diagnosis was primarily by clinical presentation and possibly chest x-ray. The disease is often called an "acid fast" illness because of the peculiar staining features of the bacteria. They stain red.

Anyhow, my Mother, being on the alert and very intelligent, knew that something was "Rotten in Denmark" and made an appointment with a pediatrician in Pittsburgh. Following a thorough history, he examined me and took a chest x-ray, which showed the primary complex of the gon's lymph nodal enlargement at the lung hilum (usually right side as the right bronchus is straighter coming off the tracher). My Mother queried, "How shall we treat this tuberculosis?" The doctor replied, "Put him to bed for a year and give him plenty of milk". I believe I stayed in bed for maybe a month or two, but thanks again to Divine Providence, I made another somewhat miraculous complete recovery. Coincidentally, I worked 3 months in a State TB Sanitarium at Sabillasville, Maryland, in the summer of 1935, prior to my senior year in medical school. While at the "San" they insisted that I have a tuberculin test and I did. My right forearm became scarlet and swelled up to double or maybe triple its normal size. This super reaction indicated that I had a very high immunity to tuberculosis (thank goodness) and a chest x-ray taken on entrance to University of Maryland Medical School in 1932 showed completely normal lungs, thanks to time and my immune system.

At this time, 1917, my Dad was working in the shipyards of the Bethlehem Steel Corporation at Sparrows Point just outside of Baltimore, Maryland. There was great demand for transport ships during the First World War to carry military personnel and supplies to France and England for the Allies. Father figured he could best contribute to the War effort in this manner.

My Mother cracked the whip in our family and was my disciplinarian. She was extremely loving and her corrections were mainly verbal arguments. She rarely lost control of her temper enough to administer physical punishment, like when I carved the bathroom window with a knife. She was really good at track and I could hardly ever escape her grasp by running away. My Father was very mild mannered and had infinite reserve and patience. He only lost his cool once, to my recollection, when he was working in the garden and I was teasing him beyond the limits of his aggravation. I ran into the house and was rescued by my Mom, fortunately, for still water runs deep. He rarely was committed to anger, but Katie bar the door when he blew it once or twice a year.

Chapter 3

My Early Elementary School Years

My first grade year was spent at Southwest Greensburg Elementary School. I believe that I was pretty much of a "dreamer" my first two years in school and didn't get the big picture of the true purpose of going to school. I can still visualize looking out the window while at my desk, not paying any concentrated attention to the instructions delivered by the teacher. I was fantasizing my participation on the playground and wishing time would evaporate and permit our play period to materialize. I didn't realize at the time how very fortunate we were to have such a lovely, understanding, imperturbable, and attractive teacher. Miss Marie Weaver, our kindergarten teacher, was the epitome of grace, caring, comforting, and happiness. Nothing seemed to ruffle her feathers. Actually, this presentation belied us into a false sense of security and didn't prepare us for the instructors in the future, who were not nearly as congenial. We had no preschool to soften the rigors and speed bumps of first grade.

In the first grade, I realized life was not really a bowl of cherries, because elderly Miss Joy Wilcox was our mentor. Although she was very competent and efficient, she was also a strict top sergeant from the old school and she commanded respect. She had a somewhat rigid adherence to her principles, rules and dictates. It was a rather rude awakening and a frightening experience which tended to acquaint us with the real, more pragmatic world. We marched to our room by Phillip Sousa's famous, "Stars and Stripes", played by a victrola. A couple of times I was vocally reprimanded for being out of line and was warned that any further disruptions would incur physical correction. Well! It happened, with my being a normal five-year-old-male gender child, that I was caught committing the unpardonable offense of pushing, shoving, and yelling loudly at the boy in my rear. I was instructed to go to the principal's office, Mr. Marsh, immediately, if not sooner. We called him the affectionate moniker of "Duck Eggs". He was a stern, cool, unfeeling, cruel, hulk of a person. He gave me a long lecture on appropriate behavior in school and admonished me to straighten up or suffer hardships. On returning to my room, Miss Wilcox decided to reinforce the principal's message verbally and added a touch of her own to indelibly imprint the lesson. She stated, "Hold out your hands, palms upward." Then she gave me five stinging whacks to each hand. I was duly impressed with her censuring process and decided that the consequences were not worth the horseplay.

At the termination of first grade, with a passing grade (unearned), mother and I moved to Baltimore, to the suburb of Dundalk, near the Chesapeake Bay to join my Father. As I mentioned, Dad had moved to Dundalk the previous year to help make ships and submarines. Dad's brother, Edward, with his wife Pearl and son Jay, lived in Dundalk, Maryland, and we had temporary housing with them. I entered second grade there and struggled mightily, endeavoring to master my multiplication tables. The adjustment to school in Dundalk was a Herculean effort for me. I was on the brink of failure, but managed to squeak through the second grade conditionally.

After this grade finalized, we moved to Hamilton, a suburb of Baltimore. But before moving, I must relate a story connected to my association with Herbert Ness, in Dundalk, a pal of my cousin Jay who was Ed and Pearl's son. Both boys were about three years my elder and we were playing in a huge field near the school and were manipulating an old rusty reaper loaded with webs and large spiders. Suddenly, Herbert screamed with pain and began to curse and grabbed his right forearm. We turned our heads in his direction and could see a small black widow spider with an orange, what appeared to be an hour glass, etched on its belly. Quickly, Jay responded and smashed the spider with a bat, which we had used to play ball. Immediately, we took Herb to a nearby brook and immersed his arm in the cool, trickling water. It amazingly relieved his pain to a high degree and cleansed the wound. Jay went to his home on the double and summoned his mother. She took Herbert instantly to the family doctor, and he applied good old iodine smack dab to the injury and bandaged the smitten arm. The doctor gave him an aspirin 5-grain tablet. Also he related to us that the spider was of the infamous Black Widow genus and recovery would consume at least a month for complete healing. The physician also emphasized the use of intermittent sessions with ice packs to the injured arm for two days and frequent office visits for inspection and dressings.

Also while in Dundalk, a community of about 5,000 people, we became close friends with the Harry Ellsworth Fisher Senior's family, which consisted of wife, Hattie, son, Harry Junior my age, and two daughters, Florence and Elizabeth. In addition we bonded with Edna and Edgar Kemp. Edna Kemp, many years later, became my Mother's brother, Robert's, second wife. His first wife, Ethel, died from arthritis and Edna's first husband, Edgar, ran off to Texas with a large plump lady.

To get back to the move to Hamilton, we moved into an apartment in the home of an elderly sea captain, Hosea Ruff, and his wife Belinda, who was really rough, gruff, tough, and very loud. She cursed like an army sergeant and had a nasty temper and crashed glasses and dishes against the wall. She really murdered the King's English, but had a heart as big as a whale.

I remember getting the mumps shortly after moving to Hamilton from Dundalk. It was a low blow and exerted a very painful impression with difficult mastication and swallowing of many foods, especially pickles, for what seemed like eons. Apparently, my immune system was defunct at that time, because I continued to get styes on both my eyelids recurrently and almost continuously for a couple of years. My Father took me to see the doctor almost weekly, but we were without antibiotics at that time and the only treatment was hot, wet compresses until the styes resolved, probably a staphylococcus aureus "Jobs" infection (Bible).

I recollect that one Christmas there I received a football. Jay and I played with it in the snow on an open field between our homes. The weather was very cold and the wind was whistling and howling a merry tune. On that Christmas I also received a station house, well constructed by my Father, along with an electric train and a bag full of my favorite licorice candy. But the real highlight that Christmas was actually the football.

I'm reminded of a trip that Jim Parker (a neighbor playmate), his little three-year-old brother, and myself took walking alongside of a small stream about a half a mile from home, following a huge rainstorm. Jim's brother wandered close to the raging brook and lost his equilibrium and fell into the water. In an instant, Jim dove into the stream and rescued his brother before you could say "Jack Robinson". It was fortunate that big brother rescued his little brother pronto, because the stream was quite swollen and moving at an accelerated rate. After this thrilling experience, we kept an eagle eye on "Peewee" (little brother) until we were safe and sound back home.

One other time, I was awe struck by a movie in Hamilton with dinosaurs as it's theme, witnessed also by my parents. I remember the word "Diplodocus" and the shrieking piano and violin music played by a piano player to accompany the silent film. While at the movie on dinosaurs, a short news commentary depicted President Woodrow Wilson as not a prime favorite, because I recall that many individuals in the theater were hissing and booing him because they blamed him for the United States' participation in World War I.

I used to tease my Mother to the brink of distraction by kicking and ruining new shoes on every tin can in sight in the street and the road while we were walking. My Mother was quite riled by this behavior and her reprimand to me was about as effective as water on a duck's back.

Upon conclusion of the "war to end all wars" we moved from Baltimore to East Liberty, Pennsylvania, a suburb of Pittsburgh. We lived temporarily with my Father's uncle (my paternal grandfather's brother) and his name was Barney Knobloch. He and his wife, Harriett (Hattie), had no children. Hattie's mother, Mrs. Haldermann, was living there also with her.

I was in third grade at that time in Woodrow Wilson Elementary School. I can recall one deleterious episode while in this school. We all had compulsory small pox vaccinations. I have never been sicker in all my life, for about two weeks, following the vaccination. My left upper arm and shoulder were tremendously swollen and painful. I had a considerably elevated temperature for several days and felt like a rung out dishrag for at least six weeks.

Aunt Hattie was a very lovely, warm, affectionate, caring, and understanding middle-aged lady. She taught me to tell time by a grandfather's clock and showed me how to make bread the old fashioned way. It smelled and tasted so wonderful and was so delicious that this is indelibly etched in my memory. She was unusually intelligent and helped me with my school homework, which was exceedingly difficult due to adjusting to a new school. She made me take a nap on the dining room lounge every afternoon and urged me to drink at least a quart of milk daily. Her dining etiquette was impeccable and superb. Her husband Barney, aged about 60 years, was an engineer. He was quite sober, quiet, cold, and of the old school philosophy that children should be seen and not heard. He and my Father were closely allied, trying unsuccessfully to invent the mechanics of "perpetual motion". Mother and Hattie formed an intimate friendship and constantly were discussing the members of each other's family.

One time Aunt Hattie was entertaining a very special, renowned and respected guest. My Mother was quite worried about my table manners and behavior in front of this guest. She promised me a big box of choice chocolate candy if I would be especially well mannered at the table and conduct myself properly to the penultimate degree. Well, I guess my behavior and table etiquette was never worse. I remember in particular chewing the celery savagely, spilling peas all over the table, and spilling gravy all over my lap. You can imagine my poor Mother's nightmare and consternation, to say the least. Needless to say, my buttocks were not so gently spanked and I did not get the prized box of candy. Surprise!.

Old Mrs. Haldermann and I had quite a contest each morning to see who could manage to enter the bathroom first. One time I locked the bathroom door and couldn't unlock it. This caused quite a bit of chaos for over an hour. Mother finally called a locksmith to spring me, while Mrs. Haldermann was chomping at the bit to use the toilet. There was a hot time in the old hometown that night, you can make a sure bet.

Hattie loved music, and one of her favorite victrola records was Rachmaninov's violin piece Souvenir, and we played it endlessly.

My Father finally obtained a job as chief of the pattern department at Elliott Company in Jeannette, Pennsylvania, 5 miles west of Greensburg, our home base. So! After one eventful, happy year at Aunt Hattie and Uncle Barney's, we moved back to good old Greensburg, to our roots at John Thomas and Emma Haines's home basement apartment for a second run.

Chapter 4

My Life – Years Eight to Thirteen

In those days of yore, schoolteachers had an appellation of Miss or Mrs. to their pupils. Practically all our elementary grade teachers were of the female gender acting the role of surrogate mothers. I remember one teacher, specifically in fourth grade, Miss Miriam Clendenon. I really fell head over heels in love with her. She was dark-complexioned, like my Mother, had a winning personality, and was very dynamic and positive. She wore the most alluring-scented perfume. She exhorted us to walk with shoulders back and gut in straight as an arrow and if we didn't, a yardstick was planted against our backs from stem to stern. Also in the morning, on arriving, the four windows at the rear were thrust wide open and we took six deep inhalations of fresh air to the cobweb depths of our lungs in unison, regardless of the weather conditions. Although being extremely sweet and affable, she commanded the utmost respect and called a spade a spade, sans mollycoddling.

I learned the Peterson writing method in fourth grade. It was a unique way of using the arm in combination with the fingers and produced very legible, speedy written words. My Father was quite an expert at handwriting and won several prizes at Seton Hill College, situated on the outskirts of Greensburg on the Jeanette Road. For some inexplicable reason, while in fourth grade, my struggles in mastering school - writing, reading, and arithmetic - ended. It was as though my brain lightened and I had a new ability to skillfully relate to my schoolwork and I developed a new explosive zest, energy, and enthusiasm. The light came on as though you would flip a switch and my grades were all in the nineties. Miss Clendenon said, "Howard, you've improved unbelievably, I think you're like Ichabod Crane and have just awakened from a long dream." Anyhow, from this time on school was like duck soup for me, and I basked in the sunlight.

My fifth grade teacher was Miss Fanny Brace and she was quite strict and emphasized obedience and no nonsense. She embodied an austere personality but was quite fair, honest and pleasant. We learned the Gettysburg Address by heart and were immunized with diphtheria horse serum antibodies. (I later became anaphylactic to horse serum and sustained a life threatening incident at Ann Arbor in 1939.) One perk Miss Brace gave us was an exemption from final exams if we students had an average of ninety on the tests given during the school year. This gesture really elevated her status as a benefactor tremendously in my estimation.

Miss Brace was quite empathetic when I would have my monthly migraine headaches and lost my stomach contents. She would put her arms around me and say, "Howard, try to relax and please don't worry for you have nothing but high ninety grades on all your tests." My Mother and Father both had severe periodic bouts of migraine, as well as my paternal grandmother, Anna, who also developed Type II diabetes, which finally summoned the Grim Reaper. After talking with my teacher and mulling it over in my mind a bit, I decided that I definitely did not need these paralyzing headache episodes and I decided I was not going to have them. Instead of internalizing stressful situations, I would externalize my feelings and attack the stressors with all my strength. Miraculously my migraine evaporated, actually forever. Fortunately, they are not hereditary but are congenital supposedly.

While in the winter of this school year I remember when sledding down a steep, long hill on Sidney Street, I lost control of my trusty Flexible Flyer and rammed full speed ahead into an iron stake near the bottom of the hill. I'm sure that I sustained multiple rib fractures, because I had excruciating pain in my right chest every time my chest moved with every respiration for about three weeks. Did I see a doctor? Do pigs fly?

I remember Armistice Day, November 11, 1918, distinctly because at around 3:00 p.m. myriads of whistles and bells blew and rang, and exploding firecrackers filled the air for a couple of hours. People were shouting vociferously "It's over! It's over."

During the summer after fourth grade, my Father undertook building a new home at 521 Foster Street, only three blocks from the Haines' home and I helped (or hindered) him during the construction. After laying the foundation, he drew up the plans and did most of the building with help from Piduti, the plumber, Paul Sindorf, the electrician, and Embler, the cement person. It was a two-story house with a cement basement and an attic, three bedrooms, parlor, dining room, kitchen, and one upstairs bathroom.

Mother had a Steinway grand piano and taught music to young pupils but refused to give me lessons because she pictured musicians collectively as alcoholics and perverts. The Hammers, first cousins Mary and Sam, Aunt Alice, and Uncle Sam, moved into a home on Oakland Avenue, just around the corner from our house at about the same time we were erecting ours. They had given us a dog, a rat terrier named Peg, who had the fur burned off her right chest in a fire. She was a very lovable creature and had an expert proclivity for chasing cats and catching rodents (hence her name). Uncle Sam had about a dozen leghorn chickens and the chicken coup was infested with rats. This was a huge bonanza for Peg, who struck them like lightening by grabbing their throats.

In the following summer, I made a visit to "Maw" Craven and her daughter, Gwen Miller's family in Creekside, Pennsylvania, about five miles west of Indiana, Pennsylvania and approximately forty miles northeast of hometown Greensburg. (Incidentally, Indiana was James Stewart's home before he scaled the Oscar heights in Hollywood.) The Millers, John and Gwen, had seven children of which Bernard, age thirteen years, was the eldest, Veretta was my age, and Cyril, the gorgeous red haired baby aged fifteen months had recently expired with diphtheria casting a pall over the home. Creekside was a small coal-mining town and Mr. Miller, the father, was a coal miner. I remember him coming home from work practically blackened like Al Jolson from head to toe, and appearing very haggard, worried, and worn out. His work was no walk in the park.

Barney had a neighborly friend, Bill Waite, his age, and the three of us palled around together. We three musketeers walked fourteen miles to the little town of Shiloctah to go fishing in a small lake for catfish. We did manage to catch five eight to nine inchers. Being a greenhorn at fishing, I sustained a painful, two-inch laceration of my right palm from the fish fins. Barney wrapped his handkerchief around my hand and put pressure on it with his thumb. We decided not to walk back to Creekside but to take transportation in a boxcar of a freight train going through to our destination. We were quite happy about making this decision until we realized that we had to jump off a moving freight going about ten plus miles an hour. However, God was with us and we sustained only minor bruises and sprains as we exited the train at Creekside.

I split my two week visit with the Millers and my devoted friend Maw Craven. Maw was a great cook and deeply religious. She prayed often and read me passages from the Bible every day. We attended her Methodist church a few times. Amazingly, Maw's daughter, Gwen, converted from strict Methodism to almost rabid Catholicism. Her son, Austin, came home from his Vaudeville performances and showed me how to make tunes on a saw and how to perform some magic tricks he did on the theatrical stage. He also was a very accomplished piano player "by ear" naturally. Shortly afterwards, Austin Craven quit the movies and came to Greensburg, married my Aunt Verna (Mother's sister), and established a barbering business close to my home on Oakland Avenue.

I remember nights sleeping under a feather tick mattress and using a bedside "slop jar" to empty my bladder as there was only a "chick sales" outdoor toilet and baby it was cold out there. Maw was extremely sanitary and kept an immaculately clean house. Austin had a favorite song entitled "The Little Wooden Whistle That Wouldn't Whistle." The theme depicted a young maiden in the courting stage and she received a wooden whistle from her Mother to use as a signal when her suitor was becoming too ardent. The system worked well until one night the whistle became plugged and wouldn't whistle.

Bernard and I became staunch friends and I enjoyed my Creekside vacation immensely. Bernard and I would go swimming in a pool of sulfur water, which was a backwater drainage system from the coal mines. Many of the miner's children also were happy participants, regardless of the repulsive brown color and repugnant odor of the water.

My sixth grade teacher was my beloved Miss Gladys Stump. She was a teacher extraordinaire, very beautiful, always smiling and cheerful, very intelligent, charming, and commanding respect of the entire class. We had about forty pupils and discipline was no problem because Miss Gladys knew how to keep us busy continuously with study, art, music classics, and problem solving. One notable event occurred towards the end of our school year. A transfer student from Sewickly Elementary, Paul Walter Seaton, joined us. His presence was a result of parental separation. He was in the custody of his father, Walter, who stationed him with his sister Minnie Klingensmith, who lived in Greensburg on Oakland Avenue, a block east of my residence on Foster Street. Paul and I became exceptionally close friends immediately. I helped him in his adjustment to the new school situation in a new neighborhood with a complete set of strangers. He became acclimated to his new environment with remarkable alacrity. I invited him to my home and my Mother established a close caretaker relationship with "Seaty". The Klingensmiths, his designated home by his father were very supportive but somewhat stiff, rigid and inexperienced. They were childless, elderly, and had no knowledge of child nurturing. My Mother had extensive natural child rearing instincts and was a superb culinary artist, which Paul Seaton appreciated greatly. We were inseparable friends for many, many years until his giddy wife terminated his life with a handgun in 1938 under suspicious and secretive circumstances. At that time Paul was teaching in Shippensburg College in Pennsylvania. I last saw him in July 1935, when I was externing at Maryland State Tuberculosis Sanitarium in Sabillasville, Maryland, close to the U. S. Presidential retreat in the South Mountains at Thurmont, where Dr. Cohen and I did autopsies on expired TB patients (galloping consumption).

During my elementary school years, I became unforgettable friends with a handicapped middle-aged man, "Charlie" Loeffler, who lived next door to my maternal grandparents. Charlie had been stricken with ultra severe rheumatoid arthritis in adolescence, and the disease was progressive to a degree whereby he was unmercifully confined to a wheelchair. His hands, arms and legs were malformed and contorted into bizarre formations with resulting frozen rigidity of function. But Charlie was truly a master of intelligence. He read classics of the day and did studies constantly. He was a great teacher and was especially gifted in mathematics. We had many sessions together and I learned how to solve many math problems and the logistics of practical problems in English structure and syntax. Charlie was very positive in his attitude toward living, despite his major crippling infirmities. He lived a saint's life and never complained of his misfortune!

My Father had a love fest for the Pittsburgh Pirates, a National League baseball team, forever and foremost. His favorite player was famous Pirate second baseman Honus Wagner, who was quite renowned in the teens and twenties, and was bowlegged as a cowboy. I saw him a couple of times when my Dad took me to Forbes Field in Pittsburg. Honus was added to the team after I had vamoosed to Maryland. Honus ran like the wind. Dad attended a World Series game when Lee Meadows, Jug Handle, Johnny Morrison, and Emil (a Submariner) all pitched for Pittsburgh. He was especially enraptured by the Homestead Grays Black Baseball Team and took me to one of their games when Satchel Paige, the greatest pitcher of all time, pitched a one hit shutout.

In 1925, my uncle, Austin Craven and Doc Wilson took me to Forbes Field to see the Pirates play the Brooklyn Dodgers. After the game we were walking across Forbes Field and Doc picked up Glenn Wright's glove and reported it to Bill McKechnie, the manager. He gave us tickets for a game with the Chicago Cubs a weekend later. We saw Hack Wilson, who was truly one of the greatest hitters of all time. Hack was short, extremely muscular , compact and built like a cannonball.

Later, I would have the rank privilege of seeing the New York Giants' homerun king, Mel Ott, the talented slugger, Carl Hubbell, the amazing screwball pitcher. Paul and Lloyd and Waner were famous brothers playing outfield for the Pittsburgh Pirates. Also, I saw St. Louis Cardinal's Frankie Frisch, manager of the "Gas House Gang" and their outstanding pitcher Jesse Haines and strikeout artist Wild Bill Halahan. I deeply regret not seeing Babe Ruth, but he was in the American League and I only saw National League teams that played in Pittsburgh. My favorite Pirates were "Pie" Traynor and Kiki Cuyler from Harrisville, Michigan.

On Independence Day, the entire Haines Family and relatives would go to various area picnic grounds: Oakford Park, Tollgate Hill, Buttermilk Falls, Ligonier Mountains, Somerset Park, and the Youghagheny Indian Battlegrounds. We would play baseball, quoits, horseshoes, and shoot off fireworks. At night we would be dazzled by the fireworks display put on by the small town of Crabtree, about three miles north of Greensburg. It would last about a half an hour and end up with a blazing sham battle, which would be literally earth shattering to my Father's spellbound delight.

My seventh grade teacher was Miss Edna Poole, who was a hard-nosed first sergeant and a rigid disciplinarian, so naturally she was not a prime favorite of the pupils. However, anyone in her class really gleaned a tremendous amount of knowledge. Her favorite subject was geography and by the time we passed her class, we knew all the state capitols, major United States cities, all the products produced and manufactured by each one of the 48 states and the square mileage of each state. She really took school seriously and gave it all her might down to the last letter; but alas, being a dyed in the wool matriarch, she was unmarried and not popular with the male gender. She was corpulent and had bulging eyes.

I do vividly remember my Mother's throwing a big birthday party on my 12th year of life. We must have had two dozen classmates. Everyone was dressed to the hilt and the young ladies displayed their Sunday best alluring makeup and essences. We played the prepubescent games of pin the donkey's tail blindfolded, revolving musical chairs, duck for apples, and, of course, spin the pie pan. Luckily, yours truly won the Donkey's Serenade and I was privileged to kiss all the girls. My designated female partner was Janie Long and I remember her at the time the popular song was "Mean to Me". She was on the bold and brazen side and therefore was not my Mother's favorite girlfriend for me. While we were busily engaged in game activities, our ice cream was purloined by a gang of rowdy boys, who believed they were slighted and wanted to make a statement. In spite of this adversity, we all enjoyed a successful party, as dear old Dad saved the day by replenishing the ice cream.

My Mother tells a somewhat humorous tale about Bud Snively and road commissioner, Bill Sovey. Bud was a very happy 14-year-old Down's syndrome boy who was very lovable. Bill was a big rough, gruff, and tough person. They were driving a truck containing mostly garbage and refuse and filled to capacity midway down a steep hill, overlooking a creek filled with solid human waste at the bottom of the 25% grade. Bill was driving the truck and Bud was designated to be stationed at the bottom of this hill to signal the all clear sign when no cars were in view, right or left. Poor Bud signaled for Bill to advance, "no cars in sight" (either way), and as Bill reached the bottom of the hill, Murphy's Law prevailed. Surprisingly, a car approaching from Bill's right crashed into his truck sending Bill airborne into the fecal creek headfirst, with garbage flying everywhere. As Bill, terrorized with fright and anger, with clothes besmirched, escaped intact from the creek, Bud kept repeating, "Umph lucky! Umph lucky!" And I reckon Bill really was! Needless to say, Bill Sovey learned a dear, unforgettable lesson.

For Christmas, 1923, my Father, bless his soul, presented me with a diminutive pool table. It served as a training game for developing me into a "sharpshooter" when in high school. It was really a blessing in disguise, for we did bet on games of "call" pool, billiards, eight and nine ball. I did win more than my fair square share of games and was able to harvest a considerable amount of spending money during the big '29 Depression period. One of my "Pigeons" was good friend and classmate Harold Holloway and our favorite location was "Sleps" Pool Hall, corner of Main and Otterman Streets. My nickname was "Ramrod" and Harold's was "Hotshot".

My 8th grade of primary school in southwest Greensburg was under the tutelage of beloved Mrs. Martz. She was a very compassionate, understanding, erudite and empathetic person, respected by all of our classmates. Her forte' was English and spelling, which she knew backwards and forewords and was quite capable of teaching to the hilt.

One of our highlights that year was the appearance of a doughty warrior, who survived the Civil War between the States. He was dressed in the full regalia of the 1861-1865 Union Army and rendered a down to earth, detailed account of the Battle of Gettysburg. He was an artilleryman, whose duty was to load cannon balls. He was of private status under Union General Buford and Colonel Caleb. They were defending the Cashtown Road near Herr Ridge on the outskirts of Gettysburg when the first shot of this battle was fired by a Confederate cannon under command of Harry Heth at 8:00 a.m., July 1st, 1863. Confederate General A.P. Hill, corps commander, had sent his two divisions under Generals Heth and Pender from Cashtown at 5 a.m. to probe the whereabouts of the Union Army, under Major General George Gordon Meade, and to estimate its strength. Lee's cavalry under his dashing General Jeb Stuart was unavailable and his army was flying blind. Some of Heth's soldiers the day before (June 30) had gone to Gettysburg to procure some shoes because theirs were full of holes from marching. The Union artillery under Buford put up an extremely doughty and stubborn resistance to the advance of the Confederate Army under the overall command of military genius General Robert Estelle Lee. Miraculously, they held off the Confederate advance for two vital hours to give the Union First Corps, under Generals Reynolds and Doubleday, precious time to advance to Seminary Ridge and engage Lee's Army head to head. The Union soldier speaking to us related all the highlights of the first three days of the battle of Gettysburg.

He had us particularly enthralled by the dramatic third day (July 3rd), which pictured General Pickett's Charge for the Confederacy against General Hancock's Corps of Union troops. The Confederate troops of 11,000 soldiers were almost completely decimated, blasted, and annihilated by Union artillery and infantry with a colossal number of deaths of their soldiers, from which the Confederacy never recovered. This was the turning point of the entire war, in combination with the colossal victory by U.S. General Grant at Vicksburg on the Mississippi River, on July 4th, 1863. Our class was mortified when, in the middle of his lecture on cannon fire, one classmate released a gargantuan blast of flatus accidentally. The soldier continued unperturbed in the least, vividly saying "Yes! Much louder than that."

I remember another embarrassing and utterly humiliating incident, circa 1922, when I went to the Strand Theatre in Greensburg to see "Birth of a Nation". This was a famous movie for the ages. Mother was having a special two-table bridge party for Dad's co-workers at Elliott Company in Jeanette. Invited were Fred Doring, Chuck Hosterman, Don Awne, and Steve Yoscak with their wives. She fixed some luscious icebox cookies and asked me to bring home, without fail, a half-pint of whipping cream from the "sugar bowl". After the movie, I did remember her request, but I put the cardboard box containing the whipping cream in my left suit coat pocket for security. When I reached home, I proudly said to Mother, "I've got your precious cream, as promised." When I reached into my pocket to retrieve my prize, guess what? To Mother's consternation and mine, I came out with a handful of beautiful white liquid. To say we were exasperated is truly the under statement of the year.

During the summer months of my last elementary school years, Mother and I would go by train from Greensburg to Baltimore via Harrisburg. From Baltimore we boarded the streetcar to Dundalk and then to Jones Creek. Cousin Jay Knobloch or Anna Stockberger would meet us at Jones Creek by rowboat and we would paddle by oars to Ed and Pearl Knobloch's cabin. Jones Creek was a small inlet of the Chesapeake Bay, which joins with the Atlantic Ocean and borders Pennsylvania, Virginia, Delaware, and Washington D.C. The Chesapeake Bay splits Maryland into the Eastern and Western Shores. We would stay a month or so and have a whale of a time fishing, swimming, hiking, camping, picking berries, and canoeing with cousins Jay, Mabel, and Anna – Pearl's Campfire Girls.

I learned to swim at age 6 years by flipping over backwards and submerging underwater. Anna Stockberger and Sister Mabel were real fish at swimming and were talented at diving. We occasionally ran into sea nettles or (vice versa) and had a painful experience, but the torture was just momentary. One thing I learned was that salt water was great for a cold and very soothing to the nostrils and sinuses by diving. We learned first rate about the habits of hymenopterae, including hornets, yellow jackets, wasps and honeybees. One time, while I was maneuvering among the abundant pussy willows near shore, I encountered a nest of yellow jackets. They flew into a rage at an imposter invading their home and inflicted innumerable stings (at least 15-20) all over my body. I dove into the water nearby and every time I came up for air, they were greeting me for about 15 minutes. It seemed like several hours. Our only treatment then was ice and, fortunately, although somewhat shocked, I escaped a major anaphylactic reaction.

We picked blackberries and Aunt Pearl made us jam, a glassful for each. We went crabbing, using rotten meat as bait and caught enough for a real crab feast. It was quite simple. All you had to do was to dangle the meat tied to a string about eight feet deep in the water and pull it up and let it down slowly until a crab caught on. Then you pulled it near the surface and netted it, but you had to be cautious of the two claws.

We often had to row across the bay from the cottage to the streetcar stop to pick up guests and visitors, although there was access to the residence by car and roadway. One special visitor to our bungalow was the McWilliams family from Perrysville, whom I remember well. They had a daughter, Lillian, about my age that enamored and delighted my heartstrings. I was with her swimming and rowing almost constantly for two days, but had to reluctantly say goodbye.

One unusual event occurred early in my 8th grade. A transfer student from Scotland presented to our class as a fellow member. His name was Jack Kinnison and he was reputed to be very high on the scale of academic ratings. He was a charming and hospitable young man with a catchy Scottish brogue, who made a profound favorable impression on all of our teachers and us. At the time, Gwineth Johnston and I were competing gingerly for class leadership by grades, and we welcomed Jack as a fellow adversary. At the end of the year the teachers voted on the number one student in our class whom they felt was most deserving of the highest honor embodying behavior, scholastics, character, and attendance. Jack Kinnison was voted that person. In general our class felt that this was an unfair choice, because Jack had only been there ½ year and his grades were definitely below Gwineth's and mine. It seemed really a snap judgment with insufficient time to assess his qualities in comparison to his classmates. I felt rebuffed at being valedictorian for nothing and being the popular choice of my peers. I convinced myself to accept the inevitable with a smile and vowed to try harder next time.

At graduation from elementary school, on that very fateful night, I pretty much decided to go into medicine for children's cause. There had been quite a dilemma for me between choosing medicine and the ministry as my lifetime pursuit and occupation, being an only kid. My love of children was the big dominant driving force. The question in my mind was how could I champion children's rights the most? The ministerial vocation could enlighten them spiritually and mentally, but the medical calling would benefit them physically, mentally and morally. My Mother and our pastor, Reverend L. E. Bair, were magnetizing me strongly toward the Creator's cause, but I felt the scales were balanced in favor of medicine. After agonizing for many days and nights and my cousin, Sam Hammer, was leaning toward being a physician, I logically decided I must please myself and not others because I must live with myself. My altruistic feelings were aided and abetted by the Friedlander children, with whom I had an ironclad friendship. They lived across the street from my home on 521 Foster Street. Popsy and Boopsy were the young damsels' names and their ages were three and four years respectively. They were striking blondes with wavy hair and heavenly blue eyes and were real live wires. They both loved to listen to animal stories and had a very keen sense of humor. Almost daily they would appear on the front porch steps and gingerly request my presence.

Mr. Friedlander, Sammy, was an excellent family dentist and he and I, with my father, would pitch quoits, (a game identical with horseshoes), in the evenings and we all took turns at winning. Sammy was a perfect blond and his wife, Rhoda, was a striking brunette. It is rather unusual that their children would both be blondes, especially belonging to the Jewish race. Across the alley, which formed the south boundary of our property lived the LaRues, a widow and three children. Robert, who was about my age, would play hockey and football with me. He later matriculated at the University of Pittsburgh and was their quarterback when they played the Washington Huskies in the Rose bowl on January 1st, 1934. Enrolled in the school of dentistry, he completed the seven-year course and became a prominent dentist from Greensburg.

One other formidable event during my childhood that took place every summer and is etched firmly in my memory, was the appearance of several circuses. There were namely: Wallace and Hagenbeck, Walter Main, and of course Ringling Brothers, Barnum, and Baily. My Father would wake me (or vice versa) at 4 a.m. and we would dress and then walk about two miles to South Greensburg to the spur of the P.R.R. Railway, where the circus established its grounds. The cars carrying the circus animals and personnel would arrive at about 6 a.m. and each car would be uncoupled and set aside in a special setting. The roustabouts, or muscle men, would pound in the iron poles with sledgehammers and set up the various tents for the administrative people, the cooks, and sundry actors and actresses. One of the first and prime duties of dire necessity was to feed and water the animals that had been without sustenance for about 8 to 10 hours since their last performance at maybe Altoona, Johnstown, or Harrisburg.

The elephants could be unchained first and fed bales of hay and given massive galvanized tubs of fresh water. The cages of the lions, tigers, horses, leopards, dogs, and snakes were exteriorized for a breath of fresh air. Clowns were the first human order of business and they were instrumental in connecting with the crowd of people by extending their hearty greetings. Lastly, when breakfast was being served the acrobats, high wire performers, bandsmen, hucksters, gamesmen, and moguls would all appear drowsy and red-eyed. We would then head for the hills and go home for our breakfast.

At 11 a.m., after all the circus unveiling and rehabilitation to the new environment had been completed and set up, came the big parade of all the animals, performers, managers, and city dignitaries. They were drawn mainly by horses in cages, auto, and by pedal locomotion. The scintillating star and piece de resistance of the parade was the calliope, which announced the beginning of the parade. People would line the streets on both sides. The clowns were the ambassadors of good will and would entertain the predominant numbers of children. Pulling those heavy wagons containing the animals was a Herculean job for the horses, especially because of the rather severe grades of our sheer hills.

There were two performances or shows by the circus – afternoon and night. My parents would usually take me in the afternoon and I don't believe I missed any one. One time, before my time I am told, there was a tremendous rainstorm the night of the circus at Electric Park, southeast of southwest Greensburg. The tents blew down; several people were killed in the excitement of the crowds and a few carnivorous animals got loose. This event caused wide spread horror and was the foundation for moving the circus location to South Greensburg, which was a much safer area to hold it. Also, there were a couple train wrecks of circus trains around the Altoona horseshoe curve and the Bessemer Mountains, which did literally devastate a couple circuses, including Hegenbeck and Wallace, and put the damper on circus travel by trains. Deterioration of the railroads also was quite a deterrent to this means of moving from one city to another.

Chapter 5

Greensburg High School

The transition from grade school to high school was a seven-league boot leap, which took a rather long struggle of acclimatization. The transformation and metamorphosis actually wasn't as brutal as it looked at first glance, and my apprehensions were laid to rest quickly. After all, the main purpose of all schools is primarily education mentally, morally, and physically with increasing levels of toughness to reach maturity. So, it was easy. All I had to do was study, study, and more study in order to attain success. Meeting 300 strange fellow grade students and half a dozen strange teachers in one sitting at one time was, to me, somewhat overwhelming. But as usual father time solves all problems. We were thrown into the lion's den, naked, at the beginning of the 1st year with no preparation. My classes encompassed English, algebra, Latin, science and ancient history and that's quite a mouthful to digest. I dug in with all my might and main and was rewarded with all A's my freshman year.

I had to walk a mile up hill to school and the reverse after 4 p.m. We would usually eat lunch from 12 to 1 in the cafeteria at school or go down Main Street to the Sugar Bowl, which meant eating on the run. The boys wore knickers and sweaters; and the ladies were attired in dresses, skirts, shirts and sweaters. We carried 2 or 3 books back and forth daily as a rule. For recreation, we had sports on weekends and that was pretty much it the first two years of high school, until I got my driver's license. Dad bought a new Studebaker Sedan in May 1927 for $1326. The garage was already built by my father, awaiting its resident car. We didn't have "dates" those first two years in high school, but we did go to movies and football games on Saturdays. There were two movie theaters, the Grand and the Manos.

All during our first year they were building many new buildings and tearing down all the old buildings. There was mud, mud, mud everywhere, about 3 inches deep. There were also constant loud noises --pounding, sawing, screeching, hammering, whistling, banging, and loud talking. We had "potbelly" stoves, coaled to keep us warm in winter the first year. Actually, it was a good experience in disguise, for we really appreciated our next three years in the plush, brand spanking, virgin new buildings. Painters, bricklayers, plumbers, electricians, and cement layers all had a field day sine parallel. It seemed like eons before the new school was structured, but suddenly there it was in all its pristine glory at the end of 1926.

Almost every Sunday we would go to church. The First Reformed Church, formed by Zwingli and Wesley, was a branch of the original Lutheran Church. We attended Sunday school, then church services at 11 a.m. and 8 p.m., and Christian endeavor at 7 p.m. We had a very close relationship with Reverend Lawrence Elijah Bair, one of the most wonderful and Godly persons that ever lived. He was wholly and holy devoted to every parishioner. He apparently had rheumatic fever in childhood, because he complained of frequent attacks of angina and had mitral regurgitation, diagnosed by Dr. Hamman. He and I had a best friend alliance and had many advisory conferences. Actually, he was quite an inspiration and hero in my high school life. Lawrence was a brilliant historian and Civil War authority.

I was quite enthralled with my freshman English teacher, Miriam Hopkins. She was well endowed with pulchritude; a striking brunette with fine, chiseled facial features, an enchanting personality, and a venusoid figure to top it off. Our first year Shakespeare play was Julius Caesar and she added her intelligence (considerable) and spice to a great story. Our first year Latin teacher (I had 4 years) was Mary Reed and she was a real peach; very understanding, charming and positive. Our algebra and trigonometry instructor was Kathy Lehman and she was talented at clarifying math for our verdant freshman class. For ancient history we were under Clara Barnhart, who had a few cards less than a full deck, and was quite unsure of herself. Breasted's history book had plenty of information to get us by. Our fifth subject was modern science taught by Mary Morse, and she was very capable, devoted and innovative.

I believe my favorite subject, no holds barred, was definitely English with dead language, Latin, a distant second. Our second year English teacher was Miss Margaret Walthour, a very affable, beautiful, and intelligent lady. I remember "Ivanhoe", "The Lady or the Tiger", and "Macbeth" were indelibly imprinted in my memory. "The Tale of Two Cities", "Far From the Maddening Crowd", and "Treasure Island" were our best books.

Our third year English mentor was Miss Cecilia Brown, a very warm, happy, outgoing, frank, and energetic person. It comes to mind that her critique of one of my themes was "bombastic, Faustian, inflated, pretentious, and hyperbolic". She really let me have it full blast between the eyes - don't spare the horses.

Our senior year prize English teacher was Miss Ethel Grace Hudson. How come they were all single? Their command of the English language struck absolute terror and fear in the hearts and minds of all male suitors. Ethel G. Hudson did inform me that she had genuine doubts about my ability to master college freshman English. That challenge spurred and inspired me on to obtain grade "A" in that special subject and I informed Ethel G. of that accomplishment. She was editor-in-chief of the "Brown and White", our monthly school publication and I was sports editor, covering all athletic events.

We had state championship teams in football my first and second years in high school. Our really top-notch games were with Harrisburg Tech and Johnstown each year. After the season ended during my junior year, we played Turtle Creek High in Greensburg for the W.P.I.A.L. (Western Pennsylvania Interscholastic Athletic League) Championship. On that day it rained like a cloud burst and the gridiron was a quagmire of mud a foot deep. We were defeated 6 to 0 when we fumbled and produced a turnover on our three yard line in the 4th quarter. Spectators at the game claimed that our star quarterback and stellar fullback, Gaurino and Hull, were engaged in extensive carousing the night before the game. Be that as it may, a lot of lachrymal secretions were shed by all the loyal fans afterwards. One highlight at the end of the first half of this debacle was a song "Let Me Call You Sweetheart" sung by a nine-year-old boy with the most magnificent voice I have ever heard. It was crystal clear, strong, vibrant, natural, and had me mesmerized. My close friend, Paul Seaton, was one of our cheerleaders and was quite a champion with the ladies in contradistinction to moi.

My Father and I took trips to Erie, Harrisburg, Johnstown, and Latrobe, Pennsylvania to see our high school warriors perform away from home. One time, during my third year, I drove our car with five classmates to Scottsdale, Arizona, for a basketball game. We thought we were big shots and got a pack of tobacco and put a big chunk in our mouths. After about an hour we suffered diplopia, vertigo, and epigastric pain and fortunately had rather violent emesis – which really cured the hangover. To enhance matters, after the game there were about six inches of unexpected snow on the ground and our car lock was frozen. We used a cigarette lighter to thaw the lock, but my hands were so numb that I dropped the key in the deep snow. After an exasperating hour of searching and agonizing, Seaty found the buried key and we were homeward bound.

On another memorable occasion we were playing Irwin in football at Offutt's Field in Greensburg. I was selling refreshments to raise money for the "Brown and White". It was near the end of the 4th quarter and the Irwin Band played "Bye, Bye Blackbird". We happened to have a black star tailback named Willie Robbins and we had the ball on our forty-yard line. Willie would get down in an attitude of prayer with his rabbit's foot at this juncture. On the next play, Willie summoned his utmost speed and ran like the wind to score a touchdown and we won with a final score of 6 – 0. Surely, the Irwin Band aroused our Willie's ire and courage to fever pitch.

It comes to mind that one Friday night before the Youngwood football game scheduled for next day, about twenty classmates boarded an open truck and headed for Youngwood. We were armed with a ton of tomatoes, cabbages, and apples and we threw these missiles all over the streets and lawns of our adversary. Unfortunately, the State Police caught up with us and escorted us to their barracks, where we were detained for a couple of hours. They recorded our names and queried us about our intents and purposes. Amongst our personage were daughters and sons of lawyers, doctors, and judges - Edie Rial, Herbie Wilson, Drake Twins, and Eleanor Snyder, to name a few. The girls were all crying copious tears, but somehow consternation didn't grip the boys. We were all discharged unfettered after an admonition to cease and desist any such raucous behavior in the future.

I passed my test for a driver's license on June 10th, 1927, a week after my 16th birthday. My parents had bought a 1927 Studebaker Sedan in May, and my Mother's brother, Uncle Bob, took me out one day and gave me one lesson in driving. My Father also learned to drive but he was up tight and jittery while driving and therefore I was delegated to do the lion's share of motoring for the family. Besides, Mother was uncomfortable and shared a lack of confidence in the senior Howard's control of the wheel.

We unknowingly believed petrol or gasoline was expensive at 10 cents a gallon and I practically never had more than two gallons of gas in the tank at one time. Every time I took the car out on a date, or with "our gang", we would take up a collection to defray the gasoline tab. We measured the quantity of fuel in the tank with a yardstick and if it was more than an inch, we would take off confidant that we had an adequate supply of gas to get by.

One of our buddies was Charles Davison, whose parents owned an ice cream parlor. Six of our group would show up at his parents establishment numbering three of each gender, - none "going steady". We did smoke cigarettes, because it was the "smart" peer thing, but we never gave one smidgen of a thought about beer, alcohol, or drugs of any kind. I guess ignorance was bliss and our parents could sleep blissfully. Our conception of being risqué and being a big shot actually was to smoke a stogie, a five-cent cigar, or to chew "mail pouch". Curfew was 11 p.m. and it was strictly obeyed to the letter or else privileges were drastically curtailed. No one carried more than 50 cents in their pocket for a "rainy day".

My closest boy friend in high school was Paul Seaton. We double dated on weekends during our junior and senior years. In reference to blonde girls, Paul had a special designation – "where there's light, there's heat". He was definitely a ladies man, true and blue, and they returned his overtures with gusto. We believed in Heinz 57 variety, and seldom ever dated the same lady twice in succession. I furnished the car and Seaty would line up our dates all over Greensburg and surrounding towns, including Youngwood, Mount Pleasant, Monesson, Monongahela City, Jeanette, and Irwin. I remember with fond thoughts, "Marty" Kennon, Carolyn Rowan, Lulu Henderson, Anne Dunbar, Betty Morgan, Betty Crock, Dorothy Calvin, "Peggy" Remaley, and Louise Stump, to name a few lovely femmes. I can associate a special song that came out at the strategic time I was associating with each particular girl friend. "I Can't Give You Anything But Love" with my ideal Marty Keenan, "Sweet and Lovely" with my beloved Carolyn Rowan, "Jeannine I Dream of Lilac Time" and "Don't Bring Lulu" with charmer Lulu Henderson, "Love letters in the Sand" with sweet Peg Remalley, "Love Me or Leave Me" with teaser Betty Morgan, "You Want Lovin' But I Want Love" with pretty Dorothy Colvin, and "Those Little White Lies" with Cleopatra Ruth Ruffner. It seems there was a deluge of beautiful, plaintive melodies in the late twenties and early thirties to complement all the gorgeous "Big Bands".

Radio was born in my verdant freshman high school year. I recall Philco, Altwater, Kent and Magnavox Radio Productions. Radios in cars were novelties and luxuries. Victrolas, movies, and vaudeville were our prime sources of entertainment in the "good old days".

Sundays were devoted to church study, walks, car rides, and visiting family relatives. In the summer of 1927, I was privileged to go to a church camp for ten days at Camp Harmony, about fourteen miles upwards from Johnstown. It was situated on top of a two thousand foot mountain at the site of the Cramahomian Dam, which overflowed at the time of the great Johnstown flood in 1888. The flood burgeoned down steep valleys, sweeping everything in its path, killing people, and inundating the entire city of Johnstown and suburbs. We took the Pennsylvania Railroad from Greensburg to Johnstown and transferred to a train from Johnstown to Gloversville and then on to our final destination. There were about fifty campers from several cities, representing their respective reformed churches. The camp activities embraced Bible study, predominately Old Testament, with swimming, hiking, vesper services, and archery. When I returned home I was expected to deliver an oration depicting my camp experiences and detailing the highlights of the study program on the "vital living" Old Testament.

While in camp I became acquainted with some unforgettable people. One of our camp mentors was Elisha Fosdick , a retired minister from Lancaster, Pennsylvania. He was a compelling inspiration and nearly convinced me that I should choose the theological profession for my vocation. If ever there was a true heavenly person, I'm sure he would be the one, for he emanated godly characteristics in all his activities. Also there was a very lovely young lady my age of fourteen, Louise Little, who was especially attractive to me but unfortunately there was not much reciprocity on her part. Most of the campers were a few years older and more mature than I – serving me as excellent guides in proper behavior.

While in high school I joined the Demolay in Jeanette, Pennsylvania. It was a youth organization, which emulated Masonic principles. At one monthly meeting in November, my Father accompanied me because of snow and ice on the roads. I drove to the meet and had a very minor fender bender in Jeanette. In those days the cars had about an inch of iron covering and you could get away with slight damage to your car in an accident. Dad drove us home and performed nobly until we were descending a precipitous hill on the outskirts of Greensburg. The car started sliding and my Father became quite agitated, steering wildly right and left. Finally we ended by straddling the streetcar tracks, headed back to Jeannette. It was a real thriller and at this juncture I supplanted Dad in the driver's seat. We reached our home very slowly, carefully, and traveling as on eggs. My Uncle Bob and Aunt Edna Haines escorted Carolyn Rowan and I to a couple Demolay New Year's dances at the Syrian Mosque in Pittsburg. Uncle Bob was an expert driver, about as safe as the safest, especially on treacherous mountain roads in the worst of weather conditions.

On one other memorable occasion in the summer preceding my senior year, I drove my date, Ruth Ruffner, and two other couples to a moonlight dance excursion from Pittsburg on the Monongahela River. We left Greensburg, 30 miles away, in plenty of time but on the Boulevard of the Allies, near Squirrel Hill, I had a minor accident, when I bumped the car ahead of me which came to a sudden, inexplicable dead stop. In braking, my problem was a wad of gum, which was glued to my right shoe on the gas pedal. This incident held us up for about a half-hour and we missed the boat and had to settle for a movie at the Goldwyn Theater. On the way home, just outside of Wilkinsburg, we unexpectedly encountered a big white horse in the middle of the road. Fortunately for the horse and us, there was a dense fog and we were motoring cautiously so we avoided the horse.

On another occasion, while coming back from a dance, we had a right rear flat tire beside a cemetery. It was grotesque and eerie, but I managed to change my spare tire. The damsel with me, Cozette Grable from Jeanette, was terrified about the cemetery and it was a bit later when we arrived to her house. Her father met us at the door and gave me a severe dressing down and wouldn't listen to a reasonable explanation. Needless to say, that was a one night stand only with Cozette, who was a devastating blonde and not really my cup of tea. On a more humorous note, I took Peg Remaley to a summer dance near Export, Pennsylvania. After each dance the bandleader would requisition a number to be played by his troops. After one of the dances, I blurted, "Love Me or Leave Me" – a famous song. The bandleader retorted, "Tell that to your friend, you brought her."

A further instance comes to mind regarding a dance at the Armory, where my maternal Uncle Frank was conducting his own big band. Mother gave me a ten-dollar bill to defray expenses and somehow I lost the money on the way to the dance. My partner was a very gorgeous redhead, Winifred Jones, daughter of the manager of the Albert Hotel, Greensburg's finest. We went to the dance anyhow and Uncle Frank bailed me out by making me a loan. After the dance, Mother and Uncle Bob picked us up and we went for a sandwich and a butterscotch nut sundae at the Sugar Bowl. Fortunately, Mother picked up the ten dollar bill from the back seat and "all's well that ends well".

During my senior year I joined a fraternity, the Omega Xi, to which my cousin Samuel Hammer belonged. It was a group of all males, all very substantial high-class persons. They were all quite friendly and held a monthly meeting on rotation at one another's home. We would talk over school problems, home difficulties, and sports activities. One of our members was Paul Rathgeb, whose family had a large dairy farm. We always relished and cherished a meeting at his place for the chicken sandwiches; chocolate milk, angel food cake, and homemade ice cream with black raspberries were a heavenly, nutritious treat for a bunch of starving adolescents. It comes to mind I was initiated into the Omega Xi at Rathgeb's farm. We were forced to swallow three raw eggs, run twice around the outskirts of the farm, asked to name twelve state capitols west of the Mississippi River, and paddled for each one we missed. I remember a few special, friendly brothers: Kenny Kile, Ed and Art Sherman, Jimmy Wohler, Ron Fox, and Jim Morgan.

In the summer before my senior year, 1928, my parents and the Fisher family from Dundalk, Maryland, on 304 Patapsco Avenue, took a conjoined vacation of two weeks at Watertown, New York, near the St. Lawrence River. Harry and Hattie were the parents, and the children were Florence, Elizabeth, and Harry Junior. We knew the Fishers quite well from previous association during the time of World War I and a trip we had shared to Atlantic City in the summer of 1920. Harry Junior, my age, and I became very close buddies and later were roommates in our first year at college. Florence, a schoolteacher, was handicapped from a severe, general reaction to horse serum rabies vaccine when she was a child. Elizabeth, twenty years old and the apple of her father's eye, was a very beautiful and winsome lass. Harry was his mother's pride and joy in no uncertain terms and I detected a slight antagonism between Hattie and myself, because Harry Junior did not exactly have a proclivity for the academics. We enjoyed a most wonderful time swimming, boating, fishing, hiking, and shopping at "Brassie Corners". One night while we were touring the countryside, the car's electricity suddenly died and we were in complete pitch darkness on a black macadam road in the middle of nowhere. We were all in a gay, festive mood and didn't panic. Fortunately, a police car came to our rescue after about an hour, which seemed like forever.

We were joined by Jack Oscar and Gertrude Maxwell Judge a few days after we set up camp at Loon Lake. Jack taught pattern making at Camp Hill in Harrisburg, Pennsylvania, and Gertrude, a very lovely lady, taught music in an elementary school there. They were childless at this period of time, but later birthed a baby boy, who had one of the world's worst cases of eczema I have ever seen. His face and features were completely covered with a mass of inflamed, yellowish, oozing, inflammatory lesions, resistant to all treatments and medications.

During my high school career, I sustained two common colles fractures of my left and right forearms. On one occasion, I was running at night on an icy pavement and my feet escalated and I fell back on my right hand and wrist and I heard a crackle and felt sudden, excruciating pain in that arm. I couldn't sleep a wink that night and the next day beat a speedy path over to Doctor Howard Hamman's office by Shanks Mare walking. Doctor Howard took one glimpse at me and said, "You look like you are in dire pain," to which I fully agreed. I related my story of woe. Howard immediately sat facing me and said, "Shake hands with me." He pulled, flexed, and extended my right wrist with a lightening maneuver and I heard a crunching sound, but there was a tremendous relief of pain at once, before you could say, "Jack Robinson". I said, "Whew!" And he replied, "You had a fracture of the radius with dislocation and I set it back in place and you will have a plaster cast covering the right wrist, hand and elbow for about four weeks." I said, "Thank you, I think." After limping in, I leaped out of his office, feeling no pain. This happened before x-rays were readily available, but he really didn't need it, because I'm sure he had experienced many previous similar silver spoon radius fractures in children. My only regret was that my pool playing was severely restricted, but I did manage to overcome this obstacle to a great degree.

On the night of our graduation, I had our Studebaker and with six other graduates took a spin about the countryside in festive celebration. There were the

Drake twins, Emily and Miriam, my buddy Paul Seaton, Frank Bender, "Shin" Ruff and myself. Miriam was with me; Emily was paired with Paul, and Shin paired with Frank. There was one new song fresh off the press that appealed to us then, "Those Little White Lies". After running out of gasoline, as luck would have it, we coasted down a steep hill and had enough momentum to almost reach a gas station. We took up a collection and managed to amass twenty-eight cents for 2 ½ gallons of gas. We decided at this time fate was sending a message and we made a beeline for our respective domiciles.

The biggest dance of the year, in no uncertain terms, was the May Senior Soiree. My partner was the lovely, pert Louise Stump, sister of my 4th grade teacher, Gladys Stump. She lived on a farm about five miles west of Greensburg, off the Delmont Road, and was a neighbor of my grandfather's brother, Lloyd Haines. The dance was in the week before graduation and it was customary to exchange gifts with your lady friend. Louise got me a cigarette case and lighter, both encased in leather. I got her a beauty ensemble, consisting of rouge, lipstick, perfume, and powder to match her complexion. At this time there was a song called, "Every Little Breeze Seems to Whisper Louise, Birds in the Trees Seem to Twitter Louise".

The males each had a little booklet containing spaces for each of ten dances to be filled in with the names of special classmates and their partners, with whom we traded dances. In 1929 we went overboard and had a big band, Kay Keyser and his college of musical knowledge. It was a good thing that we were not cognizant of the impending, tumultuous stock crash a few months later. Anyhow, it was a gala party, which broke up at 11:00 p.m. and we hurriedly bedded down for a few hours sleep. We were up at 3:00 a.m. and were off to Crisfield, Maryland, about 70 miles from home. I took three couples in the Studebaker, Seaton and Tom Jennings and our three ladies. The entourage of cars consisted of five with twenty-two couples. We had made prior arrangements for breakfast and had a very hearty one. There was one disconcerting event. Towards the end of our feast, the lady in charge announced that someone purloined a ten-dollar bill from her boudoir. She suggested that each one in our party go upstairs and come back. Sure enough, after everyone had performed this ritual, she declared all clear; the magical bill had been replaced, unharmed. We all knew exactly who did it; Bill McDevitt, who was number one bad boy of our class, a really nice person with sticky fingers.

Chapter 6

Pre-Med at College Park, MD.

My dear Mother had a whale of a time forcing me out of our home when it came time to go to college. I guess I was rather reticent and bashful and enjoyed the comforts and protection afforded by mother's apron strings. She said to me, "You've matriculated and we've paid your entrance fee and you are going to college right now, period." Mother was very determined and I could discern by the tone of her voice and flashing eyes, she was definitely not in an argumentative mood. So, I said, "Yes, dear Mother, anchors away."

Actually I was quite fortunate for my roommate was buddy Harry Ellsworth Fisher Junior from Dundalk, Maryland, just a stone's throw from Baltimore, Maryland, which is two stone's throws from College Park, Maryland. We didn't have a car at college, but shoe leather was inexpensive and the exercise was a perfect solution. Students in college really did not go for bicycles at that time period. The college campus buildings at College Park were tightly integrated and distances were miniscule. The pre-med course was telescoped and I could have made medical school in two years, but I realized my state of immaturity and decided the competition was quite enhanced. Besides, being an only, sheltered child was a bit of a handicap socially, especially for me. I was a dreamer and a reticent person by first intention.

Harry was enrolled in a business course and we would hitch hike to his home in Dundalk and back on weekends. We would indulge in loving care and excellent cuisine and charge our batteries for the coming weeks' skirmish at college.

Our school was known by the sobriquet of "Old Liners" and our song was "Keep the Caissons a Rolling". We endured the usual period of hazing and humbling by the haughty sophomores and we wore "Rat Caps" with black and gold colors. Our school designation as the "Terrapins" was to be bestowed on the University by our graduating class of '33 and I will address this issue later.

Harry's parents were as wonderful persons as I have ever met. They had a great sense of humor, and were extremely generous, relaxed, and understanding. Harry Senior would kid us after we came back from a date by feeling our scalps to see if they were wet. He would laugh and say, "I wanted to ascertain whether your lady friends had 'peed' on you." I never could fathom the logistics of this humor, but would go along with the banter. Hattie, the matron of the Fisher's, was a most loving, happy, hard working, wise lady. Harry's sisters, Libby and Florence, were also very supportive and helpful. My parents were really closely attached in friendship with the Fishers over a period of ten years. I recall one special, happy vacation when we joined them along with Edna and Edgar Kemp in Atlantic City for a weekend in July 1921.

My cousin, Jay Edward Knobloch, son of Ed Knobloch my paternal uncle, also attended Maryland University at College Park as a sophomore when we entered as freshmen. He was taking a general arts and science course and after graduation went on to become a full-fledged chiropractor. Jay was basically a regular fellow, but he was a teaser and prankster. One day, while Harry and I were in classes in winter, my cousin Jay entered our room in the dorms and poured a bottle of cod liver oil over our steaming hot water-containing heat register. You can readily imagine the horrendous emanations of odor, which ensued for several days. On another occasion, dear, sweet Jay set the wastebasket in the hallway by our room on fire at around two o'clock a.m. Fortunately, a guard was alerted in time while making his rounds and extinguished it. Luckily Jay "boy" was not detected, for I'm sure he would have been expelled from school.

We had no period of "orientation" by teachers or benevolent upper classmen to help us acclimatize and adjust to school rules and regulations. However, the president of the University had a special meeting to welcome us, indoctrinate our class of '33 and render sage advice for study.

I became acquainted and closely bonded in friendship with a fellow classmate, Charles Gassaway Spicknall. Charles was a real high-grade student, who had won a merit scholarship to Maryland because of his 4.0 average at Hyattsville High School. Beside his explicit intelligence, sincerity, dependability, and good judgment, Charles had a notable, charming personality. We formed a lasting, firm alliance through college, medical school, and even internship. We had many common goals and pledged and joined the same college fraternity, but more about that later. Hyattsville is only a hop, skip and jump from College Park (three miles) and Charles commuted to school daily. I would go home with him frequently and we often studied together. His mother, Fannie, was a warm, witty, congenial, <u>loquacious</u> person, who was always complaining about "my June dizzy spells". His father, Wilson, was truly hen-pecked up to the eyebrows, but a very, very nice man, quite generous and an arduous worker. Wilson was a proficient insurance salesman, who argued incessantly with Fannie but always lost. His two sisters, Julie and Florence, were maiden school teachers with excellent manners and understanding of human nature.

Harry and I went our separate ways when we pledged to different fraternities on the campus. He went to Kappa Alpha Southern, and I, to Eta chapter of Phi Sigma Kappa. I endeavored strenuously to get Harry to do "Phi Sig" with me, but to no avail. However, we maintained a high-grade friendship thereafter even though I moved into the frat house in November 1929.

Before being pledged, I remember a poignant incident when I was invited to dinner at the Phi Sigma Kappa house. I was seated beside the president, Johnny O'Neill, and my table etiquette was not the greatest for I had a fatal tendency to knock over liquid containing vessels. I had an inclination to talk with my hands and I would be deeply engrossed in conversation, rendering me oblivious to the real environment around me. Johnny and I were lost in discussion about student government as he was the present President of Student Affairs at the college. While we were deeply engaged in this subject, the gentleman next to me passed the gravy to me. In turn, I tried to pass it on to Mr. O'Neill and spilled it all over his lap. It was a moment of sheer embarrassment and I apologized profusely for my abject clumsiness. Johnny was extremely gracious, but fortunately the gravy had made the rounds for about twenty brothers and it had cooled. After this happening I was sure my name was "mud" and I would definitely not be invited to join the fraternity. I had made the rounds of Sigma Alpha Sigma, Sigma Nu and Beta Omega Pi fraternities, but I really preferred the men in Phi Sig by far. Lo and behold, when the invitations to join came out, I was extended an invite to pledge to Phi Sigma Kappa. Apparently, my adverse behavior was forgiven and they had evaluated me by other standards.

Harry Fisher joined with Kappa Alpha Southern, but to my elation, my friend Charlie Spicknall joined Phi Sig as a pledge along with me. It would cement an enduring friendship for three years in College Park, until we went to our respective medical schools. The Phi Sig brothers were very cordial and welcomed us with open arms, but warned us that if we were caught without cigarettes the consequences would be disastrous. Living in the fraternity house was decidedly a new experience for me. It was an association I truly needed to grow and mature in my social development, learning to give and take, and how to get along and share with others. As an only child (brat), I was sheltered to a great extent. However, I did associate with my many diverse cousins, but this was not as intimate an association as with siblings.

Our frat counselor and faculty advisor was Boris Daniels. He was a young

Russian graduate of Princeton, quite learned, affable and helpful. Danny taught us to play "Russian Bank", a card game easily mastered and somewhat similar to solitaire. He married an Alpha Omicron Pi coed, a member of our class of '33 at graduation time. She was a statuesque, pure blond, very personable, pleasant, and a real charmer. Our house manager was Mitchell Franklin and he ran a tight ship, but was fair and square. His roommate was Jim Greeley, actually a close descendant of the famous Horace. Jim had a big, red Lincoln convertible and he was the most handsome guy you can imagine. He was a real lady-killer and an immaculate dresser with the New England language accent and decor. How could any femme resist Jim? Probably none could, should, or would.

Two of my brothers were named Mason and Dixon, believe it or not. Darius McLellan Dixon was the Lacrosse manager and had his left eye accidentally extinguished by a Lacrosse ball in the year before I joined. A Lacrosse ball is almost as hard as iron and it is cradled in a long stick and hurled from player to player with the object being to get it in the crease guarded by a goal keeper. Darius McLellan Dixon was struck by accident directly in the left eye by a misdirected Lacrosse ball and had surgical removal with an artificial replacement.

An unusual incident comes to mind regarding the glass eye as being the cynosure of all eyes. Darius always deposited his unseeing eye in a glass of water before bedding down. One super hot night in June, around midnight, our brothers were returning from a sorority dance. Herb Ebe came into Dixon's room, which I shared. I was shooting the breeze with Dick Murdock. Ebe was dehydrated and breathless and before you could say, "Jack Robinson", he grasped the glass of water containing the foreign body and swallowed the eye. We excitedly told Herb he had drunk the water with Dixon's glass eye. He said, "Wow, I'm sorry but I was dying of thirst and couldn't resist drinking the glass of water containing the eye." Needless to say, we gave Herb a laxative and in 48 hours, we recovered Dixon's prize possession. All is well that ends well.

As I previously mentioned, English was always my foremost and favorite subject in high school. This continued in college. I would often study the dictionary for hours, when I had time to dream. You might say I was in love with the English language per se. Although Latin was a dead language, I was exposed to four years of it in high school and liked "Cicero" and "Virgil" especially. Math was my anathema. Spelling was always very intriguing to me and I won several spelling contests in the grade schools and was very prideful of my 100's in my compositions.

I would never accept anything less than "A" in English throughout my entire grade and high school years. As I mentioned, when Ethel G. Hudson, my senior high school teacher challenged me about college English, I accepted the gauntlet and easily obtained an A+ in my Maryland freshman English course. My teacher was Robert Hale, who was my premier instructor in my three years at College Park. Actually, my college English course was duck soup compared to my senior high school English course. Hale was a man of few words but every word was poignant, meaningful, and directly explanative - my kind of man. You can win a million dollar bet that I wrote Ethel G. a letter expounding my profound accomplishment in her life's subject. It was not to boast, but realistically to thank her for her part in preparing me for a higher challenge. One of the books we read under Dr. Hale was Thomas Hardy's "Far From the Maddening Crowd". It was indelibly impressed in my memory.

Our second year English professor was Ira Lemon and, appropriately, his name coincided with his teaching. Ira was grossly overweight; he absolutely did weigh over 400 pounds, and you can book it, believe me. We used to joke that he cried intermittently because he couldn't tie his shoestrings and was never ever able to see or find his male organ. He was as confusing with his instruction (destruction) as Professor Hale was crystal clear.

Another unforgettable professor was Edward Gwinner, my freshman algebra and trigonometry teacher. He would put equations on the board while actually dancing. He was quite emphatic with his broken English and drove home his points and conclusions with much gusto. While prancing about the room, he would point unexpectedly to one of us classmates and call out a student's full name and ask a question for immediate answer. If you were not super alert, he would revel in catching anyone in limbo. One special student in our class was the loveliest brunette you can ever imagine, Adeline Jarrell, a comely, but naive country lass from the Eastern Shore of Maryland. She was really in left field when it came to algebra, up the proverbial creek sans paddle. She and I became platonic friends and we would meet in the library to help her to understand the algebraic equations. It was an altruistic relationship, realistically, but I did enjoy basking in her charming ways. In fact, I invited her to a fraternity dance at our Phi Sig house. She accepted, but Arley Unger, one of my benevolent brothers, stole her away from me which relates loud and clear my status with the damsels (which really came in handy during WW II).

One of my first year pedants was Major George Bowes of the U.S. Army, who taught ROTC because Maryland was a land grant college, requiring two years of military training. He was a rigid disciplinarian, who knew everyone in our class by first, middle, and last name, <u>precisely</u>, after only one session. We had to know every part of the rifle, as well as being able to disassemble, reassemble, and handle it perfectly in multiple maneuvers. One special day comes to mind when we were drilling on the parade grounds and "marching in review". Our company had to be at least a half-mile away from Major Bowes' eagle eye. All of a sudden he blurted out, in a stentorian voice by megaphone, "Mister Knobloch, Howard Thomas, quit chewing gum in ranks". This was a penultimate blow to my pride and a true wake up call in front of several hundred troops. One of his surprise tricks was to encounter you one on one while at attention and say, "Present arms". You were to instantly bring your rifle up in front of you and he would grab hold of the rifle at once. If you didn't release the rifle instantaneously, he would pull you forward and you would fall on the ground. But he was a fair, square shooter, no pun intended.

One of my most enjoyable experiences happened on my chemistry final. I had never had any chemistry instruction in high school and this was my first exposure. Professor Robert White was a most eminent teacher, and we hung on his every word in class. At the termination of the course, there was a customary final exam. I studied all night before, as was my usual preparation for an important test. My instinct told me that I had aced the exam, which was taken by 400 plus freshmen and ladies. While walking to my physics class a couple days later, I met Edward Highberger, a chemistry instructor from my hometown of Greensburg. He said, "Congratulations, Howard, you have made the highest grade in the chemistry final." I replied, "You're kidding me." Mr. Highberger said, "No way, it's for real." The ecstatic news really dumbfounded and floored me. When I returned to the fraternity house, Willie Leykins met me at the door and said, "I hear you came out number one on the chem. final and we're very proud of your accomplishment." Willie was secretary of our fraternity (Phi Sigma Kappa) and also an instructor in basic chemistry. He had a proclivity for southern Maryland corn whiskey and was a very personable young man. Studying in a fraternity house wasn't a bowl of cherries because of the tremendous noise and fraternization of all the brothers after the evening meal until about 10 p.m. Then, I was able to concentrate in earnest and hit the books.

At the fraternity, we always prefaced each meal with "the blessing" so each person could get an even start. We had heavy glassware and the story was that we wouldn't purchase it unless it would bounce twice without breaking.

Christmas vacation occurred following our midterm exams, and Mr. Highberger and I rode the Greyhound Bus together to Greensburg. During the trip they played a movie, "The Grumpy Grandfather." It was an overnight ride and Ed complained of a pain and weakness in both leg calves while we were traversing the Tuscarora Mountains. After the holiday, I heard that Mr. Highberger had been admitted to our home hospital, Westmoreland General, with a diagnosis of Landry's Ascending Paralysis. He succumbed to the ravages of this disease, sometimes called an acute idiopathic polyneuritis or Guillian-Barre' syndrome. This entity sometimes complicates a vaccine reaction and is immunoreactive but its etiology is unknown.

Another of my freshman teachers was my friend, Professor Drake, the dragon of organic chemistry. He was the epitome of harshness and a top sergeant. One encounter with him would make you a quaking, quivering cream puff. He emanated the true "fear of God" to a "T". I'll never forget our first surprise exam on which I garnered a big fat "43", but the class average was a "40". It was a shocker and a real alarm of things to come. I struggled valiantly to sweat out a B-minus for the course and felt quite happy to come out alive in one piece.

Another first year professor was Dr. Pearson in Zoology and Vertebrate Anatomy. He was an elderly, dried-up prune of a man and our class nicknamed him a fitting sobriquet, "The Bug". One of his instructors was a huge giant of a man, who I'm sure was suffering from a malady of the anterior pituitary glands. It is known as Acromegaly or Gigantism, whereby all parts of the human body are magnified. One of the specific areas is the maxilla and mandible, which appear as a Lantern Jaw: or a grossly enlarged jaw. One morning I appeared in his class and endured the height of embarrassment when he called me aside and informed me surreptitiously that my fly was gaping. I offered no excuse, but my face was never more scarlet.

My Public Speaking teacher, William Bobs, was a real gem of a person. His favorite word was "Sfiggeringktum" which means with a burst of super, energetic zeal, to put your heart and soul into an undertaking. One time in the middle of a speech, my mouth became so dry I couldn't talk, masticate, or swallow. I had to leave the room and ran to the fountain at the end of the hallway to quench my overpowering thirst. He recognized my embarrassing plight and thereafter we had a pitcher of water and cups immediately available.

If I live to be 150 years old, I'll never forget the Physical Chemistry class. It was by far the most difficult study course ever, barring all medical school subjects. Our professor was excellent for clarity, explanations, and expression, but it was rank memory and very confusing with all of the illogical, complex "laws". It was at most insensible and the problems were compound, comminuted, and incongruous. Our greatest fears were concentrated in the final examination, which was the basis for the entire grade. All the poor engineers were duty bound and imperatively required to pass the course to receive their degree and diploma. We were all in the same boat, up the proverbial creek sans paddle. There really was only one way for me to hurdle this obstacle, namely by committing to memory all-important portions of the textbook and lectures. I figured for sure that I had flunked the examination, but wonder of wonders, I garnered a B and said a prayer of thanks to Jehovah and my lucky stars. Several pre-med and engineer students, unfortunately, didn't receive a passing grade and were compelled to repeat the course in the summer. The pre-med course wasn't exactly a "bed of roses", however by consolation; anything worthwhile means blood, sweat and tears. The reward is, however, sugar sweet.

For recreation, we were in close proximity to Washington D. C., only ten miles to the west and south of College Park, and a mere forty miles to Baltimore. Cars were rare and most college students, for some querulous reason, did not use bicycles. So the course of least resistance was by hitchhiking via automobile. Quite often we had to ride the "Rumble Seat", a popular conveyance means. As it was open, it was really air conditioned and "refreshing" but a bit uncomfortable when it rained.

Most of our fraternity dances were held at frat and sorority houses, at hotels, and country clubs in the DC area. My first big dance was on New Year's Eve, 1930, at our brother Phi Sigma Kappa house at George Washington University. My buddy, Harry Fisher, had set up a comely, hefty, and very attractive Baltimore lass for me. We double couples all toured to Washington on the evening of December 31st and had supper at the Phi Sig house. After our repast we had a Mint Julep and went to the Mayflower Hotel, the locus for our dance. The Phi Sig brothers were in a festive mood and offered us a couple libations of good cheer to cement our friendship and to relax us for dancing. Popular songs in this era were "Stardust" by Hoagy Carmichael, "When the Blue of the Night" by Morton Downey, "Take off Your Skin and Dance Around in Your Bones", "St. Louis Blues", "Tiger Rag", "Carolina Moon", "Sweetheart of Sigma Chi", "Love letters in the Sand", "Button up Your Overcoat", "Autumn Leaves", "Goodnight Sweetheart", and "Dream a Little, Dream of Me". Along about midnight with the revelry in full swing, Polly, my date, whose chest would put Dolly Partons to shame hands down, decided to go downstairs where another big band was playing. Polly was definitely feeling no pain and about at the middle of the stairway she slipped and headed strongly for a nose-dive over the balustrade to the next level, fifteen feet down. My heart stood still, but I instantly clutched her and pulled her back to safety. From then on she drank strong coffee and walked outside where the temperature was well below freezing. We had a 6 a.m. breakfast at the George Washington fraternity house and headed back to Baltimore. As we neared our destination, we suddenly saw a human body lying alongside the road. Harry was driving his family car and asked me what we should do. We decreased speed and our first inclination was to stop and render help. However, we decided negatively. There had been several incidents recently describing similar situations where the Good Samaritan had been brutally assaulted and robbed. Therefore, we wisely decided to continue our trip home. Needless to say, Polly Robinson didn't recall one iota of her harrowing narrow escape from a critical fall at the hotel. I took Polly to one of our Phi Sigma Kappa dances the following spring. Her brazen behavior with the two Powers brothers after the dance was quite unacceptable and this ended our friendship.

One of my very best friends in our fraternity was George Matthews. George helped me immeasurably to get adjusted to the rigors of fraternity life. Being an only child did have serious drawbacks and disadvantages socially. George had four older sisters, of which two were in training at Baltimore Mercy Hospital, Mary Ann and Catherine Louise. George had learned how to deal positively with the ladies through life with his ever-loving and charming sisters. I was invited to George's home in La Plata in southern Maryland for the weekend. It was in the fall of my sophomore year that I met George's girlfriend's sister, Evangeline Lyon, with a sobriquet of "Cubby". Agnes, Cubby's sister, was George's steady femme and they lived in Hughesville, Maryland, about twelve miles from La Plata. For me it was a "blind date," and actually I was really dazzled and blinded when I was introduced to Cubby, almost speechless in fact. She was a striking, petite brunette and just about the most pulchritudinous lady I have ever been privileged to meet. It was a double date with George and Agnes. Truly, Agnes was almost as lovely and beautiful as Cubby, but definitely more mature. George was about the nicest, affable person you could ever imagine, but he would never win a beauty contest. We went to a dance at Leonard Town and I believe I had no more than one dance with my escort, as she was so popular and attracted all the eligible males like bees to honey. I couldn't blame the young men for congregating about us as she was truly a knockout and she was garbed fit to kill, with a plunging neckline, as I recall. I saw her several times thereafter, at home in the company of George and Agnes with her parents in the next room. Her mother was quite attractive and of noble bearing. She had given birth to nine dead baby boys, due to an RH incompatibility, of which the biochemistry was unknown until 1944. She deserved an A+ for effort, certainly for her staunch belief in Catholicism. She was determined to have a son and the father concurred. He was an elegant, intelligent, handsome, tall businessman. He owned and was proprietor of a general merchandise store in Hughesville.

I distinctly remember a fraternity dance at the Chevy Chase Country Club in Washington, D.C. in my junior college year, attended by Cubby, Agnes, George and myself in May 1932. As usual, she was dressed like a beauty queen, and she wore a white rabbit fur jacket. We had a wonderful time at the dance with big band favorite, Woody Herman and his "Musical Lumber Jacks". Hughesville is about fifty miles from Washington, D.C. and by the time we had a repast at the club and arrived in Hughesville, the sun was rising. Cubby slept on me, the driver, during the ride to her home and when we arrived there my suit (tuxedo) was completely plastered with rabbit hair and I looked like one. Cubby was quite frail and delicate and certainly was under five-feet tall. She married one of the local suitors shortly after I left College Park and died a few years later of tuberculosis. She is firmly cemented favorably in my memory always.

We pledges were initiated into the Phi Sigma Kappa fraternity at Maryland on March 8 and 9, 1930. We each were responsible for bringing a specific animal or bird to the initiation locale behind the college campus. I was designated to bring two barnyard swallows, which I felt was assignment impossible. However, my good friend, brother, and fellow pledge, Dick Murdock, came to my rescue. He invited me to come home with him to Mount Airy, Maryland, one weekend and it was a piece of cake to obtain the swallows from their roosting nest on the barn ledge at his farm home. Just before our frat induction ceremonies, Dick and I went to his home, where we received the most regal hospitality. On Sunday, Dick went to the barn and gently grasped two resting swallows. He inserted them into a box, punctured with holes for oxygen and containing a small cup of water and birdseed. On our ride back to College Park, I noticed that the birds were making a terrific ruckus as though intensely combative. Dick answered my query about this relationship by stating that they were of opposite gender and apparently this boggled my mind until I thought; now I know why there are so many divorces.

The pledges all met at 8 p.m. Saturday with their designated live animals. There was one discrepancy; Ramsay brought a cow instead of a goat, the hazard of being a big city boy. We were given credit or debit for our farm products. The debits received three paddles delivered generously by our dear brothers to be. We walked about a mile to a small pond, which was lightly frozen. They had built a roaring fire and we were instructed to remove all our clothing. This was rapidly accomplished and we gathered about the fire. Then the grilling questions began. Our fraternity chapters were 100+ spread over the entire (then) 48 States at various colleges and learning institutions and we were expected to know each one designated by a particular Greek letter. Our chapter was Eta, or the fifth one, which was founded in 1865. Our designation was "Brothers of a Social Circle". We were given points for correct answers and debits for incorrect ones. Fortunately for me, having been blessed by a fairly good memory, I saved my gluteal muscles several whacks. Then we were told to immerse our whole bodies in the pond after the ice was broken and return to the fire to dry. The next step was a blindfold and we were given a brick to hold in our hands. A cord was tied around the brick with one end and the other end was loosely tied around our reproductive organ. After a few minutes, we were told to drop the brick at the count of four, or else. Jerry Geary, our president counted agonizingly slowly and at the count of four all but two pledges dropped their bricks. I figured the active brothers had endured this procedure so I dropped mine. Fortunately, as perpetrated, the strings were all cut in the middle before the bricks dropped and an immense sense of relief pervaded. Needless to say, the pledges that held their bricks received the consequences. Next we were arranged sitting in a circle straddling one another with our legs to the outside and our hands placed on each other's shoulders. We were each given five (not fresh) eggs and commanded to break the eggs over the person's head to our front, one at a time. I was in front of Murdock and Doyle was in front of me. Then the brothers dumped feathers all over us and we were told to dress. Next, they related to us there were six hidden messages in trees nearby with instructions on how to retrieve them. After we obtained all the messages we were to turn them into the frat house. A final message was to be gathered at the Riverdale Post Office about five miles southwest of College Park. At this juncture our beloved brothers left us to stew in our collective juices without a flashlight. By a stroke of genius, Charlie Spicknall had hidden his Essex automobile just back of the college campus. He knew our environs like a book because he lived in Hyattsville, which was only a stone's throw, 3 miles from College Park. While Charley went to get his car, we tried to extricate the feathers from our bodies and wash our faces. With the help of Charles's Essex for travel and light, we did garner all the messages, which were about a mile apart, and then we found the final paper at Riverdale and returned to the Phi Sig house. However, we kept the lifesaver car a secret. The brothers were waiting for us at the house when we arrived. They could not figure out how in the world we could be there at 3 a.m. with mission accomplished. It was a perplexing enigma, for we were expected to arrive at 6 a.m. or later. Anyhow, we took showers and changed out rags for nice dry clothes.

Our next order of business was to get branded by burning alcohol with the letters Phi Sigma Kappa on our breasts. Then we had a hearty breakfast, thank the Lord. The last part of the initiation was the formal didactic ordination and ritual, which was mainly verbal and which consumed about two hours. The only sticky part for us was at the end. We were blindfolded again and, one at a time, were told to stand on a high chair. Then Brother Mitch Franklin had us feel a board full of large iron spikes 6 inches high. The board of spikes was placed on the floor in front of our chair and we were instructed, while standing, at the count of five to jump on the board. In the meantime, before jumping, the iron-spiked board was replaced with a similar rubber spiked board. Then the bandage was removed and the countdown started. I decided it was a hoax and jumped, but was mightily relieved when I felt the soft rubber spikes on my soles. This part of the ritual was to reveal what depths of help we would render to a brother in distress. So this ended our nightmare and we felt like we really deserved to be in the Brothers of the Social Circle, truly a "baptism by fire".

Due to my undying love for football, I decided, with urging by Johnny O'Neill, class and Phi Sig President, to go out for football manager. Our team was coached by a powerful personality, dynamic Curley Byrd, who was an influential person second to none at Maryland College. His teams never really established a superlative record, but usually split even for the season. We played Duke, North Carolina, North Carolina State, Virginia, Virginia Military Institute, Virginia Polytechnic Institute, Navy, Yale, Kentucky, and Western Maryland. All these were typically played in one year. My adversary in competition for manager was Whitey Herzog, a very affable, capable, and striking blonde young man in my class. I gave it my best shot for 2 years, but then conceded the job to Whitey because I had decided to go to medical school after 3 years of college. I believe Whitey and I were about even in our endeavors for manager when I made the decision to withdraw. Curley was built like a stallion and the best looking Don Juan you ever saw and all the ladies he confronted had round heels. His reputation in public relations was unparalleled. I really would have preferred to go out for the team, but my weight was a meager 125 pounds and that would get me nowhere except in the mortuary. My special contribution in football was my modest dropkicking and I honestly could drop kick the ball between the goalposts from the fifty-yard line. On one Saturday, after a game with the Duke Blue Devils, Harry Fisher and I hitched a ride to Baltimore (40 miles) with the school president, Harvey Pearson. He was quite hospitable and took us to our final destination of Dundalk.

I sent my laundry home every 2 weeks for my wonderful Mother to wash. She would return it with an added bonus of cookies, doughnuts, and cakes, which I shared with my fellow brothers. I didn't forget my high school sweetheart and corresponded regularly with Carolyn Rowan, with whom I felt strong feelings of romance. But distance was a strong deterrent and there were so many beautiful co-eds available. However, I must say, notwithstanding, I unabashedly did bury my head in my books primarily and my grades were A's and B's throughout. There was one affable young lady in my English class, Emma Gibbons, who caught my eye, and we did go to a couple dances in Washington D.C. On another occasion my fraternity brother, Bill Bishop got me a grudge blind date with Helen Randolph, with whom he was quarreling in a steady relationship. She was a lovely high-class beauty, but the atmosphere was charged with electricity and our association was "one night only" and out.

We held a Mother's Day tea party at the Fraternity House in May, 1932, and all out mothers participated, including mine. My Mother was on pins and needles when I poured tea for the moms, because I had a gross affinity for spilling liquids at critical times and places. However, this time I displayed perfect control and her fears were completely unfounded. She said many times during my childhood, "That darn kid (meaning damn brat) always spills the beans." No secrets were sacred.

A most unforgettable character in the frat house was our "counselor" preacher, Elijah Brown, an aged black male. He gave us advice and monitored out activities generally and was the best natured jokester with a buoyant personality. When we were down in the dumps, Elijah was always there to soothe our bent-out-of-shape feelings.

One incident worthy of note was a run-in I had with Jerry Mason, one of my frolicking good-time brothers. Mason had just come back from the red light District of Columbia one evening when I was pouring my brains out over quantitative analysis and was deeply engrossed. He had been to a house of ill repute, had had many beers, and was in a euphoric, non-insultable mood. He came over to me and was truly disruptive, to say the least. He disrobed and started flicking pediculi pubic bugs all around me. In spite of my protests, he continued his misbehavior. I arose and grabbed him by the shoulders and threw him over my back and he landed flat on his back on the floor. He immediately retreated, apologized, and I resumed my study. I strenuously advised him to shower and he quietly complied.

During the summer vacations, while in college, I worked for my Father at Elliott Company in Jeanette, Pennsylvania. I made 35 cents an hour demolishing old wood patterns. My Father was the foreman of about 45 well-trained pattern makers, who had learned the trade over a period of several years. They were all real professionals, but behaved immaturely in many ways, like playing tricks on one another and newly hired men learning the basics. Henry Kimmel and John Sykes were two of the characters who really inducted me in the initiation process. Dad had a real talent for reading blueprints and exerted excellent control over these men. I worked in the pattern storage, preservation, and destruction department. The patterns were made for dehydrators, heaters and engines. My duties entailed breaking up old patterns and driving the crane to position the patterns.

I loved onion and limburger cheese sandwiches, which irritated John and Steve Yosczak because of my "mild" offensive breath. The storage area was rat infested because we ate our lunches there. Occasionally we would line up with paddles and execute huge rats almost the size of cats.

One of the "tricks" Steve Yosczak pulled on me was during a date I had with a Jeanette girl named Cozette Grable, an ultra gorgeous and sophisticated blonde. I escorted Cozette to a movie in Jeannette (named after H. Sellers McKee and founded in 1810). After the movie we got into our '27 Studebaker

Sedan and my eyes lighted up like a 200 watt electric light bulb when I envisioned a large, red, French, tickler condom on the knob of my gear shift. At that time the gearshift consisted of a two-foot rod planted in the middle of the front seat, with a billiard-sized ball at the top. The gearshift was situated between the driver and the passenger. To say I was mortified and embarrassed is stating the situation mildly. Actually, I was speechless and Cozette blushed unrestrainedly. There was no option but to remove and discard the condom, which I did expediently. We had a chocolate nut sundae as I recall hazily, and then I took my friend home. My intentions really were to make a big hit with Cozette, but, undoubtedly, I flubbed the dub. Vaguely, I believe, there was a cacophony of laughter from an unusual source as we left the theater.

One other instance of romance in the summer of 1931 gained my scrutiny, front and center. There was a terrific blonde lady extraordinaire in Irwin, about 12 miles from Greensburg that caught my attention. Phyllis Hockenschmidt was a devastating "light" headed femme I met at a dance in Oakford Park on the night of my birthday, which, coincidentally was her birthday as well. I gleaned this fact when my partner and I exchanged dances. In spite of a threatening admonishment from her partner (a football hero), I damned the torpedoes and dated her. Phyllis was a very calm, cool, and collected, somewhat plump, beauty queen, crowned in a recent beauty contest. Her father was an astute engineer who owned a welding company and graduated from the University of Pittsburgh. He played college football for a couple of years. He quit cold turkey after a complex comminuted fracture of both the tibiae when he endeavored to tackle Jim Thorpe, the great, all-time, all-American of the Carlisle Indians. He told me that his leg injuries never really healed completely. Phyllis and my chemistries apparently didn't match and after a couple of summers, we drifted apart. She later married Jim Baughman, a character, who was involved in a country club dance fracas of despicable description. He emptied his colon in the rear seat of a rival's car at the dance.

In late May of 1932, Charles Rhinehart, one of my friendly fraternity brothers, invited me to go with him to his home in Hagerstown, Maryland, after school had terminated in the summer of 1930. "Rhiney" took me to a local tavern in Hagerstown our first night and only night at his home. I remember this night with a passion. Rhiney was known particularly well for sitting up sleeping excessively on weekends and many evenings in the fraternity house. He was rough and tough and had a heart of gold. He was very outspoken, a man of few words and surely laid his cards on the table, face up at a pub. Rhiney ordered twelve bottles of "bootleg" beer; so naturally, I ordered twelve bottles of "bootleg" as well (this was during prohibition). Well, my staunch friend drank several bottles of this "bootleg" and was going strong, as he was well experienced in worldly ways, while this was my first experience with beer. I naively drank about six bottles and became pale, green, and severely nauseated. My good friend was well aware of my plight and said "Knobby" come into the men's room. I staggered to the commode and Rhiney gave me the "Heimlich Maneuver". Well, I erupted ala Mount Vesuvius and beer came up everywhere like an explosion. I had a heavenly feeling of relief and thanked my Good Samaritan for his deliverance. The next day, after bidding fond adieu to Rhiney, I took the high road (National Highway) by hitching rides to my beloved home in Greensburg.

In my junior (third) year in college, I was forced to make a decision to choose my medical school. My two choices were university of Maryland in Baltimore and George Washington in Washington, D.C. Therefore, I applied to both medical schools. Each school granted me the courtesy of an interview, which I consummated. I was accepted by both schools and selected Maryland. Actually, I was invited to attend the medical school at Maryland at the end of my sophomore (second) year at College Park, MD, but declined because I knew I was way too green and immature. It would be insurmountable. One other reason I chose Maryland was that my very good friend Harry C. Bowie had selected Maryland for his medical school. We had been together for three years at College Park and had taken practically all the same classes. Harry was from La Plata, Maryland, the same city I visited with George Matthews. Harry's mother (Bowie) was widowed and managed a grocery store. Harry had a sister killed in a tornado, while in first grade and she was mourned intensely by his Mom. My great friend, Charles Spicknall, decided to go to George Washington. My frat brother, Darius McCellan Dixon, a year ahead of me was one of my sponsors at University of Maryland.

One of the most memorable events that happened to our 1933 graduating class at College Park was the naming of the University of Maryland as the "Terrapins". As mentioned previously, the first year in medical school doubled as the fourth year in college. I received my Bachelor's Degree from the class of 33 at College Park when I completed my initial year in medical school. For some inexplicable reason, this practice was discontinued. Now there must be 4 years preparatory before entering medical school. To begin the "Terrapin" saga, our '33 graduation class at College Park was required to give (as all graduating classes did) a parting present to the University. As described previously the Great Depression of '29 had drastically curtailed everyone's financial status to the vanishing point. Therefore, who could help us any more than the number one man at the University, Curley Byrd, and the all-powerful benefactor? Our class president went directly to see Curley and delineated our sad situation in detail. "Curley" responded positively, after pondering our plight. He said,

"I have a farm on the Eastern Shore of Maryland and on it meanders a small stream, which is well populated with Maryland's famous turtles, the so called "Diamond Back Terrapins". "One of my former fullbacks on the '23 football team runs a foundry in Boston and I believe he will cast a turtle likeness for you in galvanized iron for your class to give the University as an outgoing present." Ted White, our class president accepted the live "Terrapin" with overflowing gratitude. He and Harry Hasslinger our vice-president were off to Boston with the historic turtle by automobile post haste. There was an overnight stop in Scranton, Pennsylvania, along the way north and the turtle got loose several times in the car and hotel. He was reconnoitered each time and finally they reached Boston. They met Jim Stanton and he graciously condescended to cast our Terrapin. The casting was not without its price, which was torture, but not the animal's life as it lived on for many years. Anyhow, the perpetrated deed was completed and Ted and Harry were College Park bound with the inanimate iron turtle. This cast was presented unceremoniously to the University President. Prior to this donation the mascot of the University was the "Old Liners" apparently a hangover from the Civil War days. The battle song was "Keep Those Caissons a Rolling Along". Upon the receipt of our present, the council of the University decided to adopt the nickname "The Terrapins" for University sports. The vicissitudes of the "Terrapins" included a purloining by the University of Virginia students in 1948 and several aborted attempts by other schools. However, it always returned back to its home. Finally, in 1982, the University of Maryland decided to go all out and construct a massive duplication of the original diminutive "Terrapin" and dedicate it formally. It was a statue of a turtle at least four feet in diameter, mounted on a near four-foot tall base, which was encased in cement. There is <u>no</u> danger of this one being stolen. I attended the dedication ceremony in 1983 and our class members were feted by the president, Kirwan, at a special dinner and fanfare, recognizing our '33 class donation to the University. The "Terrapin" now is recognized as "Testudo", which is the Chinese name for turtle. Incidentally, the Chinese worship the turtle as being a deity. Testudo is revered by the Maryland students now and signifies an omen of good luck. He (she) occupies a prominent position on mid-campus and every time students have a test or examination, they trip by Testudo and either plant a kiss or commit a laying on of hands for favorable fortunes. Maryland is well known for many premier qualities: horse racing, beautiful women, oysters, crabs, Japanese Cherry blossoms, and Diamond Back Turtles, commonly known as Terrapins. Their turtle soup is also a delicacy.

Doris and I did attend the twenty-fifth reunion at College Park in October 1958, along with Harry Fisher and his wife Elizabeth Akehurst. We saw our football team vanquish the Duke Blue Devils 27-20 with our star halfback

"Chet" the Jet Hanulak dominating. That night we were privileged to dance to the heavenly music of big band Tommy Dorsey. Later, I did attend the 50th and 60th class reunions at College Park when we dedicated "Testudo" permanently.

Our one all-American sports star was Bozey Berger in basketball and baseball. We were Southern conference champions in basketball in 1932. Bozey went to the big leagues in baseball and played in Cleveland, Ohio, for a few years as a first baseman. We did have National Lacrosse Champions for a couple years also.

Chapter 7

University of Maryland Medical School

It was with a strong feeling of confidence and a burning desire for all out success that I entered the University of Maryland Medical School. Foremost in my mind was my unfailing advocacy for infants and children with medicinal measures to help them. Harry Clay Bowie and I were consumed with considerable ardor; fervor and compassion to roll up our sleeves and dive into medical means to render help to our fellow people. Mrs. Bowie and my mother became close and devoted friends to help their sons matriculate at medical school. We all got together and searched diligently for a habitat to live and dine. We did succeed in discovering a temporary home on Park Avenue, about a mile from school. We nailed down a third floor room with board at the Percival ("Gunboat") and Marlene ("Tweet-Tweet") Gunby Residence. He was a huge hulk, cross-eyed, middle-aged, bald man and she was a tall, slim, painted, pseudo redhead, strongly perfumed doll. They were affable and we accepted their living terms of $50.00 a month. Unbeknownst to us, we were to discover that this was the medical fraternity house for Phi Rho Sigma. A half-dozen plus members lived on the second floor. Morton Downey was their leader and he was an elegant, personable person, who exuded convincing charm from head to toe. We were also pursued as possible candidates for Nu Sigma Nu and Phi Chi. We were "between the devil and the deep blue sea," but after a few weeks of battling this quandary, we decided to go bare (negative). Our freshman roommate across the hall was Phillip Gregory from Bar Harbor, Maine, a very likeable, droll man who decided to join Phi Rho. We were left holding the bag, so after two months, we decided to move to another location. We found a convenient room with board on Eutaw Place, run by a real nice, convivial man. It was a wee bit farther from Lombard and Greene Streets, the locale of our University and University Hospital, but a "bird in the hand" convinced us to move in. The renters here were not medical students, but all were academically involved in art, music or accounting, so we were all in the same boat, striving for vocational supremacy.

I recall vividly our first walk to class; we had no car or cycle. The walk was about 15 to 20 minutes. About a block from Davidge Lecture Hall, there was a grave two paces from the sidewalk on Greene Street. The headstone (very common) was overgrown with weeds, but being in such an uncommon site, we had to check it all out. To our utter amazement, this was the grave of our famous Edgar Allen Poe, the one and only. It was inconceivable that such an illustrious person would have such a tawdry grave in the midst of the downtown hubbub of Baltimore. Surely, such a renowned personage of "Quoth the Raven Nevermore" deserved a much more prominent resting-place. I first learned about Poe in senior high school while under the erudite tutelage of Miss Waltour. We studied Poe's autobiography in a book called, <u>The Dreamer</u> and I was indelibly impressed with his turbulent life as a vagabond and his demise from tuberculosis. His grave is now located inside the grounds of Westminster Presbyterian Church on the corner of Greene and Market Streets, circa two blocks from Davidge Hall. A mysterious admirer for the past 27 years commemorates each year of his birthday by placing a half dozen white roses and a bottle half-filled with cognac on his grave at 0230 AM on 12/21. My elder son, Tom, and I visited his gravesite during our 1996 get together and celebration of my sixtieth medical school class reunion; and we took several pictures.

One of our first duties after matriculation in September, 1932, was to have a complete physical examination by our student physician, Doctor Harry Carey. I was elated to find out that my childhood tuberculosis had completely disappeared with no traces on the X-ray of my chest. We all passed our physicals with flying colors except one, William Schmieler. He was OK physically, built like a stallion, but he had some weird, unusual habits and antics. He would walk up and down stairs on his hands. He would go outside the Phi Chi house in the middle of the night and let out blood-curdling, "Tarzan" yells which would call forth the police force and be unproductive. One time my Uncle Bob (mother's brother) came to Baltimore in June '34 to pick me up for a trip home. Schmieler went to Greensburg with us as he lived nearby in Kittaning. Amazingly, when we reached the top peak of Sideling Hill, which is incidentally the high point of the Appalachian Mountains, Schmieler got out of the car while we were cruising slowly. He gave a prodigious "Tarzan" yell, one of his loudest, and started running down the mountain alongside of our car. I thought my Uncle Bob was going to go into shock and he exclaimed, "My God, what was that?!" I retorted, "Just one of Bill's patentable "Tarzan" yells." Well, Bill met us at the perigee (bottom) of Sideling Hill and said, "Sorry, guys, but I just had to get some exercise." Bill's girlfriend from Kittanning would occasionally meet him and we knew exactly when, for he always sang his theme song "When it's June in January". Coincidentally, when we were taking our obstetrics exam in May, 1936, Bill's wife Felicia was birthing their first baby, Helene. Bill had to "sweat out" not only the exam, but also his fatherhood. When asked a question, he would always give a vague, double answer. Actually he had a brilliant mind and was an astute student.

I'll never forget our initial class in anatomy, proctored by Dr. Luther E. Little, an instructor. He was in the general practice of medicine, but had a special interest in dissection. Luther was a jovial prankster and a man of few chosen, concise, and precise words. His first question as he addressed our opening session was a blunt, "How many of you guys (we had one female) can wiggle your ears?" About a dozen hands reached for the sky. He promptly replied, "Gee, I didn't know we had so many jackasses in your class." Shortly, thereafter, he rendered a brief lecture and admonished us to get packing and remove the skin from the arms of our cadavers, "Carefully."

There were four persons assigned to each cadaver. Our four were Bowie and I on the right side and Bieren and MacCaulay on the left side. The odor of formaldehyde strongly permeated the atmosphere, as they were kept in a huge tank of this vile liquid as a preservative. We were not apprised of the manner of obtaining these "bodies". We surmised that they were preeminently former sailors, corpses who were killed in fights and drunken orgies, and unclaimed homeless bodies without family or friends. Our cadaver was a little, middle-aged man, who had perished from the ravages of tuberculosis. We were given a female body to dissect in the second half of our anatomical course.

Our first semester's work consisted of anatomy, chemistry, and histology. Uhlenhuth and Figge were the two acting anatomy professors. Davis and Picorney were our histology professors, and Wylie was the chemistry chief. Realistically, we had an entire first year of anatomy, which included neural anatomy in the later half of the year. When we went to a theatre or restaurant, patrons and consumers within a radius of twelve feet would evacuate the premises due to the acrid aroma we emanated.

Dr. Uhlenhuth was a uniquely stern, uncompromising disciplinarian of the old school, sink or swim version. He was massively built physically with a bushy head of gray hair and presented a very ominous personality. Dr. Figge, on the other hand, was a small, diminutive person, quite relaxed, good-looking, and friendly. He was our champion and refuge in the storm of hypertensive anatomy. His research was devoted mainly to salamanders, but he always seemed to be in a happy, jovial mood. Specifically, I recall one particular dance with my to-be wife, Doris, at the Belvedere Hotel in my senior year.

Figge and his lovely wife traded dances with us. He was an elegant dancer and seemed to be quite enthralled with Doris' charms.

Our histology professor was Dr. "Ducky" Davis. He was bald and looked like one of our evolutionary ancestors, about 4' ¾" tall with a high pitched, squeaky voice. When we got agitated and started to engage in noisy conversation, he would rush out of his office and in a menacing voice would forcefully state, "Gentlemen, this is a histology lab and not a playground. Get back to your microscopes and apply your excess energy there." He gave us a surprise, unnerving exam one day during the Yom Kipper celebration, which was celebrated by our Hebrew members. They compromised almost one-half (honestly) of our entire class. We were disgruntled because the Jewish population was exempt from the test due to their holiday.

Another event early in the course happened to me. I was called in to Dr. Davis' office, solo, out of a clear blue sky and was subjected to a quiz by him, one on one. He had me look into a microscope and he queried, "What do you see, young man?" I knew it was a salivary gland that we had begun to study. "You are right," he said, "But what is the name of the secretion in the gland?" Truly, I did not know, but the bell saved me. The phone rang and he answered to the tune of his wife's dulcet, mellifluous voice. They engaged in conversation about a list of foods that he was to bring home for supper. There was a slight disagreement and argument over the menu, which gave me time to look at the open book on his desk. Luckily, I had a chance to survey the description of the salivary gland and discovered the magic name of the secretion before his tete a tete with his spouse (better half) ended. He came back to me and said, "Pardon me, sir, but I believe I questioned you on what the glandular secretion is named." I replied, "Yes sir, it is Zymagen Granules," to which Dr. Davis said, "That's right, exactly! Don't ever forget it." And I never did.

We poured over the books day and night with utmost diligence, but occasionally we would trip the light fantastic on Saturday might. One reminiscence stands out flagrantly. One of my classmates, Pembroke, from Annapolis, Maryland, convinced me to double date with him in October 1932, with a Gaucher Ladies College student. Her name was Peg Doubleday and she was from Tarrytown, New York. Peg was a truly perfect blonde goddess with fine chiseled facial features, beautiful skin, and golden hair, the real McCoy. I was speechless for a while and thought I had ascended to heaven with a "blinding" date. Peg was a great, great granddaughter of Abner Doubleday, Civil War general and famous for being the inventor of modern day baseball. Coincidentally, to further imprint my memory, a song called, "Peg O' My Heart," had just originated. Being in a bit of a fog, I can't exactly remember, but I believe we went to a movie at the Rialto. The picture we saw leaves a vacuous blank. About a month later, I escorted Peg to a fraternity dance at the Belvedere Hotel and this time my mind was as clear as a bell (belle). I saw her once more in the spring of '33, when she invited Bowie, my roommate, and I to a Gaucher party at the Troutman's Department Store residence on Cold Spring Lane. Peg was never lovelier, but she did have a steady boyfriend and it was curtains for me. I do remember, reluctantly, one occasion with Peg as my partner, she had reserved a room for after the dance, but I demurred – the story of my life.

One other time our first year, Bowie and I were invited to a party given by Roland Bieren's (my dissecting co-partner) girlfriend. This was another Saturday night escape from the formaldehyde laden air. There were several couples and the cognac was flowing freely for some reason. Bieren's girlfriend became enamored of me, but I was not especially attracted to her. She told me all about the puppies her dog had had and wanted me to go upstairs to see them, but I resisted. I recall that when someone filled my glass with cognac, I would pour it in someone else's glass and pretend to be imbibing. Maybe this happened 4 or 5 times. I winked at Bowie and motioned toward the door about 10 o'clock and we were homeward bound. I've never indulged in alcohol as my father, bless him, served as a perfect example. He would have one ounce of Jim Beam once a year, at twelve o'clock New Year's Eve. Well! Guess what? To my amazement, Bieren's girlfriend dropped in to see me at our residence on Park Avenue the next day. Bowie, Pembroke, and I were outside engaged in conversation about our anatomical dissection. She boldly approached and interrupted our discussion and asked me to go home with her. I blushed (they told me) and demurred negatively and told her I couldn't due to my arduous study schedule. My friends taunted me unmercifully and I retorted, "You're just jealous."

They tell a wild story about "Ducky" Davis, the anatomy professor, before Uhlenhuth assumed the chairmanship. Dr. Davis was rendering one of his unique lectures on bones in the human body one morning to a freshman class several years ago. He was demonstrating the bones of the pelvis and was holding up an entire pelvis by the right femur with his right hand, and said, "Gentlemen, I have in my hand one of the greatest specimens of anatomy." His left hand was in his pocket. At this point, an "astute" student in the rear of the room ejaculated, "Which hand, Doctor?" And all the classmates in the room convulsed with laughter. Whereupon, Dr. Davis, sternly shouted, "You'll flunk, you'll flunk!" But, unfortunately, he couldn't discern which gentleman blurted out the query. I was uncannily adept at imitating Dr. Davis' high-pitched, squeaky voice and would mimic this tale complying with numerous requests.

An associate professor of anatomy, Monte Edwards from England, was very unique and clairvoyant. He was indeed the smoothest, most knowledgeable, understandable instructor we ever had. His speech was flawless and flowed sweetly, like honey, without interruption. He knew his anatomy to perfection and could transmit it likewise with the King's English.

Our chemistry professor that first year was the venerable, scholarly Dr. Wylie (Wily) and similarly to Monte Edwards, was distinctly one of our best. He was something of a trickster and one of his entrapment questions was "What is the Alkaline Tide?" It stumped everyone and the simple answer was "fruit juice", which is converted from acid to alkali in the urine. He related a very practical and cunning solution to freezing rain on a car's windshield at night. He was returning home from a party in Annapolis with his family one night and this eerie situation (fogged windshield) occurred in the middle of nowhere. He stopped the car pronto and remembered he had some buttered sandwiches, which were given to him by his host at the party when leaving. He smiled to his wife and applied the butter to the windshield and proceeded home fearlessly. The butter reduced the surface tension and prevented freezing on the glass, allowing him clear vision.

Our Dean was Dr. J.M.H. Rowland, a very distinguished, elderly obstetrician, who had compiled a textbook of renown on obstetrics, used in medical schools worldwide. We revered him as a master and shining light to emulate.

One important event confronted me head on early in my first year in pre-medicine, and that was my father's surgery by the one and only Dr. Walter P. Dandy, Johns Hopkins neurosurgeon at Union Memorial Hospital on Charles Calvert and 33rd Streets in Baltimore. Dad had severe migraine headaches for a lifetime and was a champion worrier, a contributing factor definitely. By a quirk of fate, his mother and wife also suffered these devastating headaches, but not so blatantly as my poor father. Dr. Hamman, our family physician, had tried all his tricks of magic to assuage my father's migraines, but came up empty handed. So, being a Johns Hopkins graduate, he implored Dr. Dandy for a consultation to render a helping hand in an emergency predicament. Dad did go to Baltimore and was scheduled for immediate surgery by Dr. Dandy to relieve his migraines. The operation was to sever the two superior cervical ganglia at the base of the brain, which was purely experimental, devised by Walter Dandy. However, it was "any port in a storm." It is really amazing that after surgery, my father's migraine was appreciably ameliorated. But, as is usual in medicine, one credit is counterbalanced by a debit, and he developed Horner's Syndrome. The seeming cure had its counter reaction. Horner's Syndrome is an ornery condition where a person can't salivate and has a dry mouth with marked difficulty chewing and swallowing. The operation was a success and the patient survived, but the consequences were somewhat disastrous.

According to the human genome, I should have inherited blazing migraine headaches, but I was superlatively determined not to, and I didn't. Having seen the devastating effects on dad and mother was more than enough to mold my mind. I firmly believe migraine has a lot to do with lifestyle, with much worry and internalization of feelings and emotions as causation. I decided on a course of active externalization by bowling, participating in sports, and not being passive like a shrinking violet. In other words, by being positive at all times and not getting ulcers. My philosophy is express yourself and don't keep your feelings pent up. Instead, give ulcers if necessary.

One of our casualties during our first year in medical school was Johnny Fissel's demise. Johnny was truly a wonderful friend. Johnny was of French ancestry, always smiling and very congenial, an all-around positive fellow student. The dagger was our global disease enemy, tuberculosis. Our class was heartsick for weeks. It was a real tragedy, an only son engaged to a wonderful girl and a really superlative student. His best friend was Salvadore Pentecost, fellow classmate, and I thought we'd have to bury Sal along with Johnny. We had known Johnny for three fun years at College Park and our bonding was almost as Damon and Pithias. But life is not a bowl of cherries, as the saying goes, and this was one of the pits of life. It is said that, "Only the good die young", a hard, true lesson.

During my first summer vacation in 1933, I felt compelled to engage in a productive effort to earn money to enhance my parent's contribution to my schooling. Fortuitously, my Uncle Frank, mother's brother, had been managing a business called "Cappies Crab Cakes" for a couple of months, and had built up a sizeable clientele. He had been making crab cakes with considerable help from mother, and then peddled them to the beer parlors to sell. Actually, there is nothing tastier than a combination of beer and crab cake. Anyhow, Frank was leaving as I was coming and he convinced me easily to take over his budding, established business. Mother would order fresh crabmeat from Crisfield, Maryland, (Eastern Shore) by air. She would mold the cakes by hand, deep fry, drain, and then cellophane wrap them. My duty was to canvas all the beer establishments in the environs and sell them the crab cakes. They were about the size and shape of a one-pound hamburger. Crab cakes were quite the novel delicacy to our landlubber folks in southwest Pennsylvania. Regardless of their overwhelming appeal, people must taste and eat them to appreciate their irresistible goodness. My mother had had extensive experience in handling crabmeat with her longtime exposure to the Baltimoreans, who thoroughly know the utmost about preparing seafood from the cradle. Besides, she was intuitively a natural and expert cook with topnotch training by her mother and my father's mother.

In order to whet the appetites of the managers of the beer establishments, my close buddy, Paul Seaton, and I would pay them a visit on weekends.

Paul was a born salesman and he would go into the bars in all the surrounding towns around Greensburg and set the hook. He would rave about "Crappies Crab Cakes" and give them one to eat. On Monday and through the rest of the week, I would go into the bars with the crab cakes and their person in charge would say, "Yes, I have had requests for these and the taste is great." I would sell him a dozen cakes for $2.00 and he would sell the patrons the cakes for 25 cents apiece. We had a booming business going and the only drawback was that we couldn't supply the rapid demand. Dad made a special contrivance to mold the crabmeat into a cohesive cake that wouldn't break up. I made enough money to pay for a $200 semester in school.

There was one particularly ludicrous happening during our second year in Physiology. We were working intensively with frog experiments and a classmate was pithing his frog over the sink. Pithing involved destroying the spinal nerve cord by inserting a rod down the entire spine. This maneuver was necessary to ablate any response by the frog's nervous system. Our mentor was a lady instructor and she was making the rounds to check the progress of each student in our class. When she saw Ted over at the washstand, she made a beeline to him and in a very loud, excited, stentorian voice shouted, "Mister Weems, you know you're not allowed to pith in the sink." Naturally, there was a spontaneous eruption of sustained laughter in spite of her endeavors to restrain our reactions. Her face turned crimson and she realized her "faux pas" and hurriedly vanished from the room.

Harry Bowie and I lived our second year of medical school at a house managed by Bidwell Cranage. Bidwell was a fellow classmate who had flunked his first year in medical school, the year we entered. He was the son of a famous shipbuilder in Bay City, Michigan, and his grandfather was the venerable Dr. Virgil C. Tupper, an eminent surgeon in Bay City and Bidwell's sponsor. I became acquainted with Virgil in his retirement and learned that he played football for the University of Michigan in the rough and rowdy days when an entire team consisted of 12 players and there were no pads or helmets. Bidwell really had no business being in medical school because his heart and brain were not attuned to medicine. Bidwell was a man of considerable intelligence and ingenuity and had produced a few worthwhile inventions. He performed nobly as a house manager and was adept at fixing household problems with his hands. He worked arduously in all his spare time to keep the house running smoothly, mostly at night, and as a result, his schoolwork and study suffered immensely, causing him to fall asleep during lectures. This conduct was totally unacceptable to our teachers, resulting in his flunking out of school after the first semester. In addition, Bidwell was courting a nurse, Mary, at Women's Hospital and they finally were married. Bowie and I roomed together at the Cranage House on the third floor with Thompson across the hall, and with Fichtner and his family on the second floor. Evans, a dental student, was in the crow's nest, above us, and he was the ultimate womanizer. We also boarded there for breakfast and dinner, so it's easy to understand why Bidwell, in spite of a gargantuan effort, failed school.

During Christmas vacation, 1932, I invited Mary Ellen Kelly from Indiana, Pennsylvania, to be my houseguest at our home in Greensburg. Paul Seaton, while a student at Indiana Teacher's College, had introduced me to Mary Ellen the previous summer on a double date and we had become lukewarm friends. We enjoyed sharing the holidays together to a minimal degree. My parents and I drove Mary Ellen to her home in Indiana and on the way back to Greensburg, mother divulged a secret. Mary Ellen had purloined my father's robe that Margaret (my mother) had given him for a Christmas present. I was flabbergasted because her parents and sister were outstanding and benevolent people with lofty social and religious morals. I wrote to Mary Ellen when I returned to Baltimore and asked her directly to explain her behavior with dad's robe. She returned a nasty epistle denying the theft and that was the termination of a not so beautiful friendship.

Chapter 8

Sabillasville, MD.

I motored from Hamilton to the state TBC Sanitarium on June 10th of 1935, reluctant to leave my true love Doris Mathilde Meyer, and excited to meet my new medical adventure with much greater responsibilities, encompassing human lives. Sabillasville is approximately 60 miles from Baltimore, located in the beautiful Catechin or South Mountains. It is in the vicinity of Camp David, our U.S. president's retreat and playground. It seems that TBC Sanitariums are all located in pre-eminent, mountainous areas to emphasize spiritual loveliness, fresh air, sunshine, and happy feelings. It was all that Dr. Spencer depicted, and then some. The Western Maryland Railroad had a station there to accommodate visitors and patients. In other language it is somewhat comparable to the "Garden of Eden".

My duties there encompassed making daily rounds of the patients of the doctors I was covering. The regular physicians were taking a month's vacation. Another extern from Johns Hopkins Medical School, between 3rd and 4th year, shared patient assignments with me. We were actively engaged in doing pneumathoraces, our primary duty, to collapse lung cavities, promote healing, and wall off the acid fast organisms to prevent transmission via the bronchial tubes to other humans. We would inject air into the thoracic cavity to compress the lung daily. We had to employ the utmost care to prevent puncturing the lung or heart.

My fellow student partner was John Stallings and he brought his wife, Edna, with him. Dr. Victor Cullen, a graduate of Hopkins was the man in charge of the hospital and Doctor Benjamin Cohen was our immediate supervisor. The food was absolutely gourmet, the best institutional nourishment that I have ever enjoyed, but Union Memorial's repast was a very close second. We took frequent chest X-Rays to follow the effectiveness of our air injections and we held intensive X-Ray review conference each Saturday morning. We would perform autopsies at night in a mortuary parlor in nearby Thurmont, Maryland.

The staff has a mandatory rule that everyone without exception have a tuberculin test, the first thing on the agenda. I told them that I had childhood tuberculosis, which they viewed with a jaundiced eye, and proceeded with the test on me. Well!! I derived a tremendous outward reaction from the intra-dermal injection overnight on my left forearm. It was swollen at least twice its normal size, quite inflamed, and painful for a couple of weeks. Dr. Cohen said, "You're a lucky man, for this is a reaction of immunity, meaning you have a huge resistance to any future development of TBC." I didn't quite agree with Cohen, but after 2 days of bed rest, I was able to function 100%.

Doris dispelled my loneliness and malaise by coming to visit me via the Western Maryland Railroad my first weekend there. Dr. Cohen said again that I was a lucky guy in that anyone who would take that train to Sabillasville must surely be in love with me. Cohen was a very intelligent, young bachelor, who always laid his cards on the table face up and called a spade a spade. He was honest to the point of brutality. In fact, Doris visited me to my sheer delight every weekend that I was there staying at a home in the village Saturday night. I would take her back to Hamilton in my trusty '27 Studebaker. Once in a while, on the return trip, I would get somnolent and would pull over on the roadside for a little siesta. One time on returning to the Sanitarium on a Sabbath night, I misjudged my gas reserve and consumed all the gasoline in my tank. This happened in the middle of nowhere. I walked up a steep hill and luckily, to my utter surprise, I could see the Pimlico Racetrack dead ahead. I climbed a 12-foot fence surrounding the track. There was no barbed wire, fortunately, and I walked around the racetrack to the opposite side. The track was deeply pitted by horses' hooves and muddied by a recent rain. It was pitch black and I thought "What if someone guarding the horses caught me red handed?" After climbing the fence to extricate myself from the racetrack, I walked a couple of blocks and it was my fateful day. Lo and behold, a gasoline station was staring me smack dab in the face. The man in charge of the station was really obliging and let me have a carrier with two gallons of gasoline. I ambulated about a mile back to my car with the gasoline, put the gas in my tank, and returned to the station to fill up the tank with the precious fossil fuel. I wiped the perspiration from my forehead and said "Thank you, thank you Lord". I promised the Lord faithfully to never enter the racetrack again without a ticket.

One Sunday afternoon, after a sumptuous dinner, Doris and I were resting in my quarters when the telephone rang. The operator stated that I had guests, Paul Walter Seaton, my childhood buddy, and his wife, Frances. They also had brought a " date" for me and wanted to take me to dinner. I politely demurred the invitation and told him that Doris was with me. This was unfortunately and unknowingly the last time I would see my dear friend Paul. About two years later, during a family quarrel, his wife shot him "accidentally" and killed him. I was shocked when I was apprised of his death by his Aunt Minnie Klingensmith. At the time of his demise, Paul was teaching at Stroudsburg College and I still mourn his life being snuffed out while he was in the prime of his productive age. I always regarded Frances as a light-headed, loose cannon. She was the only child of a millionaire and a real spoiled brat but cést le Guerre.

About the middle of July I was asked to go to Mount Wilson, the Sanatorium in Pikesville on the outskirts of Baltimore. Apparently, they needed a physician there to help Dr. Smith, who required a replacement for his only physician helper who was on vacation. However, I had no objection to being transferred because the location was much closer to Hamilton and my sweetheart. Before I left the State Sanitarium the doctors, nurses, and patients staged a picnic at Caledonia State Forest Park, between Chambersburg and Gettysburg, in Pennsylvania. We had a wonderful party and I got dunked trying to jump over a rivulet that I misjudged for distance. We had loads of culinary delights concocted by our supreme chef at the Sanitarium. One of our exploratory walks took us to nearby birthplace of former President James Buchanan. He was a bachelor who directly preceded our Union Savior, "black slave liberator", the one and only President Abraham Lincoln. My duties at Mount Wilson were similar to those at Sabillasville, but with more responsibility.

Before leaving the State Sanatorium, Dr. Victor Cullen requested a meeting with me. He really put me through the paces, reading X-Rays and examining several patients, to test my diagnostic abilities. After an interminable time, he said "You are going to be an excellent physician and I'm going to recommend you to the powers that be at Johns Hopkins Hospital for internship there."

At Mount Wilson, I met the doctor in charge, Doctor Roland Smith, and nurse, Louise Steigerwald. They had about fifty tuberculosis patients in various stages of the disease, but generally not quite as ill as the ones at the Sabillasville facility. They also had splendid repasts and we also had a rest period after the noon dinner. We didn't have movies nightly as at the South Mountain Sanitarium. I slept on a high hospital bed and received many night calls for chest pain, cough, headache, vomiting, hemoptysis (lung hemorrhage), fever, and night sweats. I usually ate breakfast with Miss Steigerwald and we would discuss the state of affairs regarding each patient on the serious list.

I recollect one patient in particular, Danny Krivitzky, a fourteen year-old young man who developed miliary tuberculosis and was complaining of a blinding headache. I did a lumbar puncture and unfortunately, the tap revealed tuberculous meningitis, which killed him that night.

One time, Dr. Smith invited Doris and I to dinner at his residence. After a hearty meal, we were engaged in pleasant conversation when Mrs. Smith screamed suddenly. I followed her gaze and amazingly there was a huge, fearsome recluse spider about the size of my hand on the floor near me. I quickly grabbed a newspaper and rolled it and crushed the critter with a prodigious blow, disseminating spider limbs all around. We left shortly thereafter when the hospital required my presence for orders for a new admission.

One incident I should mention is one regarding a 44 revolver that I was examining in the staff office. Frank, a patient friend, was standing nearby when the gun accidentally discharged and the bullet missed him by a hair. I had a sinking feeling, thinking of the enormity of the situation, and apologized profusely. It put the fear of God into me and since that day I've had tremendous respect for guns. Always use the safety latch when not hunting. They are made for one purpose only, and that is to kill, and I have avoided them like the plague.

While at Mount Wilson, Doris and I motored to Greensburg one weekend in August for Doris to become acquainted with my family and vice-versa. My parents liked Doris very much, but were disdainful and disappointed about her Catholic religion. They made no bones about it. On the way back to Mount Wilson, Doris and I had a disagreement which left us unsettled. Doris stayed overnight with Miss Steigerwald in her apartment. Steigerwald laid me low the next day and I was quite contrite.

Chapter 9

Fourth Year Medical School

I was accepted for an internship at Baltimore City Hospital at the beginning of my fourth year at Maryland Medical School. It was a full year assignment taking medical care of about 60 cancer patients with diseases involving all body organs. My duties entailed performing urinalysis and complete blood counts weekly on all persons. Also, I was assistant to the resident surgeon on emergency cases at night. My compensation was complete room and board, and gas allowance for my car. City Hospital was just outside of Highland town, about ten miles from the medical school. I made the round trip daily in a faithful old Hupmobile, bless its soul. Gasoline mileage was minimal, but it never failed me. Harry Bowie garnered a position as extern at St. Agnes Hospital in southwest Baltimore for his fourth year. We hated to part our staunch friendship. School expenditures were burdensome and our poor parents deserved a break and reward for their unfailing support in times of acute financial distress. Our tuition had been raised fabulously from $200 to $250 each semester.

I was smitten relentlessly by the love bug and was romancing Doris in all my spare time. Doris' father, Johnny, had a steady lady friend, Jeanette Cobb. She was a nurse at Union Memorial Hospital and had an apartment around the corner from her place of employment. Jeanette truly, as I live and breathe, was one of the most dignified, distinguished, and memorable personages it has been my privilege to ever know. She embodied all the positive attributes you equate with nursing. Her empathy, kindness, and compassion were really outstanding and surely a godsend to her patients. Her roots were traceable to the famous Cobbs of Atlanta, Georgia. They were governor, house, and senate members of the elite class. I was privileged to visit her with Johnny and Doris often when I had my first year internship at Union Memorial. This was especially true the following year of 1936/37.

One happening occurred on a Sunday at dinner at City Hospital, when I invited Doris to be my guest. Our food there was high class and we had a delectable standing roast with all the trimmings. We had vanilla ice cream and chocolate cake (my favorite) for dessert, including butterscotch topping. We were sitting at a table surrounded by several interns and their wives, and were engrossed in concentrated conversation. There was a gravy bowl. The butterscotch bowl was along side it, both yellowish brown. Unconsciously, without looking, I took the gravy boat and mistakenly poured it copiously smack dab over my ice cream. Needless to say, everyone's attention was transfixed directly on me. My response was, "I prefer gravy as topping for all my ice cream, always!" I proceeded to swallow my innovated aberration with relish. Everybody cast a doubtful stare in my direction, but I was calm and deliberate and believe me I pulled off my act.

Doris and I used to take long strolls up Charles Avenue and our favorite rendezvous was beneath a statue of George Washington at Park Avenue. It was located across the street from Peabody Music Conservatory, where my Mother took piano and voice lessons during our stay in Baltimore during World War I. George's statue exhibited a large protuberance in the midsection of his body, showing him holding a book while standing on top of the pedestal about fifty feet above the street. It was daringly suggestive and every individual who gazed at the statue would say, "No wonder they claim Washington as the father of his country."

It was here that we were truly in love with each other and absolutely nothing would intervene to separate our relationship. However, in the spring of 1935, our love was subjected to a test of fire. Doris' old boyfriend, Junie, from Pittsburg came out of the blue to Hamilton to see her. He proposed marriage and had offered her his grandmother's ring at one time two years previously. They had been in love and he had promised that he would return when financially favorable and claim her as his bride. There was a song at the time, "I've Got This Old Feeling", and Doris said this feeling pervaded her mind when she first saw him at the door unexpectedly. She called me on a Saturday, while I was engrossed in work at City Hospital. She related Junie's appearance. I was urgently compelled to rush over to her home, but she wisely cautioned me to "cool it". She said she would meet me the next day and we would work it out. In the meantime, she put Junie "on hold" pending the outcome of our meeting on Sunday. Doris and I did meet and bared our thoughts and feelings to the nth degree. After several hours of agonizing and professing strongly our innermost feelings of love, Doris made a decision in my favor. Her Father, Johnny, had considerable influence in the matter and decided in many respects that I was the one and only. The crisis terminated and probably, fortunately, I never did see Junie.

I applied for a first year internship in December of my last year in medical school to Union Memorial as number one. I also applied to Church Home and to Baltimore City Hospital. I didn't apply to University of Maryland Hospital on purpose, because I felt I was well acquainted with their physicians and I wanted to work with the Johns Hopkins physicians. I wanted to ascertain their ideas, methods, and teachings. Diversity is the staff of life, and Maryland was family practice oriented. Hopkins was more for research and specialization. Union Memorial Hospital was attended almost entirely by Hopkins doctors and this would fulfill my desires and goals.

Hallelujah! I along with classmates Stu Franklin, McCauley, and Sunday were accepted as general initial year interns at Union Memorial Hospital. It was with exceeding jubilance that I accepted my appointment. They had many premier and famous physicians who cared for their patients there. Union Memorial Hospital was founded just after the Civil War, hence came the name. There was Hopkins Doctor Dandy and neurosurgeon J. M. T. Finney, surgical physician in charge of all expeditionary forces in WW II. Also, there were Finney's two sons, George and James, surgeons, Reinhoff, surgeon, Staige Davis, pioneer anesthesiologist, and D. C. Whatron Smith, renowned pediatrician. The intern training there was unparalleled in 1936 A.D..

Graduation exercises were held in Baltimore at the coliseum across the street from the Baltimore and Ohio Railroad Station on May 30, 1936. Dr. Pincoffs, Professor of Medicine at Maryland, was the principle speaker. Five of us received certificates of honor out of the one hundred graduating students in our class. Howie Davis, from the Eastern Shore of the Chesapeake Bay, was our number one and Bowie, I, Kolodner, and Kroll followed in the ranking. We were ecstatic to receive our M.D. degree after four years of arduous blood, sweat, and tears. My Mother, Doris, Johnny, and Cobbie helped me celebrate the ultimate triumph of my young life. Pincoffs threw down the gauntlet and challenged us to continue our success by rendering honorable medical services to our fellow humankind as embodied in the Hippocratic Oath. Afterwards, we deployed our exuberance by going to the Chesapeake Restaurant and having a crab fest. We consummated graduation rites along with the nurses by going to Byrd Stadium in College Park to receive our sheepskins on June 2, 1936, one day before my birthday.

I neglected to mention the mountain we climbed just prior to our graduation. We had to take a trial by fire, a bevy of twenty examinations during "Hell Week" on all the subjects and medical categories we had studied during all four years. One special incident comes to mind. While we were sweating out the obstetrics exam, Schmieler (Pecks bad boy) was sweating doubly as his wife was in labor that Saturday at University Hospital. She delivered a bouncing baby boy as our test culminated. We toasted George with a glass of imaginary champagne (water). There was also one melancholy note to our emancipation from study. One week before graduation, one of our classmates died with sub acute bacterial endocarditis. Unfortunately, this was before antibiotics were known. Danny was one of the sweetest, dearest, angelic persons you can imagine. He was quite frail and fragile, but we were all shocked and flabbergasted at his death. It put a pall and damper on our spirits and graduation activities. The next day was June 3, my 25th birthday. There was a conglomeration of uplifting days to counteract our grief.

I would be remiss not to relate the hows and wherefores of the circumstances revolving around my historical meeting with my future wife, Doris, while a third year student. We met fortuitously March 15 (Ides), 1935, one evening. One of my colleagues, Bruce Irving approached me after a pathology exam and said "Howard, you've been hitting the books pretty hard and I believe you have earned a dulcet break. I would like to introduce a lovely lady to you that I have been dating. Really, she and you were made for each other." Bruce was adamant to the third degree and after a couple weeks of haggling and harassing, I broke down and acquiesced. Bruce escorted Doris to my residence one evening. I was dressed in my regal study clothes, knickers and a sweater. We met, shot the breeze for a few minutes, and parted. I was favorably impressed and telephoned her the next evening, requesting a Saturday night date. She demurred for a couple moments and then said "Yes. I had an engagement, but I'll break it." The next evening Doris came to see me and brought a mellifluous weapon – my favorite food to die for – a batch of BROWNIES! Our friendship was double sealed. Bruce ended up being a psychiatrist in D.C.

Chapter 10

Union Memorial Hospital, Baltimore, MD.

My benevolent, gracious and all-caring parents bestowed upon me an extremely practical and useful graduation present, a new Plymouth automobile of vintage 1936. It cost the fabulous sum of $600 plus our pitiful, decrepit and worn out '27 Studebaker, which almost died a natural death as we reached the final destination for the trade-in. The Plymouth sedan was absolutely and positively the ultimate gift possible. I told my mother that I would reimburse her and father as soon as my medical practice would come to fruition. Where upon she with alacrity responded, "Howard, you needn't pay us back for your gratuities, but promise me faithfully you will put any and all of your children through college and the initiation of their life's profession." I gladly acquiesced to her promulgated proposal and followed through with my end of the bargain to the nth degree later even notwithstanding that she had only one child and I had four.

It was with deep reluctance that I separated from my bosom partner Harry Bowie. We had a kind of a Damon Pythias relationship with never a hitch through four years of the roughest and arduous years of our young lives. We had struggled and agonized valiantly like twins for a common goal and succeeded to the maximum degree. Harry also obtained a premier, class A general, rotating internship at St. Agnes Hospital in South West Baltimore. He majored in surgery, doing five years internship, and became an eminently successful surgeon with an office suite on Charles Street in Baltimore.

Union Memorial Hospital is and was located at the confluence of Calvert and Charles Streets with Thirty-Third Street which runs east and west. It originated in the Civil War era as a permanent, massive building of brick, cement, stone and granite which presently stands intact. There have been several additions since my heyday, but essentially it embodies the three floor structure original plan. (I made rounds there with a visiting physician during my 1986 class reunion.) For some controversial reason a majority of hospitals in the U.S.A., in the first third of the Twentieth Century, frowned disapprovingly regarding married interns. This prejudiced attitude was fortunately and logically on the verge of appropriate revision to the opposite frame of mind. Actually, married interns are undoubtedly more stable, focused, serious, and dependable because they are, in the main, the number one, unfettered support for their family. Anyhow, I decided to take the marriage plunge toward the termination of my first year intern duty, damn the torpedoes and the unknown.

Each intern had a specific call number. My call number of clicks was 4-2-2. Our rotation series consisted of 2 months each of pediatrics (Peds), laboratory, emergency, anesthesia, medicine and surgery with 24 hour duty daily. The chief resident clinician managers were Doctors McCoy and Jenkins for pediatrics, Merkel for laboratory, Morgan for emergency, Frewing for anesthesia, Goetz for medicine and Johns for surgery. They were our immediate superiors. Also there was a bevy of supervising doctors in practice to complete the hierarchy of succession. "Red" Smith was resident chief of obstetrics and we had one month on this service in combination with lab. On pediatrics Dr. D.C. Wharton Smith was head of this department, Dr. Baetzer headed medicine, J.M.T. Finney headed surgery, and Staige Davis was the pinnacle doctor in anesthesia (in fact, he was one of the fathers of anesthesia).

We unflinchingly and veritably "busted our butts" on each service. There were fifteen basic interns, including myself. We made rounds of our assigned patients three times daily and performed all CBC's, urines, sedimentation rates, gram stain smears, transfusions, intravenous, collections of blood for the lab, cross matches, cultures, and lumbar punctures, comprising the majority of our services. We each had an individual / single room with telephone and a valet who was in charge of our shoes and uniforms. We received no remuneration but the food and meals were out of this world for hospital fare. We had steaks three times a week and squab every Sunday. Besides our three daily, delectable repasts we had a second super supper at 2300 (11 PM) for those nurses and interns working the "swing" shift. Out interns were a motley lot, coming from Maryland (4), Virginia (4), North Carolina, Florida, New York (2), Tennessee, Mississippi, Pennsylvania, and Missouri. We had no feminine doctors, with the exception of Eleanor McCoy, on the entire medical staff including our entire governing physician faculty. Dr. Borden was chief ear nose and throat (ENT) surgeon and Dr. Looper (loop the loop with Looper) was an occasional, undesirable operator. As a group of first year M.D.'s, we revered Dr. Gray, an eminent surgeon, as a paragon of virtue with undefiled character. He was a model of what a surgeon <u>should</u> be.

There was one super, duper surgeon at Johns Hopkins Hospital and that was Rubin Reinhoff, who would rankle us to the core with his super arrogance.

He married Hugh Young's daughter. Hugh was the father and kingpin of all urologists forever in Baltimore. Dr. Reinhoff strutted as though he was God's gift to all Baltimore surgeons. He was born in Leningrad, but was educated at Johns Hopkins Medical School and affiliated with Hopkins and Union Memorial as his base hospitals for his practice.

My connection with Reinhoff occurred when I was serving on the surgical service. I had a young lady of thirty years with malignant hypertension of sudden onset from Chilicothe, Ohio, which was about 46 miles due south of Columbus. Funny, I should remember this city, but the name is rather unusual and rings a bell (after 75 years). After considerable testing and head scratching, my final diagnosis was a tumor of one of the adrenal glands, which rests on top of the kidneys and secrets adrenalin. Dr. Reinhoff in consultation concurred with my diagnosis and elected to do an exploratory operation. After my patient's surgery, Rubin related that our diagnosis was confirmed and he had definitely extirpated a tumor from the right adrenal gland. However, our pathologist, Dr. Merkel, punctured our balloons and blatantly stated that the specimen removed at surgery was a glob of fatty tissue. I felt completely deflated but coincidentally, as though by a miracle of fate, her blood pressure came down to near normal anyhow.

There was an organization of Hopkins senior students called the "Pithotomy Club" that performed vaudeville-like, <u>frank</u> characterizations of their professors each year. One of the character portrayals in May, 1937, concerned my friend Dr. Reinhoff. After a high build-up with dialogue praising him to the sky as one of the premier elite surgeons of the world, there was a long pause while Reinhoff was basking in the adulations. The speaker stated, "We have had a famous artist, a budding Renoir, paint a picture 4 by 4 feet of Dr. Reinhoff dedicated to his superb excellence as a surgeon and we will unveil it now." After much further hype and commendation, the curtain was pulled and guess what?! The canvas displayed 1/2 of a black horse; the southern half of the horse facing north. Enough said!

Another memorable event I recall was an encounter as scrub assistant with a <u>real</u> honest to Jehovah surgeon, Doctor J.M.T. Finney senior. He was in his later years, but performed operations with superb manual dexterity and celerity. There was a mutual patient of ours suffering a tumor of the right axilla. I was distinctly honored to be his assistant at surgical excision of this tumescence. My duties were to hold retractors, pressure bleeding vessels, and clear the operative field of any obstructions (blood). The tumor had woven itself around the axillary arteries and veins and invaded the axillary plexus of nerves to the arm, forearm, and hand. It was like an octopus, actually an intricate and complicated total mess, to say the least. I was dumbfounded at his unbelievable ability to untangle this tumor from all of its octopus-like arms. He didn't hesitate a second, but went at the Herculean task calmly, as though it was duck soup and his daily routine. Amazingly the tumor was extricated in probably a little more that 1/2 hour. The tumor was about the size of a large plum with several extensive roots and projections, but it fortunately turned out to be non-malignant.

The piece de resistance during my twelve months at Union Memorial transpired shortly after I began my internship. This major incident occurred in August 1936 on the pediatric service monitored by chief resident Eleanor McCoy M.D., a University of Virginia graduate and assistant resident Jim Jenkins, a Yale graduate. Six year old Mary Frederick was a patient under my care and she was critically ill with erysipelas. Erysipelas is an infection of the skin with a group A Beta hemolytic streptococcus organism which causes strep throat and rheumatic fever. The disease, a flaming red rash, covered both of Mary's legs, abdomen and chest. Mary had an unrelenting fever of 106 plus degrees, was in total misery, and, I believe, she was at Brink's door. I contacted Dr. McCoy and expressed dire concern for Mary's life. There really was absolutely no effective treatment for erypipelas and we were stymied, up the creek without a paddle. I said, "Eleanor, is there anything we can do to alleviate Mary's lethal situation." Eleanor replied after considerable cogitation, "Yes, there may be something" (as her pupils dilated with excitement). Perrin Long just returned to Johns Hopkins from London, England. He's been experimenting with a 'sulfa' drug, injecting group A Beta Hemolytic Streptococci into mice's peritoneal cavities. The mice he treats by intravenous 'sulfa' live and the mice injected with normal saline solution die. It's the same organism that Mary is battling. I'll give him a call stat."

Dr. Eleanor McCoy called Dr. Long at Hopkins Hospital and after a brief summary of Mary's illness, he said, "I'll be over right away." About ten minutes later Perrin Long was in the pediatric suite of Union Memorial Hospital. He explained the properties of the new experimental drug 'Sulfa' and its ability to kill many gram positive bacteria, including strep, staph, meningococci and pneumococci. He said, "Take Mary into the treatment room." In this room we performed transfusions, intravenous, lumbar punctures and all special procedures. He said, "Place Mary on the table and put a bedpan under her for she will have a red bowel movement. I will give her this ampoule of 'Prontosil' intravenously, but slowly."

The mission was accomplished and the patient did have a red stool almost immediately after the injection. Perrin stated after the treatment, "Here's an ampoule of powdered Prontosil, give this to Mary subcutaneously this evening after dissolving it in a pint of normal saline solution.". We thanked

Dr. Perrin profusely for his emergency service and he thanked us for his opportunity to carry on his research.

That evening Mary's mother visited her and I described her status as critical and unchanged. I related all the details concerning the new 'sulfa' drug which Dr. Perrin Long had administered intravenously and the infusion of Prontolin which she was having now. "We are earnestly hoping and praying that this entirely new, experimental medication will reverse the disease and pull her out of the woods," I said. Mrs. Frederick was exceedingly grateful and thanked me profusely and said, "I know you are doing your utmost with an all-out effort."

The next morning, I anxiously made rounds in Ped's early to ascertain the results of our "new" medicine for Mary. I was utterly dumfounded to find out that her rash had disappeared and her temperature, and vital signs were completely normal. Mary was smiling and her eyes were razor sharp. She was enjoying a sumptuous breakfast. It was one of those believe it or not stories that ended positively, thanks to dear Perrin Long's research.

I at once called Dr. Eleanor McCoy and Dr. Perrin Long to relate the happy news. "It's a miracle, Mary has risen from the pearly gates," I said. It was most unusual for us to proceed boldly with a new experimental drug without even consulting with the mother beforehand, a drug which to my knowledge had never been used in the United States. However, it was a desperate measure to save a human life. Maybe mice are much more human that we give them credit for. The drug we used for Mary had been manufactured by a company in Great Britain. The news of the miraculous antibiotic properties of sulfa quickly spread world wide. Shortly thereafter, we were using it for strep throat, pneumonia and impetigoes as well as meningococcic meningitis. I know for a fact that it was employed for a case of meningitis at Sydenham Hospital (contagion) in Baltimore and it proved to be curative.

I saw Mary one more time after her discharge from Union Memorial Hospital at Children's Hospital of Philadelphia (CHOP) in the fall of 1937 when I was a resident intern in pediatrics. Mrs. Frederick brought Mary to visit me there, in the city of the Quakers and "brotherly love". She gave me a book entitled, "An American Doctor's Odyssey," which I treasure immeasurably and keep in my library. She also bestowed a big, wet, juicy kiss on me as she was leaving. I can still see Mary's image and often wonder her whereabouts and lifestyle. Incidentally, Domagk, a German scientist, discovered sulfa circa 1868 and it apparently lay dormant, incognito until Perrin Long began his research with mice. I should have published a paper on this new miracle drug to combat the pernicious strep organism, but somehow I didn't realize the magnitude of the medication.

There was a vicious epidemic of acute severs gastroenteritis in infants in July and August during my tenure on the pediatric service. I was giving transfusions and intravenous restorative fluids by the dozens day and night. Most of our patients were very young, in the 6 months to 1 1/2 year old range. It was a virulent and lethal infection despite our intensive efforts in treatment. Correcting electrolyte deficiencies and anemias were our primary objectives. Cultures by the dozens came up empty, and we concluded that the infecting organism must be an intractable virus. The main reason this rotavirus attacks infants around 6 plus months of life is because at this age the neonate has lost the vast majority of his or her maternal antibodies endowed by the mother during the intrauterine inhabitance before birth. The mother bequeaths gamma globulin A to the baby from previous encounters with this same identical virus during her infancy and childhood. The afflicted infant at 6 to 12 months is trying desperately to form antibodies in the bone marrow to conquer this fulminant organism, but being its initial exposure to this ravishing gastroenteric infection, the baby is almost totally unable. Our mortality and morbidity rate was dishearteningly high. Sometimes the veins in these little ones were almost microscopic due to severe dehydration, anemia, shock, and weight loss. Unable to do phebotomy, we resorted to infusing subcutaneously in the back or thighs or, as a last resort, in the inner ankle cut down to canulate the saphenous vein. We probably lost fifteen / twenty infants to the grim reaper in the two months while I was on pediatrics, despite all heroic efforts to the contrary. We were virtually up the creek sans paddle.

One of the dramatic highlights of my freshman year of service in Union Memorial Hospital was my medical experience with my patient Eddie McClain, age 7 years, while working in medicine under Dr. Folz. Eddie lived in Washington D.C. with his mother, Evelyn Walsh McClain, daughter of John Walsh, owner of the richest silver mine in Nevada. He struck it rich when he stumbled on the mother silver lode while exploring for gold. The patient's father was hospitalized in a mental institution in the D.C. area with a diagnosis of schizophrenia for several months at this time. Evelyn Walsh McClain possessed the renowned "Hope Diamond," a ten / twenty carat jewel, and proudly, stupidly displayed it at several of our confrontations. Its dazzling unique beauty now rests in the Smithsonian Museum in Washington, D.C. and is on public display.

Evelyn was somewhat haughty and liked to flaunt her powerful wealth by taking over every room on the third floor at Union Memorial for her retinue of hired maids, guards, and lackeys. She rebuked the hospital food and had all meals catered by the famous chef at the Belvedere Hotel. Apparently the fame and reputation of Union Memorial as a medical Mecca had been the deciding factor for Eddie's admission to Dr. Baetzer's and my services.

The admitting diagnosis was fever of undetermined origin. Symptoms consisted of chest pain, unremitting cough, weakness, anorexia, weight loss, headache, and fever of 103 degrees Fahrenheit for two weeks. Logical, differential diagnosis dictated an acute infectious disease with septic ramifications. Undulant fever, tularemia, pulmonary TBC, typhoid, pneumococcal pneumonia and mycoplasmal pneumonia were prime diseases to be provisionally considered. His W.B.C. was mildly elevated at 14,800 and there was an increase in polys of 82%, indicating a sub acute infectious illness. I ran several blood, urine, throat, and nasal cultures and came up empty. Chest X-rays were indicative of pulmonary inflammation generally with no specific infiltrates. Sputum culture gram stain, TBC stain and pneumococcis typing equally exhibited negative results. Examination of gastric fluid after overnight coughing paroxysms and the purified protein derivative TB test likewise were non contributory. We really blew a gasket in an all out, no holds bared effort to nail down a definite diagnosis, but we were stymied at the crossroads of futility. To my best diagnostic soul, I firmly, unconditionally believe Eddie was suffering from undulant fever or brucellosis. It is caused by brucella mellitensis bacteria and is contracted by eating contaminated, uncooked food or unpasteurized fluids, most notably milk. He gave me a history of having drunk unpasteurized milk and raw hamburgers.

At least we knew what diseases he did not have. We treated him with our newly discovered, first antibiotic sulfa medication, and I do believe it did ameliorate his sickness somewhat. Nowadays treating brucellosis with our multi-big league antibiotics is like shooting fish in a barrel.

One time Evelyn, while visiting him during my rounds, told Eddie she had salvaged a feline animal from the jaws of death. Eddie became quite agitated and rose up in his bed exclaiming fervently, “No, Mother, not another God damned cat!” Actually, with this remark, toxoplasmosis, a protozoan disease, crossed my mind. I believe, with the exception of good supportive treatment, we must give his natural immune system the credit for any progress in conquering the disease that Eddie made in the two weeks that he was hospitalized.

There were a couple of encounters with my good friend and next door roommate, George B. Morse, during my first year as intern at Union Memorial. It happened late one summer night, when I returned to the hospital after dating my sweetheart, Doris. Usually, in order to gain entrance to the Intern Quarters, a person would have to enter the main entrance, check in, walk through a long corridor on the east first floor, and unlock a difficult dial lock. This night I was in a mellow mood and was overwhelmingly tempted to take the easy, direct route to my room. I had left my window slightly ajar as we had no air conditioning and it was no hassle to scale the back wall, open the window, and enter my room on the first floor. The only obstructions were bushes at the base of the wall, which were generously endowed with pickers. I decided all lights were go and I mounted the wall and was opening the window when I was startled by a loud stentorian voice challenging me. Instantly I recognized George's voice, "Who goes there?". I shouted back, "It's me you damned fool." I entered my room and there was Morse, dressed in pajamas with a loaded, cocked 38 revolver. I was looking down the barrel. Apparently my clumsy movements had awakened him and he thought he was being invaded by a burglar. I apologized to George and promised on scout's honor never to repeat this foolhardy entrance again.

George was one of our sharpest, most intelligent interns and a true friend. He was mature and cognizant way beyond his years. He took advantage of the $50 recompense for giving a pint of blood. Fortunately, he was a universal, type "O" donor and was in demand as a donor for hematological products. George somehow was aware of the bonanza gleaned from donating 500 cc of blood. He volunteered a pint of blood monthly for the entire year netting $600, enough to purchase a brand, spanking new Plymouth automobile. He was no worse for wear and tear following each transfusion, probably due to very healthy bone marrow.

Money in 1937 was as rare as hen's teeth and dinosaur eggs. I recall an instance when I borrowed $2 from George to obtain a marriage license. He graciously acquiesced on the condition that I repay him within a month at 10% interest. He was all heart with strings attached. However, I did pay him back with money earned by pool shooting and ping pong matches in our recreation room. We also had a tennis court, but I cannot claim any great shakes in tennis games. Another source of financial income, if you were lucky, was in the poker games which were held at least once weekly. Stakes were necessarily low profile, however. There was just good natured banter and innocent, pure fun. One of our interns, "Rev" Pearson, was especially ecclesiastical, hence his nickname, which really fit him like a glove. His manner was befitting a minister to a "T" and he was continuously upbraided and harassed. Nevertheless, he treated us like water on a duck's back. He was truly a man of few words and sober as a judge, married with several children. We also had a bit of fun and merrymaking with our real drinks of Mint Juleps. We had these at special parties at the time of the Pimlico Horse Race, two weeks after the Kentucky Derby. One bar advertised - If you can drink two Mint Juleps and stand afterwards, they are on the house. And believe you me, there were no winners.

My memory recalls a dynamic incident when I was on emergency room duty. My phone rang about 3 a.m. while I was fast asleep and the nurse in the ER (emergency room) summoned me ASAP in an agitated and tremulous voice. Immediately I jumped into a shirt, trousers, and slippers and made it to the emergency suite at the other side of the hospital. The nurse directed me post haste to an elderly man dressed in a tuxedo, bleeding like a stuck pig from a large deep gash in the forehead. I at once grabbed a kelly forceps and after a couple minutes' pressure to the wound, ligated a good-sized artery which was pulsing bright red blood. After obtaining stasis of bleeding vessels down to the aponeurosis (skin layer next to the skull), I called Dr. Morgan, my immediate superior monitor. He told me to proceed at once with suturing of the wound and he would check it in the morning, but no aspirin because of bleeding.

As I started suturing the subcutaneous tissue, I could smell a very strong odor of high octane alcohol emanating from the gentleman's mouth. Indubitably, I placed half dozen subcutaneous sutures and about a dozen skin sutures for closure. I applied a pressure bandage to the wound and then tried to extract some history from this inebriated fellow. He had fallen down the stairs from the mezzanine floor of the Belvedere Hotel and fortunately had not sustained any neurological deficits from the head injury. Needless to say, he did not require any local anesthesia. We observed him for an hour and a gentleman with him volunteered to see that he got back to his hotel room intact. He was from Charlottesville, Virginia, and was attending a medical convention for dermatologists. Further history revealed that he was the professor of dermatology at the University of Virginia Medical School. Boy, did I take a hanging in effigy beating from the four fellow interns from Virginia the next morning. They criticized me unmercifully for having the audacity to perform such a difficult operation on their prized professor. Actually, after inspection by Dr. Morgan and a dermatologist from Hopkins, I was commended for doing a satisfactory job under verbal pressure.

Another unusual happening involved our Assistant Chief of Medicine, Dr. Aaron Wolfe. Aaron was not the most brilliant internal medicine M.D. and gossip was that he exerted considerable "pull" to gain his lofty position in the hospital. On his every day morning rounds he habitually had each patient stand erect at the bedside. On this particular morning at about 7 a.m., he had a decrepit old man stand up facing him. Aaron said, "Good morning Mr. Jones, you're looking wonderful, a picture of good health today." About a minute later the inevitable happened. Mr. Jones keeled over and fell to the floor with a dull thud and dropped stone dead. No amount of resuscitation by Aaron and the accompanying nurse would restore his life. The timing of his demise was perfect and all the interns had a "field day" twitting Aaron even though it was an act of God. The post mortem exam clearly proved that Mr. Jones had succumbed to a massive coronary infarction and saturnine attack. Dr. Wolfe was completely exonerated.

Fellow intern Jim Bradley, an M.D. graduate of Cornell University Medical School, was involved in an unfortunate incident in an ugly confrontation with a nurse on the obstetrics floor. The nurse had done the unforgivable act of pouring ether on a parturient birthing mother to prevent delivery of her newborn until the doctor arrived to deliver her. Bradley, on arriving at the scene, became overly incensed at the inherent dangers to the mother and baby and spontaneously exploded with a barrage of expletives and curse words directed at the nurse. The nurse reacted with a few choice words of her own, and the situation was reaching a combative stage when fortuitously intern David Dodd happened along and quenched the fire. The nurse, feeling severely affronted, reported the incident to her superior and from her to Dr. Frost, chief hospital administrator. Bradley reported to Dr. Murray Copeland, chief of all interns. The hospital board members called a meeting of all parties concerned and the situation was discussed and reviewed in detail. Finally Dr. Copeland took the floor and stated in a commanding voice, "Intern Bradley was just performing his duty and I must say I wouldn't give a damn nickel for any intern who didn't lose his temper once in awhile. Here we are dealing with two lives or death. Case closed." And it was closed, for Murray was quite forceful and I don't mean maybe.

Dodd was our fastest intern. He practically ran while walking or vice versa.

Another noteworthy happening encompassed Dr. Staige Davis one early morning while on emergency duty. I was called to the ER around 2 a.m. to see a young man with a compound, multi-fractured femur caused by an automobile accident. I gave him a hefty slug of morphine and began debridement shortly thereafter, while flushing the wounds with huge amounts of normal saline solution. Meanwhile the nurse alerted anesthetist Staige Davis and orthopedic surgeon, Ed Johns. He was taken pronto to surgery for reduction of dislocated fractured bone fragments and suturing of wounds under anesthesia. My job was to hold the leg and pass instruments. We were having tremendous resistance from our patient as he refused to go to sleep. After about twenty minutes of Herculean struggling, unable to get to first base with the operation, the light came on. Our problem was that aging anesthetist and venerable Staige Davis was dozing and had forgotten to turn on the gas machine. After simple correction of this problem, the patient relaxed and fell asleep. We all stayed awake and the operation was smoothly performed to completion.

We had an enormous intern party on Christmas Eve at the recreation room of our quarters. All of us invited friends, wives, sweethearts, and guests. It was a gala, festive affair, the party of the year. We had a huge punch bowl of liquids that packed a Joe Louis sock, loads of sandwiches, potato salad, stacks of Maryland fried chicken and various and sundry hors d'oeuvres. I invited my betrothed, Doris, and she was there.

The punch bowl was "off limits" to me because I was on call for obstetrics. At the beginning of the celebration there was no activity in O.B., but as luck would have it, along about the witching hour, two mothers in labor were admitted. The party was abruptly over for me and I found a trusted intern, Stuart Sunday, who volunteered to take Doris Meyer to her home for me. Actually, it was only a hop, skip, and a jump to her home in Hamilton from the hospital.

After saying my regrets and apologies to my darling, I excused myself and scrambled post haste to the obstetrics floor. On arriving there I could discern that there was a predicament evolving. I was confronting two mothers at about the same stage of labor who were "going to town" and proceeding rapidly with no holds barred. They were 24 year primiparas (first baby) showing a little bloody discharge and about a 3 to 4 centimeters dilated cervix with active labor contractions about 15 minutes apart. They were almost like twins, blondes with similar appearing husbands, all a twitter. I was all alone with my responsibilities for the resident intern "Red" Smith and the referring clinical doctor were both unavailable and celebrating the holidays. I was prompted to say a little prayer asking the Lord to give me strength and support.

At about 3:15 a.m. the first mother delivered a gorgeous, healthy 6 3/4 pound baby girl and immediately after the placenta came out, there came an urgent call to come ASAP to the other mother's bedside in an adjoining room. She was "crowning" (head showing on the perineum) and after donning a clean pair of sterile gloves, I guided the head exteriorly. Then the shoulders were gently externalized and the body came out slowly with ease. The second baby turned out to be a beautiful 7 1/2 pound boy. Fortunately both babies came out crying and needed no CPR or resuscitation. The placenta looked normal and both newborns were wrapped securely in warm blankets and placed in cribs on the side to supine position to negate aspiration of meconium. As soon as the heads were delivered the noses, mouths and throats were gently suctioned to clear the airways.

We all heaved a tremendous sigh of relief after the ordeal was completed. Nurses, patients and, most of all myself, were relieved and we offered a heartfelt prayer of thanks to mother nature. After the babies were safe and secure, I bedded down in an adjoining room and fell instantly into the arms of morpheus. I awoke around 7 a.m. to the heavenly and angelic singing of the nurses, who were caroling throughout the hospital on Christmas morning. Emotional shivers like electricity pervaded my body for they were singing my favorite carol, "Hark the Herald Angels Sing." Aroused, I went to the dining hall to breakfast.

We had a high class of patients sometimes but the majority were from the broad middle class. One notable reminiscence was of a fortyish man who had emergency surgery for gastric ulcer with massive hematemesis, which is downright life threatening. He was an ideal patient, no hassles, questions with impossible answers, or demands and always cheerful. He asked me if I liked brandy and I answered in the affirmative whereupon he presented me with a 4/5 pint of Five Star Hennessey (the ultimate) at discharge.

When we were on the medical service we were required to make seven o'clock a.m. rounds and do venipunctures on all patients needing lab work. Somehow the nurses designated me as "one stick Knobloch" to give reassurance to the persons from whom we drew blood.

We did have our fun moments with an occasional dance with orchestra for the nurses and interns. One of the most memorable pair of dancing partners was Dr. Eleanor McCoy, Pediatric Resident and Dr. Bill Jenkins, Assistant Pediatric Resident. Eleanor was at least 70 inches tall whereas Bill was really stretching reality to reach 60 inches in height with shoes on. But in spite of this prominent Mutt and Jeff differential, Bill could swing Eleanor around with the utmost of ease.

Another one of our most beloved and revered monitors was Igor Primacoff, chief of the medical department. He was a very astute clinician and diagnostician. "Primie", as we all called him, was a natural born teacher that could analyze and put all the signs and symptoms together in a neat bundle, leading to a logical, coherent conclusion which was invariably correct.

"Primie" was modest, humble and unassuming. His relations with patients, nurses and interns were always most gentle, kind, and professional. After leaving Union Memorial, I saw "Primie'" in Vancouver, Washington, in 1942 at Barnes General Hospital while in the Army. He had been inducted in the Medical Corps as a Major, but shortly after arriving in Vancouver was stricken with intermittent claudication of the lower extremities and had to be discharged from the Army. It was a sad, low blow to me for I held him in high esteem.

We did have a mild epidemic of Beta Group A Hemolytic sore throat amongst the nurses, interns and hospital attendants in May of 1937. It was traced by cultures to contaminated milk by someone who had an acute strep throat. The milk was drunk from large steel pitchers that had been refrigerated overnight and had incubated the pathogenic group of strep. Fortunately, sulfa was in vogue and the budding epidemic was immediately quelled before it could create serious complications.

Throughout the year I would occasionally visit Jeanette Cobb, registered nurse and girlfriend of John Meyer, Doris's father. Her apartment was just around the corner from the hospital and we would all convene there on free time weekends. We had a gala Christmas celebration with gifts galore. Cobbie took me to a sumptuous crab fest dinner one Saturday before my marriage.

Doris and I were married on April 2nd 1937 in the rectory of Saint Boniface Church by a priest because I was <u>not</u> a Catholic. The one paramount church rule that galled me to distraction was that I couldn't marry Doris unless I signed over the birthright of all my children to Catholicism and had them all baptized in the Catholic religion. This was an extremely <u>bitter</u> pill to swallow as I was truly a devout protestant from the cradle. However, love conquers all and I was madly in love and figured the problem could be solved later amicably.

I was never more wrong, as I realized later. This would have required one of the marriage team to unconditionally surrender his or her religious rites. We were both only children. She was an only grandchild and quite headstrong, very immature, and not about to willingly surrender her religious indoctrination.

My parents and none of my family were present at my marriage, and that occurrence sent a strenuous message of disapproval. Present at our wedding ceremony were her father, Johnny, his girlfriend, Cobbie, and Doris's Uncle George and Aunt Nettie Gibson. Anyhow, damn the torpedoes and we were married.

As I have previously mentioned, George Morse loaned me $2.00 to obtain a marriage license and I do believe that I did reimburse him. I took advantage of the $50.00 recompense offered for "donating" a pint of blood to pay for our honeymoon. We each took off work for a post marriage celebration trip for a weekend to Atlantic City and the Boardwalk. The fifty bucks neatly covered hotel lodging and meals and a Saturday dancing splurge. We did plan to not have any children for a couple of years using a combination of ovulation rhythm, barrier devices, and coitus interruptous. We were successful, for our first-born Susan arrived on March 9th at 8:00 a.m. in 1940, at Marquette Michigan's General Hospital.

The interns did get together an Abner Doubleday game of old-fashioned baseball. We practiced arduously for several weeks before the May Day game at Baltimore's Babe Ruth Stadium, in proximity just a few blocks, east on 33rd Street and home to the Baltimore Orioles. Our team was beaten by several runs. The opposition had a bunch of home-run sluggers and they stole the show. Nevertheless, it was a chance to have some fresh air, sunshine, exercise and good clean fun.

We had no gymnasium, but there were two tennis courts begging for action. One of the ludicrous, but painful happenings on the court occurred when brother intern Stu Sunday missed a 125 mph fast tennis ball with his racquet. Luckily, it struck him above the right eye, but it rendered him a dandy raccoon eye, which was quite swollen and black and blue for a couple weeks. It stood out like a beacon light. Stu wasn't hurt and withstood an avalanche of taunts nobly. It could not have happened to a more impeccably dressed person for he always presented an immaculate appearance a la "Little Lord Fauntleroy." A flush hit directly on the eye globe could have ruined his vision.

Along about November of 1936, I had to be thinking and planning where I would serve my next year's internship. I decided it would be wise to consult my astute pediatric resident – Dr. Eleanor McCoy – and I did. Eleanor asked me point blank, "Where would you like to go?" And I replied, "To some pediatric center in Philadelphia or Pittsburg, if possible." She said, "I know the chief resident at Children's Hospital of Philadelphia (CHOP) and I will gladly write to him and inquire if there is a position in pediatrics available there - for a "hard working" intern." I readily agreed and replied, "I'll be anxious to hear from you of further developments in the near future" and I thanked her immeasurably.

About two weeks later McCoy called me to her room and related the good news to me that there was an opening for a house officer in pediatrics at Children's Hospital of Philadelphia. I should write to Dr. Joseph Hennigan, Chief Pediatrics Resident on 18th Fitzhugh and Bainbridge Streets in Philadelphia and confirm a meeting date with him on December 28th, 1936, at CHOP. It was a done deed and my future fate in pediatrics was unalterably fixed.

Doris and I decided to spend Christmas in Greensburg with my parents and use it as a vaulting point to Philadelphia for the strategic meeting with Dr. Hennigan. Vividly, and with a bit of trepidation, I remember the evening of December 27th when we departed Greensburg bound for the big city on the Delaware in Pennsylvania. It was almost dark, stormy, and windy with snow showers and a wind chill of zero Fahrenheit when we "hit the road." Driving was an unnerving, monotonous, and tedious experience and staying alert and sharp was a chore. Surely the Good Maker was with us all of the way as we traversed the mountains, then drove through Harrisburg and onto Lancaster where we decided to call it quits for the night. The toll, super highway was treacherous, especially descending steep passages, but I decided to take them easy and to always follow a big truck in low gear. We reached Lancaster at around 11 p.m. somewhat exhausted and obtained lodging at a recommended hotel. After a hearty breakfast following sleep that "knits up the raveled sleeve of care" (As You Like It), we proceeded undeterred to Philadelphia and our final destination.

My meeting with Dr. Hennigan was positive in all respects and I was practically assured of a position as house officer for the coming year of July 1937 to July 1938 at Children's Hospital of Philadelphia. After our marriage in April, Doris wore her paternal grandmother's wedding ring. Doris's father staked us to an apartment on Eutaw Street, just north of North Avenue, which was fairly near Union Memorial Hospital. I was kidded inhumanly when the bride went to work on Monday morning after our marriage weekend in Atlantic City and the groom luxuriated in bed on a day off hospital duties. Upon signing up for my year in pediatrics at Children's Hospital of Philadelphia, Doris went to Philadelphia in April '37 to search for an apartment for living quarters for a year for us. She was persistent. After a couple days fortune smiled and her efforts were rewarded. She nailed down a nice apartment on Locust Street just off Rittenhouse Square, not far from CHOP.

I might briefly mention some other occurrences in 1936 tied in with relationships formed at College Park, Maryland in pre-med days. I ran into my old Phi Sigma buddy, George Matthews in the fall of '36, while shopping. We exchanged pleasant greetings and George related that he had tied the knot with Agnes Lyon recently and that her sister, "Cubbie", whom I had dated, was engaged. I in turn told him that I was engaged and was planning to wed in the spring. He also extended a dance invitation at a Mercy Hospital affair as his two sisters, Mary and Marie, were in nurses training there. I demurred the invite regretfully as I was on call that night.

Also, Jerry Geary, Phi Sigma Kappa president during my tenure at Maryland, dropped in unannounced to see me at Union Memorial Hospital. After our relations in the Phi Sigma Kappa House at College Park in my pre-med years, he was rather impressed and surprised that I had my M.D. degree and was interning. Jerry and I were not the best of friends but we had a mutual respect for each other. He had a flower establishment in Baltimore and was thriving, but was in difficulties with Uncle Sam for tax evasion.

I pricked my right thumb with a hypodermic needle accidentally when I was endeavoring to aspirate "laudable" pus on a cervical abscess of a little girl in the fall at Union Memorial. An abscess developed on the digital phalanx of my right thumb. The gram stain smear and culture on the neck abscess yielded a diagnosis of staphylococcus aureus; so we knew "N" sulfa medication would kill it. However, it did not faze this virulent organism and we had to resort to applications of continuous massive hot, wet packs of normal saline solution. But after a week of hot packs, the stubborn abscess was unresolved, and we resorted to surgical incision and drainage by Dr. Weaver under nitrous oxide (laughing gas). This final attack did the job. There is an old maxim in medicine and that is, "If it's piss or pus, let it out."

Anesthetic art was highly and meticulously emphasized at Union Memorial, although it consisted mainly of good old ether, chloroform, and avertin. Avertin was by rectal preoperatively followed by ether inhalation. My instructor was Jim Frewing and he was extremely competent, sensitive, and practical. Anesthesia is a very delicate and difficult procedure with little margin for error. It means that you are balancing a person's life in the palm of your hand. Avertin was an ideal drug for usage to control tetanus spasms and I used it several times in practice later on. Fortuitously, by the Lord's unfailing and unerring hand, I had no untoward anesthetic problems.

Chapter 11

Children's Hospital of Philadelphia, PA.

Children's Hospital of Philadelphia was one of the first purely children's hospitals established in the United States, probably around the time of my birth. I was a "House Officer" there from July 1937 to July 1938. As interns, we rotated on four services of two lead pediatricians each. The hospital was located in the worst possible, scurrilous, run down, poor, crime-ridden section of Philadelphia. Actually many children's' hospitals have similar locations because this is where the sick patients, the traumatic patients, the infectious disease patients and the mentally ill patients live. The address in which intensively ill and wounded children lived was excellent for teaching purposes for interns and staff. It's a natural with having five practical varieties of patients which illustrate all the diseases in medical text books – a fertile and unmitigated wealth of material for starved interns to unleash their vaunted expertise of didactic medical acumen. Saturday nights were especially noteworthy for serious gunshot wounds, emergency poisonings, choking incidents on foreign bodies, severe lacerations of all body parts, and acute respiratory infections. Many nurses coming back from dates were assaulted and had purses snatched on these nights. The nurses' home was adjacent to the hospital.

Our chief pediatric president resident was Jim Hanks, who had his Peds experience at Baltimore City Hospital. The associate pediatric residents were Helen Aff and Lion Perlman from Columbia and McGill Universities respectively. There were six other house officers including Evelyn Smith from Johns Hopkins, Kochendorfer from the University of Pennsylvania, George Clammer from Pittsburg, George Burnett and Dave Pewterbraugh family physicians in private practice, and Marian Hotopp from Harvard.

We all rotated on four services as previously stated. These services consisted of 1: Joseph Stokes Jr., pediatrician-in-chief working with Bill Guiness; 2: Mitchell Rubin and Milt Rappaport; 3: Irving Wolman and Pop

Reilly (private practice in Camden, New Jersey), and 4: Charlie Chapple and George Lyons. We served 2 ½ months on each service and 2 months in the dispensary (out-patient emergency), all teaching physicians at all times everywhere. Interns were all medical doctors. All our instructors and supervisors had hospital based offices and were readily available at all times for consultation and assistance with puzzling problems. We were encouraged to conduct research of a practical nature with our patients, such as how many had palpable spleens. We were responsible for cross matching and rendering all transfusions. Also we were expected to run all the CBC's and urine tests on every patient and also enter daily progress notes in the records.

We each had our own room on the second floor of the hospital, including refrigerators with pop and edibles. We received no stipend and were required to furnish our own uniforms, hand-me-downs from previous residents. There was a telephone in the hallway which meant extricating ourselves from delicious slumber and bed to answer the call.

There was a problem with answering the phone during our first two months of service. The newborn and neonate nursery was next to our quarters and there was no air conditioning. They blasted forth a cacophony of loud howls for their bottles frequently. It was beastly hot in July and August (about 90 degrees Fahrenheit) and of course we had all the doors and windows wide open to capture every little zephyr accessible within a mile. After working a 10 to 12 hour day, we slept very soundly and often couldn't hear the phone ringing. The ringing was also drowned out by the crying babies and that meant that the nurses would have to come into our rooms and literally shake us into reality and consciousness.

My wife, Doris, sought employment and was fortunate to obtain a job as secretary and medical assistant for Dr. Tom Walkling, a general surgeon. He was a pleasant and efficient man with a great personality and soothing bedside manner. We also had ample sustenance and living expenses from wonderful "Johnny", Doris's father, to fill in the vacant spaces. Our apartment comprised two large rooms, a combination kitchen and dining room, utilities and combination living room – bedroom, and a bathroom with tub. The bedroom had a folding bed / couch and was imbedded in the wall. It was totally adequate for our needs and we were as happy as the veritable "bug in a rug".

Doris developed a lasting friendship with Barbara Jones in the next door abode. "Barb" did visit us later in Marquette, Michigan, and I met her flight at Sault Ste. Marie, Michigan, when she came. My spouse also met me frequently for the noon-time hospital meal and sororitized with "Evie" Smith and Marion Hotopp in close relationships.

We often had gift tickets to the Philadelphia Symphony, which we relished, although I must confess I occasionally did succumb to a brief slumber when the music became saturnine (dull). We frequently took rides to the great park, zoo, and visited the historical landmarks and surrounding countryside. Evie Smith had an "old flame" in Easton, Pennsylvania, on the Delaware River, only an hour's ride away and we escorted her on a journey to Easton one weekend.

We were challenged medically to care for an infinite variety of quite acutely ill slum and inner city children. We had a preponderance of rheumatic fevers, strep throats, pneumonias with emphysema, rickets, scurvy, and critically ill prematures. One ward was filled with 40 to 50 "red hot" cases of rheumatic fever in the early stages. We performed numerous thoracenteses for critically ill staph and pneumococcal pneumonias. We also saw numerous vitamin deficiency infants. In addition, we envisioned many cases of tuberculous, meningitis, "snowstorm" military pneumonias, acute osteomyelitic nephritis, and cervical glandular abscesses. The Lord had adequately prepared me for this ordeal of fire by wisely subjecting me to primary pulmonary tuberculosis as a child. This illness auspiciously protected and immunized me against this dreaded disease (phthisis, scrofula tuberculosis). Unfortunately, we also had to treat a plethora of cases of meningococcal, pneumococcal virae and influenzal meningititis, <u>nakedly</u> and without any antibiotics or magical bullets. We also saw our share of polio and encephalitis. Furthermore, we had our full quota of chronic diseases such as rampant anemias, malnutrition, dental caries, hydrocephalus and juvenile arrthritides. We were armed with a cap gun when we really needed a cannon to fight and battle these gigantic goliaths. I should mention that measles, mumps, chicken pox and all contagious diseases including acute infectious diarrheas were also rampant and grossly uncontrolled. Actually, we were children facing men's and women's work face to face, but we gave it all we had, including blood, sweat, tears and warmth of heart and soul.

One of my most embarrassing experiences came in the spring of '38. I perpetrated an "innocent" joke on my wife, which backfired with a bang. In a jovial moment I called her at work and feigned being a Doctor Brown, who was referring an adolescent with acute appendicitis to her Doctor Walkling for probable surgery. Before I could tell Doris I was kidding, she hung up and for over an hour her line was busy, busy, busy. I knew she was valiantly and continuously calling Dr. Walkling in all possible locations to relay this message. Finally with perspiration pouring from all parts of my body and intense guilt feelings of anxiety, I did persevere and was able to tell Doris that I had given her a fictitious story about the appendicitis and I apologized to high heaven. That evening I traded calls with Dr. Burnett (he was very understanding and sympathetic to my plight) and I took a bouquet of flowers and a box of candy to my forgiving wife. I also called Doctor Walkling personally and he was very, very forgiving but warned me to think before acting in the future. It was an indelibly etched lesson in my corpus callosum (memory). In addition, Doctor Walkling invited Doris and me to dinner at his home, but there hangs another tale.

We did honor his dinner invitation willingly and my face was crimson when I was introduced to Dr. Walkling. We did enjoy a sumptuous repast of t-bones as I recall, and my favorite devil's food cake. Coincidentally, this was the night of the Schmeling and Joe Louis heavyweight championship prize fight. We were all glued to the radio including the doctor's lovely wife, Emily. There was a huge sigh of relief when Joe Louis put Schmeling into dreamland with a knockout punch in the first round. After our delectable dinner, I was feeling intense pain in my extreme lower back (spine), and Dr. Walkling forcibly said, "Let me have a look see, Howard." Following a detailed examination in his study room, he said, "Howard, sorry, but you have a pilonidal cyst abscess at the base of your spine. Sit in a tub of hat water several times a day to evacuate the pus. It isn't life-threatening, but it's damned uncomfortable."

I followed his instructions to the letter, including some good old aspirin and had immediate heavenly relief. We had a Dr. Little, who did only child's surgery without any charges. His mother had left him one million dollars inheritance on the promise that he would never charge anyone for his medical services. It was advantageous because he had zero economic restrictions and was under no pressure to "buy his baby shoes" with meager pecuniary funds. In other words, he was his <u>own</u> man and could call his shots without any bias financially. On one of his visits to incise and drain an acute cervical abscess on one of my patients, I conversed with him regarding my pilonidal abscess. He advised immediate surgery to open it up high and wide to discharge all the purulent debris. He scheduled me for such an operation and Dr. Stokes assigned me a bed in – of all places – the <u>nursery</u> of the hospital, no pun intended. The operation was successful, but healing had to take place from the bottom outward. This was a mighty slow and painful process, meaning the taking of warm sitz baths in a tub for an hour twice daily for a minimum of six months. I saluted and said "aye, aye" and buckled down to the task. The end result was as Little predicted – perfect healing.

Jim Hanks, our chief resident physician, was a tall, gangly, extremely thin, hungry man from Anderson, South Carolina. He had a Southern drawl you could not cut with an axe. He had roving, crocodile-type eyes and was as sharp as a razor blade. He never missed one of our errors and cracked a stern whip. We really didn't appreciate Jim's methods until the year's end, when we realized he had taught us and developed our pediatric training immeasurably.

Helen Aff and Lyon Perlman, our two assistant chief residents were the opposite of Jim Hanks. Helen was from New York City and Lyon was from Montréal, Canada. They had a pittance of sense of humor. They were quite relaxed, lenient and understanding. They were quite supportive and instructive for rounds with us on all our patients, and we had daily presentations of cases with the entire staff for an hour after the noon meal.

Occasionally each professor, while on his service, would invite Doris and me to their homes for a dinner. Joe Stokes, a true Quaker, invited all the interns to his home for a dinner (hotdogs) and in May, 1938, he invited us for the day to his cottage on Lake Louise in New Jersey (about 25 miles east of Camden, across the Delaware River from Philadelphia).

There were some unforgettable songs that came out about this time. Some of these were: "Where and When", "In the Middle of the Night", "You Hit the Spot", and "Goodie, Goodie". We also celebrated a Christmas Party in our intern quarters and Dr. Milt Rappaport attended. We had a variety of snacks and some spirits to oil the wheels. At this time "The Big Apple" dance was in vogue and a few of us were trying to perform this dance. Milt, who weighed at least 300 to 400 pounds, joined us and somehow lost his footing and fell supine on the floor. He was feeling no pain from imbibed spirits and couldn't arise. We struggled with all our might and main for an interminable period of time and finally somehow managed to get him on two feet. That was the finis of "The Big Apple". Milt was a real expert at doing intravenous cannulation of the very tiny ill infants with their collapsed, microscopic veins.

There were two notable visitors during my year at Children's Hospital of Philadelphia. My dearest Mary Frederick came up unannounced from Baltimore with her mother one Sunday afternoon in September, to visit with me. She looked lovely and healthy. It was a wonderful reunion to reminisce about our close encounter with Saint Peter's pearly gates. Mrs. Frederick showed her genuine appreciation by giving me a book called <u>An American Doctor's Odyssey</u>, which I still possess and adore for what it represents. Apparently, Mrs. Frederick found my whereabouts and decided to show off Mary's salubrity. In addition, I believe that Mary contributed greatly to my final decision to make pediatrics my life's work and also to incorporate the theme of this book into mine.

Another visitor was my friend, Jerry Kinzel, who interned with me at Union Memorial Hospital the previous year. Jerry came to see me in July on a Saturday at noon when it was literally hot enough to fry eggs on the sidewalk. The natives were restless and some agitated human threw a baseball bat through the windshield of his brand-new Chevrolet when he approached the hospital about a block away. Jerry was non-plussed and braved the wanton display of Northern hospitality. I commiserated with him, but he said "Never mind, I have a reliable insurance policy." We enjoyed reminiscing about our many mutual experiences during our intern year in Baltimore.

Another harrowing tale occurred on a hyperthermic Saturday night in August of 1937. Business was unusually slack on this night and a bunch of us interns convened. We decided someone should go to the "Brown Bomber Bar" and pick up a six-pack of beer. Lucky Jim Hanks was the designee to retrieve the libation. I say lucky because he was exempt from paying for his share. While he was gone we thought we heard guns firing nearby. The Brown Bomber, named for heavyweight champion Joe Louis, was only two blocks north of Children's in an extremely tawdry section of Philadelphia. Jim obtained the beer and when he returned to our quarters, he looked unusually pale and worried with dilated pupils and disheveled hair. He related a very scary story. When he was ½ block from the hospital, he heard gunshots whizzing overhead and dropped prone on the pavement for a couple minutes. After recovering his composure, he proceeded hurriedly in a semi crouch to the hospital. We shuddered and rewarded him by giving him first dibs on the beer. We thought of that heavenly aphorism, "But for the grace of God there lies John Wesley".

A humorous event happened in the emergency room while I was on call one evening. A little two year old African-American boy with an earache entered the ER I responded and while examining his mouth and throat, he bit my right forefinger. I couldn't extract my finger and it was downright painful. I gently tapped him on the forehead with my ostoscope and he instinctively opened his mouth wide from surprise and I removed my finger with gusto. His mother responded, "Doctor, does you think you has fractured his skull?" I laughed and said, "Absolutely not. There's no mark on his forehead." I assured her that an X-ray was unnecessary and told her to return if there was any problem. The ear turned out to be benign and before he left the earache was gone, thanks to the tap on the cranium.

I turned another hurdle on the way to medical practice in April of '38 when I was successful in passing the Pennsylvania State Boards in Medicine, enabling me to practice there and in forty five other states. Luckily, I had been out of school only a couple years and wasn't too rusty, but I did buckle down to a couple months of study and preparation. The exams were administered at the University of Pennsylvania Medical School.

Our superintendent of the hospital was Susan B. Francis, a la Susan B. Anthony, an unforgettable character if there ever was one. She was fiftyish, a spinster, very sober, stiff as a brick wall, tolerating no foolishness or horseplay. She invited all the interns to her apartment on the third hospital floor to witness and celebrate the coronation of Queen Elizabeth II of England in, I believe, August of 1937, a Sunday evening. She had a movie of this earth-shattering event to show us. It was a command performance and woe to the poor intern who rebuked her invitation.

We had to dress up to the hilt and observe our best Sunday etiquette. Wives were permitted, so Doris unwillingly came along. Susan was dressed in funeral black with black earrings and necklace. She served us tea, crumpets, and itsy, bitsy one bite sandwiches. Conversation was stilted and reserved and we were prisoners for what seemed like ages (only two hours). After we were emancipated from her tentacles, we loosened our collars and we all went down to Hammachers famous Crab and Seafood Restaurant on the waterfront and had a gourmet feast.

An ominous situation developed one Friday evening in July, early in my internship. I was getting ready to sign out after an arduous day's labor and I decided to take a shower. The shower was directly across the hall from my room in the intern quarters. After undressing, I removed my Hamilton wrist watch that my grandfather had given me when I graduated from medical school. The watch was a sacred symbol of honor and a highlighted prize of my graduation. I took my shower and when I came back to my room the watch was gone. My clothes were intact. I was heartsick and diligently searched everywhere. But, alas, the watch was nowhere to be found. I checked in all the other rooms and discovered only one other person in a room at the end of the hall, George Clammer, a fellow intern. He was feigning sleep and "awoke" when I rapped on his door. I told him about my missing watch and asked him point blank if he had seen it or if anyone had entered the quarters while I was showering. He steadfastly said no to all my inquiries. I know for <u>sure</u> George was the guilty culprit who absconded with my irreplaceable watch while I took a shower. He was the only person in the quarters and I remember seeing a shadow for a fleeting second in my room as I showered. I advertised in the Philadelphia Inquirer Newspaper offering a handsome reward, but came up with negative results. I thought I would case his room when he was gone from the hospital, but I was thwarted as he kept his door locked. Sad, but true, I never saw the watch after the fateful shower.

We would often have rotating externs from the University of Pennsylvania and Old Blockley (Pennsylvania) hospitals serve a few months at Children's Hospital of Philadelphia. They would get a little taste and exposure to pediatric clinical hospital experience. One particular extern from Old Blockley, "Okie" Kitamura, five years removed from Japan, was quite overbearing, arrogant and self-centered. He was hypercritical of American medicine, especially our therapy and treatment, lab, and X-ray facility at CHOP. He bragged about Japanese might and military prowess as compared to our puny Armed Forces. He predicted a mighty conflict would probably take place in the not so distant future. Apparently he was well aware of the Japanese buildup for the attack on Pearl Harbor while we were asleep.

One of our more brilliant instructors was Charlie Chapple, a very sharp guy, bubbling with good cheer and loaded with friendliness. He was a graduate of the University of Michigan and had interned and tutored in pediatrics at the University of Michigan Hospital for several years before coming to Philadelphia. He was so affable I don't believe he had any enemies. He related that one time when his car was parked on a steep hill in front of his home he forgot to turn his front wheels against the curb. The emergency brake failed and his poor car ran backwards down the hill and totaled.

Charlie was experimenting with helium gas when I was under his able tutelage and, as you know, helium distorts the voice into a high-pitched weird sound. He asked me point blank where I was planning to intern the next year. This was in November. I said "Pittsburgh, Buffalo, or St. Louis" with resounding conviction. To which he replied, "Howard, why don't you apply to the University of Michigan Pediatrics. They have a marvelous program with excellent instructors, probably the best one in the country." After cogitating a couple of days, I decided to take his sage advise and I applied to the University of Michigan Department of Pediatrics. I then put this application on limbo mind-wise. Lo and behold, about two weeks later I received a letter of acceptance to the U. of M. Pediatrics Department. I was quite elated and excitedly contacted Charlie. I said, "Charlie, I received my letter of acceptance to the University of Michigan Pediatrics." Charlie at once lit up like a Christmas tree and replied, "What are you going to do about it?" I hesitated an instant and slowly said, "Oh, oh, I don't know." Charlie emphatically blasted out, "Well, take it you damned fool!" And I did, to his sheer approval. That, folks, was how Charlie chose my career at the University of Michigan.

My year at Children's Hospital of Philadelphia was very valuable in teaching me how to deal with acute, emergency children in the slummy areas with unbridled freedom to follow my own dictates. University of Michigan Hospital would be pretty much diametrically opposite. They had mainly chronic cases in pediatrics such as cancer, rare diseases, and preventive medicine.

Doris and I packed all our meager belongings in our doughty old Plymouth sedan. We left CHOP packed to the rafters on Friday, June 30th, pointing our car to Ann Arbor, Michigan. This was the travel day of liberation for all the interns going to their respective new locations to continue in the pursuit of the Holy Grail of pediatrics.

George Burnett was packing his suits in his car but discovered two suits missing when he was fully packed. As previously mentioned, this Philadelphia district was not exactly a "Shangri La". His car was "securely" parked inside the hospital courtyard, surrounded by a 6-foot iron fence. In spite of all precautions, someone managed somehow to abscond with Burnett's suits. Clearly, these unemployed people had developed the purloining art to a high degree and nothing would deter them.

We went to Greensburg, Pennsylvania, on the last day of June to bid my parents adieu over night and then set out for Ann Arbor early on Saturday, July 1. We arrived in the city of our destination in the early p.m. and found parking spaces at a premium. It was a perfect day weather wise and Ann Arbor was jostling and bustling with verve, busy as a bee merchandise wise and traffic up to the rafters..

Chapter 12

University Hospital in Ann Arbor, MI.

After grabbing a bite to eat and imbibing some coffee at a local bistro, we set out earnestly to find an apartment for rent in Ann Arbor. At last our efforts were rewarded and we found a neat little apartment suitable for two persons on Huron Street near the University Hospital. We were ecstatic to discover such a fitting place to hang our hats, but we were running out of gas in our tanks after a somewhat exhausting journey from Greensburg to Ann Arbor. It was about a 450 to 500 mile jaunt. We moved all our belongings into our new home and paid one month's rent to a pleasant, welcoming landlady. We slept like two logs our first night over in Michigan, the Promised Land.

After a refreshing siesta overnight, I called Franklin Mellencamp, chief pediatric resident intern, and arranged a meeting to get oriented and acquainted with my brand new surroundings and duties. I met Frank at University Hospital at around 10 AM, Sunday, July 3; and he was quite warm and friendly. I knew immediately we would mesh gears. He was a happy, incisive, smart man of few words.

We took the grand tour of the pediatric wards, which were subdivided, on three floors. During our "rounds," Frank querulously approached me and questioned me. "You're Howard Knobloch, aren't you?" To which I replied, "Why yes." Then he said, "Well, you will have to take a little trip" Frank said, "to Traverse City." With my mouth wide open. I stammered, "Where is that?" And, he stated hesitatingly, "Why, a little north of here." While we were checking out the babies, I discovered a map of the state of Michigan and after searching diligently for minutes, I located Traverse City about 170 miles northwest of Ann Arbor. Traverse City was located on the northeastern shores of Lake Michigan. I swallowed hard and got up enough courage to ask Frank, "When do I have to go there?" And the startling answer was, "Can you go this afternoon?" To this I weakly said, "Why yes." This shocking turn of affairs was completely foreign to my awareness.

It was almost noon when I entered the intern quarters on the second floor. One of the interns looked up with knitted brows and said, "Why on earth are you looking so sad?" My reply was, "Oh, hell, I have to go to Traverse City today!" His emphatic answer was, "Why you lucky bastard! Traverse City is the most beautiful spot in Michigan, especially now!" This was at least a happy note of consolation, but I was highly worried about how Doris would react to this radical change of events. I thought the best policy was honesty and I would lay it on the line with the cards face up. When I got to our abode I related verbatim all the details of my meeting with Frank. Doris immediately crashed with a flood of tears as I expected. I assured her our trunks would be taken care of, pronto, when they arrived from Philadelphia and would be forwarded to Traverse City. I originally thought Frank had called it "Transverse City".

We settled with our landlady, who graciously returned our apartment deposit after we explained our mandatory change of plans. We grabbed a sandwich and milkshake and were on our way. We arrived in Big Rapids about 7 PM and decided to stay there for Sunday night. Refreshingly, we made our destination, beautiful Traverse City, about midday the next day. At the children's clinic alongside Munson General Hospital, we met Mark Osterlin, the James Couzens/University of Michigan clinic head. Mark was effusively happy to see me and laid out the red carpet for us. The good news was that the Cherry Festival and parade were to begin the next day. The bad news was that Mark and Helen, his wife, were taking off tomorrow for a month's vacation and lucky me was in full charge of all the in-hospital patients plus all the daily out-patients.

Our first priority was now to establish a residence. Mark did give us a big lift by steering us to "Mama" Shields' Boarding House" on Fourth Street. Doris and Mama Shields immediately fell head over heels in love with each other, enabling us to relax and settle in with comfort and a happy mood.

An explanatory dissertation is in order at this juncture. James Couzens, a man of great renown and philanthropy with a hearty soft spot for children, especially the poor and handicapped, had endowed three Michigan children's centers. The centers were located in Detroit, Traverse City, and Marquette. Couzens was born in Chatham, Ontario, on August 26th of 1872, and died October 22nd of 1936, the year I graduated from medical school. Father, James Couzens, and mother, Emma Clift, were immigrants from England. He was raised in a stern Presbyterian household and lower income family. He was a newsboy, stirred smelly boiling vats of soap for his father and went two years to Business College. James migrated to Detroit in 1890 and performed as a railroad checker for Michigan Central. In 1895 he established a relationship with Henry Ford, the great automobile icon. He was an astute accountant and kept Ford's business solvent. While working for Ford, he and Henry had a disagreement in 1919, which caused dissolution of their association and Couzens settled for 30 million dollars. In 1898 he married Margaret Manning, a devout Catholic and they had five children.

James had a burning desire for politics and became mayor of Detroit in 1918 to 1922. He brought about "Municipal" ownership of Detroit's transportation system in 1922, and also in the same year was appointed as a Republican to fill the unexpired term of U.S. Senator Truman Newberry, who resigned because of a scandal due to election irregularities. He served 14 tempestuous years in the Senate.

James was abrasive, strong-willed, bulldog stubborn and uncompromising. His mayoral campaign saying was: "I will reward no friends and punish my enemies". He gave $650,000 to Harper Hospital for a nurse's home and also $650,000 to the University of Michigan for a nurse's home. His great philanthropic gift was 30 million dollars, endowing the three children's clinics in Michigan. He also donated money for a biological and chemistry lab, erected next to Detroit Children's Hospital. His prime interest was in help for the maladjusted child through psychiatrists, psychologists and psychiatric social workers. He emphasized that helping children was a matter of "absolute justice" and he was very sentimental about the plight of deformed children. It is said that he suffered actual pain at the sight of a crippled child.

Couzens expressly stated that the three children's clinic's funds were to run for 25 years only, which was from 1929 to 1954, and that was all. Actually, he wanted desperately to remain completely anonymous for all his magnificent donations. In 1919 he also bestowed 1 million dollars for crippled children. His everlasting poignant motto was, "New services for health, new implements for self-discipline and an enlargement of scientific knowledge have come into being with our assistance. And we have entered into the lives of hundreds of thousands of children to their happiness and advantage." At the clinic in Traverse City, we had a very astute, devoted psychologist to assist us with behavioral, attitude, and personality problems in our young patients.

Dr. Heidemann had preceded me as Resident Physician from Detroit Children's Hospital. He and Mark Osterlin were not on the same wavelength by a long shot, due to his overbearing super ego as commented on by Mark. There were seven Residents in Pediatrics at the University of Michigan in Ann Arbor, including myself. Three of us were in the Traverse Children's Clinic for 4 months apiece, and four of us were in Marquette Children's Clinic for 3 months apiece. I had no idea in the world concerning this arrangement until I locked horns with Frank Mellencamp.

Out-patient and in-hospital patients at Traverse City were managed at

Munson General Hospital and referred by general family practice doctors in the environs. We had quite an epidemic of shiga and salmonella diarrhea during my tour of duty at Traverse City. My treatment consisted mainly of intravenous (IV) fluids and transfusions and this regime was eminently successful. As I recall, we didn't lose a single child to the Grim Reaper. At the end of my tenure there, I, by Mark's request, presented a dissertation on "Treatment of Diarrhea" to the County Medical society. The presentation made a favorable impression. We also had a couple cases of tetany hypocalcium, especially in the newborns that were treated by IV calcium chloride with dramatic success. Transfusion is a very valuable tool to counteract anemia and enhance immunity by furnishing valuable antibodies, hemoglobin, nutrients, and iron.

Mark Osterlin, my mentor and trainer, was an extraordinary administrator but woefully weak on diagnosis and academic treatment of acutely ill children. We hit it off nobly and he designated marked authority to my judgment and jurisdiction in the treatment of all acutely ill infants and children. Actually, he had not realistically kept up with new medical advances by study, medical seminars and actual direct head to head contact with pediatric patients. Mark had a ravenous penchant for winemaking and wine quaffing. He was a happy-go-lucky type of personality and he would spend hours stomping barefoot on crates of grapes in the cellar of his home on the Peninsula.

The Michigan Peninsula was a strip of land about six miles wide and twenty miles long, which jutted out into Grand Traverse Bay and separated the east and west arms of the Bay. Mark was originally from Norwalk, Ohio, but attended the University of Michigan Medical School and had his pediatric residency there. Mark also was hooked on the pipe and was an inveterate smoker. His wife, Helen, was a flaming redhead with a temper to coincide, making Mark tread the straight and narrow path. At our Pediatric Clinic we had a highly qualified psychologist, Miss Jones, who worked diligently with Mark to treat all the behavior problems. The problems were usually from disruptive families, as you might deduce.

Doris worked gratis as Doctor J. Jerome's secretary. He was an orthopedic surgeon and quite a character, addicted to alcohol. He was not dependable and would completely disappear for stretches of 24 hours plus on occasions. Doris did form a rather binding friendship with a bachelor dentist, Sam Stein, who served the state mental institute patients. We would take excursions with Sam to the sand dunes on the east side of the peninsula for companionship and relaxation.

Sam was a personable, felicitous hulk of a man and he invited us to his home in Detroit. I remember coming through Saginaw on the road to Detroit and also tasting Gefilte Fish as my first experience. Sam also made a mask of Doris after several sittings and did a very respectable job.

Doris also formed a close relationship with Josephine, a social worker at the State Mental Hospital, where we partook of our dinners and became acquainted with the psychiatrists who worked there. I remember one person in particular, who was wholly capable, maintained his sanity and defied expression of the average mental health physician's personality. He was a rare levelheaded psychiatrist with feet planted firmly on terra firma. William Hyslop and I harmonized with our thoughts and feelings in major medical issues.

During our four months of living in the heart of the cherry country, the "garden spot" of Michigan, we made numerous safari trips to the surrounding environs. Glen Lake nearby is considered one of the ten most beautiful lakes in the world. Sunset or sunrise on both arms of Grand Traverse Bay, viewed from the peninsula, is an almost awe inspiring vista. Frankfort, on Lake Michigan, is a quaint jewel dedicated to fishing, sailing, and swimming. I am mindful of my first swim encounter there. I foolishly dove into the water from a pier and sensed an entire body numbing paralysis for a couple of frigid seconds. It literally took away my breath and I got quite a razzing from my spouse. She had the last laugh! I associate a poignant song that was popular then with Glen Lake, and that is "Red Sails in the Sunset."

Doris's Aunt Dolly and Uncle Jack Noll from Clarksburg, West Virginia, came to see us for a visit in July. They were indelibly impressed with the sheer and unbridled beauty of all the panoramic views surrounding Traverse City. They lived in the coal country of West Virginia near Clarksburg where Jack was a supervisor of a large mine. The sand dunes and the cherry country were especially appealing to them, as well as the hypnotic sunrises and sunsets over the Grand Traverse Bay.

Teaching pediatrics to the nurses in every hospital I have interned in, and practiced in, has always been my intense desire and duty. Innumerable teachers have supported me over the years and I feel strongly that my duty is to pass on the knowledge I have accrued to help anyone in need. Besides, teaching enables me to keep up to date on the subject being taught and the satisfaction of rendering help to those who require assistance. So, I did instruct the Munson Hospital Pediatric nurses with special one-half hour lectures twice weekly on the common acute illnesses of babies and children. Subjects covered were meningitis, pneumonia, cryptic fevers, dehydration, diabetes, pneumatic fever, arthritis, and behavior problems. Medicine and pediatrics at this juncture was evolving strongly in the direction of prevention modalities. The aphorism, "An ounce of prevention is worth a pound of cure," consists of words no truer spoken.

Speaking of pneumonia, I did have a round of viral pneumonia just prior to departing this haven. I dared fate and had a farewell swim in the bay in spite of near freezing temperatures. My big chill led to viral pheumonitis, which, fortunately was rather moderate. My recovery was ensured within a week with rest without antibiotics.

Being an avid baseball addict, I was in mourning for my beloved Pittsburgh Pirates of National League vintage. While driving in the boon docks one late September afternoon during my recuperation from the acute pulmonary infection, I was listening intently to the radio broadcast of the Pirates and Chicago Cubs baseball game. The scenario was nothing but the highest voltage with all the marbles on the line. These two teams were in a virtual tie in percent of games won and lost for first place, and this was the last game of the season with winner taking the National League Championship. I was totally on pins and needles because the game was in the extra eleventh inning, tied at four runs apiece. My Pirates had just batted run less in their one-half inning and the Cubbies were now batting. There were Cubs on first, second, and third bases with two outs and Gabby Hartnett, Cub catcher, was at bat. He had a 3 ball 2-strike count and the Pirates' best pitcher was on the mound. I was earnestly praying and pleading for just one more big strike to end the extra inning. Larry French wound up in the almost darkness at Wrigley Field in Chicago (no lights then) and smoked the ball with all his might. It came over the heart of home plate and Gabby launched a prodigious, mighty swing with all his strength. There was a loud crack of the bat and the ball went way over the outfield brick wall, covered with ivy. The homerun killed the Pirates and my fervent hopes for a Pirate National League Championship for 1937. I can't remember who the announcer was, but I believe he gasped and swallowed his chewing gum, and so did I!

We were very sad and reluctant to leave Traverse City, Garden of Eden that it was, and all the binding friendships we had made there. It was a most happy and eventful four month's tour of duty and we had no realistic idea of what exactly to anticipate in our next eight month's stay at Ann Arbor, University Hospital.

Chapter 13

Completion of the Ann Arbor Internship

There was a heavenly bonus awaiting me when I returned to University Hospital in Ann Arbor on October 31st, which helped welcome me with open arms. I received the life saving check of $100.00, rescuing me from the ranks of poverty. I had forgotten that as a second year resident I received the monumental remuneration of $25.00 per month, and I had served 4 months away from the Mother lode.

Finally I became reconciled with my fellow residents. There was Arthur ("Pinky") Keller, M.D. from the University of Pittsburgh, Donald Bourg, M.D. from the University of Michigan; Ward Chesley, M.D. from Wayne State University; Fred ("Phearless") Palmer, M.D., from the University of Michigan; Bill Wilson, M.D., from the University of Pennsylvania; and Freddie Fehlman, M.D. from the University of Illinois. Along with yours truly, we comprised the "lucky seven" residents, a gang of rough, tough, full of stuff hombres.

The chief of the Pediatric Department at University of Michigan was D. Murray Cowie, M.D., a converted internist and first official Professor of Pediatrics there. Associate Professors of Pediatrics were Louise Schnute, M.D., a mighty astute and rigid lady of few words and Harry T Towsley, M.D., who really didn't have to work. He married Grace Dow, daughter of Herbert Dow, founder of Midland Dow Chemical Company and sister of Eldon Dow, the great, renowned architect. Harry and Grace lived in a unique house built by Eldon and there was a big tree and a swimming pool located in the living room. Harry would become President of the American Academy of Pediatrics in 1955. We interns would have monthly academic meetings in Harry's house. He was a superb host, but, honestly, a highly touted teacher too. Harry had a brother, Wilbur Towsley, M.D., who was a family physician practicing in Midland, Michigan. Harry loved to hunt deer, and he and Wilbur would go on deer jaunts every year.

D. Murray Cowie had an office in Ann Arbor. He practiced a combination of adult internal medicine as well as pediatrics and shared his office with John Law, M.D. He was a pediatric professor of near equal pediatric rank from Emory University in Atlanta, Georgia. When John Law first appeared in Ann Arbor, he put on a magnificent show to impress his new colleagues. He had a big white escort Cadillac with a black chauffeur and paraded through all the streets of Ann Arbor. John was a wee bit arrogant and loved to exhibit his southern hospitality. Cowie was his diametric opposite. He was humble and down to earth in feeling and dealings.

Murray was intensely interested in pediatric research and especially devoted to contagious diseases. There was an entire building dedicated strictly to contagion called, "The Pest House." Upon entering this "sanctum sanctorium", you were compulsorily required to don cloth boots, long gown, cap, mask, and gloves, besides walk through a bath of disinfecting fluid containing chlorine. Talk about isolation! This was the rank epitome of isolation in all its pristine glory.

When I was in charge of contagion (2 months), I was privileged to treat just about every infectious disease in the books, yes, even a case of smallpox, which was practically extinct then. This patient was so plastered with pox lesions that you could hardly put a pinpoint between the pustules. He was in a stupor and near death for several days, but somehow we managed to defeat Mr. Brink with the Creator's magical healing propensities.

One of the internal medicine interns, Bob Hoobler, son of pediatrician Sidney Hoobler, came down with a fulminating case of chicken pox. He too was covered with vesicles, just like a blanket, but he survived after two weeks of intense suffering. A few years later, Hoobler became a professor of internal medicine at the University of Michigan.

Another instance of the deleterious effects of varicella occurred in June of '39. One of our prized pediatric nurses got spliced and on the very first night of her honeymoon came down with a florid case of chicken pox and was admitted to my service on the contagious ward. Her husband laughed and said, "Doc, here's a bottle of champagne for you. It won't do us any good, but maybe you can find some usage for it." Apparently, the pox bug had inoculated his bride by a child on her service at an "inopportune time." She must have led a very sterile childhood.

Dr. Cowie became famous for his instigation of "iodized salt" to prevent thyroiditis along about 1928. Thyroid goiter was a common illness around the Great Lakes because of deficient salt sources (incidentally, Detroit is built over an ancient salt bed!). Along the coastlines of the United States there is salt water galore, containing sumptuous, enticing seafood too.

Cowie was generous and invited the staff and interns to his cottage on a picturesque lake in the Irish Hills west of Ann Arbor. It was a gala affair and notable for the time at which Doris became pregnant with our first child. Shortly after this party, Doris and Martha McGuire drove to Baltimore to see her folks. Doris couldn't figure out why she was so nauseated when smoking during the trip to Baltimore, especially in the early morning. But, it didn't require a rocket scientist to figure it out shortly after she returned with the pregnancy test.

When we returned from Traverse City, we were lucky to find an excellent apartment on the southeast corner of Ann and Fourth Streets, but it was a little beyond our limited budget. However, fate intervened and we discovered a Public Health Nurse, a Michigander, Martha McGuire registered nurse, at one of our dining out suppers at the Michigan Union. She also was looking for a rental abode and we struck a deal with her. There was ample room and bedding facilities in this apartment that we had our eyes on. So, we decided the three of us should share this second floor apartment until July 1, 1939. Doris and Martha were a perfect fit, so we nailed down this homestead. Martha was single, but she became enamored with a stalwart, studious, nice oncology intern, Arthur Siwinski, M.D., around March 1939. Martha and Arthur did tie the marriage knot in June of '39, just before we departed for Marquette in the Upper Peninsula of Michigan for my Chief Residency year.

Doris had a huge melanotic melanoma on her right mid, external upper arm. It was quite ugly, dark, and foreboding and seemed to be getting blacker, larger, and heavier. We decided immediately to engage Dr. Gilbert, M.D., and Professor of Oncology at the University. He advised prompt surgery to remove this tumor by ablation and excision. The tumor dimensions were roughly 2 by 2 inches - in a circular pattern, truly life-threatening. Doris and I went to the hospital dispensary - tumor clinic on a Saturday afternoon in April, where Dr. Gilbert eradicated the benign (thank God) melanoma under intravenous analgesia and local anesthesia. Doris was a real dyed in the wool soldier and withstood the procedure with amazing fortitude and bravery. It probably affected me more deeply than her for I had a definite squeamish feeling during the surgery. We rested over the weekend, but you can't hold a good woman down, and she was up and at 'em on the following Monday.

Being a fanatical football sports nut, I avidly attended the November, Michigan football games in Ann Arbor at the mammoth stadium, built in 1926 by the revered "point-a-minute" Yost. I was mesmerized by the great feats of all-American tailback, Tommy Harmon, and his running mate, peerless Forest Evashevski, who did all the blocking for him. I remember the time Harmon made a long touchdown run against the Southern California Trojans in Los Angeles and an ardent Trojan fan came out of the stands and tried to tackle him in the end zone. Another time, Harmon was stacked up against P.G. Riblett, University of Pennsylvania's all-American running back with much ballyhoo preceding the contest. I was at the game at Yost Stadium in Ann Arbor, and I remember watching from the eightieth row while Harmon dispelled all questions regarding his utter superiority over Riblett, football-wise. Michigan vanquished Pennsylvania in a touchdown victory of five to one.

The Elliott brothers, Pete, quarterback, and Jimmy, linebacker, were also stellar players. Harmon, in spite of all his ability, could never score against the powerful Minnesota Golden Gophers. After World War II, I procured season tickets to all football games played in Ann Arbor every year from 1946 through 2000 and three of my children were University of Michigan graduates. My college graduate school was Maryland, but my football heart almost belonged to Michigan, even when Michigan engaged Maryland in football at Ann Arbor. Actually, I belonged to the University of Michigan Alumni Society.

There were two tennis courts adjacent to contagion and there hangs another tall tale, which is engraved deeply in my cognition. One of my best friends, Vincent Sender, who was a red-headed, first year intern in internal medicine at University Hospital, was my tennis partner playing the outer court. Vincent was a Mormon from Salt Lake City, Utah, and a rank amateur tennis player similar to myself. We were engaged in a relaxed game for fun one gorgeous May Day afternoon and I was serving. Somehow I knocked the ball over the high fence (it wasn't easy!) and completely out of the court. Naturally, I had to retrieve my ball, so I skirted the right side of the court. While searching for the ball in the tall weeds and underbrush, I fatefully stepped on a large nail spike. It penetrated through my tennis shoes and became deeply imbedded in the ball of my right foot distal to the second metatarsal (phalangeal joint). I let out a vociferous yelp and hopped on my right heel back to the court where Vincent met me. While lying on the ground, Vincent, with a mighty jerk, extracted the spike from my foot. There was a paucity of bleeding and the endorphins from my brain ameliorated the pain temporarily. He called emergency from a phone on the court and they picked me up by ambulance and transported me by stretcher to the emergency room.

They called surgery for consultation stat. Surgery responded tout de suite and advised surgical removal of the tract of the nail and injection of tetanus antitoxin. I protested vehemently because I knew I was anaphylactic to horse serum. I had been tested with skin pricks to about forty allergens, including horse serum in diphtheria antitoxin and found to be extremely reactive to the Shick Test and diphtheria toxin. The allergy doctors told me, to never have any injection containing horse serum, without exception, because of possible fatal anaphylaxis. I said to the surgical physician, "I agree to surgery to ablate the path of the nail, but please skip the tetanus antiserum containing horse serum." One of the surgical residents countered by saying, "Parke Davis pharmaceutical has come up with a tetanus antitoxin containing bull serum instead of horse serum, to obviate any reaction." I took his statement with a big grain of salt but was badgered into condescending to the injection of bull serum by miniscule injections after the operation. They gave me a healthy slug of morphine and took me to the operating room without hesitation.

After the surgical exploration, "bull serum" injections began every twenty minutes. I didn't have any immediate reaction to the serum, but in the middle of that night, I awakened. I couldn't breathe or swallow or talk and had a vice-like feeling in my chest. I grabbed the alarm bell at the bedside stat and rang for the nurse. She appeared immediately, thank God. I grasped my neck and pointed to a prearranged syringe of adrenalin lying on the dresser and she picked up the syringe in an eyelash and jabbed my arm with alacrity, administering the life-giving contents of adrenalin. Within seconds (it seemed like ages) my chest relaxed and I could breathe, swallow, talk, and the stomach pain abated. I expressed heartfelt thanks and said, "I think you have saved my life." To this she said, "Think nothing of it, I do this every day." Apparently the "bull" was a horse as you've probably guessed. The honest truth was that it was horse serum.

I knew that I was anaphylactic reactive to horse serum, which had sensitized me as a child in first grade when we all were compulsorily given active diphtheria antigen intramuscularly. It contained horse serum, and it was a preventive immunization because two classmates had been victims of diphtheria. Furthermore, I had about fifty allergen skin tests a couple of months previously at the U. of M. allergy clinic, and they showed a 4 plus reaction to horse serum and egg white. The allergist, Dick Lowrie, M.D., stringently warned me to avoid horse serum. However, the same night of the tests I ate 3 fried eggs and had no reaction. This goes to prove that with allergy testing, you can have false negatives and false positives. Subcutaneous injection allergen testing is more accurate but can only be done by a doctor with adrenalin at his fingertips, in a syringe, ready to go instantly. This means that blood testing is truer than skin testing.

Following my experience with the bull serum, I was covered with myriads of hives of all sizes. My entire body was like a giant hive. I have never ever had such intense and unbearable itching in my life for several days. They gave me almost constant soda baths and Benadryl until the cows came home, but only time could really ameliorate those nasty hives. As a sequel to the "bull serum", Doris became impregnated with our first child about two or three weeks later. As you can imagine, I took an unmerciful avalanche of teasing amongst my fellow interns.

There was a deleterious practice of thymus irradiation practiced at Ann Arbor when I first arrived there. The purpose was to shrink the thymus to prevent pressure on the trachea and to avoid strangulation. At Children's Hospital of Philadelphia we learned that this practice was unnecessary and actually harmful because the thymus was later revealed to be a most important organ involved with cellular immunity. Also, later on, there was a strong feeling that irradiation could lead to possible cancer of the lungs, larynx, or thyroid. The main, probable culprit here was the Obstetrics Department, which was headstrong about using this mode for any respiratory difficulty in the newborn. This thymic irradiation practice was discontinued shortly after my arrival at University Hospital and I like to believe that my pressure had a positive affect in stopping the heinous, antiquated procedure. Pediatrics and obstetrics always seemed to be at odds with each other with medical issues.

One special case stands out in my mind. I was on call on Christmas and was summoned to the emergency room on the double. It was a well nourished eight-month old baby that was dead on arrival (DOA). There was a history of violent abdominal cramping over a three-day period with hematochesia (gross bleeding) from the rectum for two days. This was compounded with constant vomiting. Two doctors had seen this baby and had both missed the boat. The doctors were now unavailable. Postmortem confirmed my clinical diagnosis of intussception. The poor mother was crying her heart out and I felt so helpless. There was absolutely nothing I could do but commiserate with this inconsolable Mother.

Ordinarily, diagnosis of intussception is made by abdominal swelling on the right side, blood on the rectal finger, and intermittent severe abdominal pain every couple of hours. The child also shows great fear and is usually motionless between attack spasms. The cause is usually ileal ilium telescoping of the cecum into the ascending colon. Diagnosis is clinical plus barium enema or air inflation enema at that time (before Ultrasound or CAT imaging). Sometimes the enema will resolve the telescoping but if there is any question (delay), surgery is the order of the day.

Cystic fibrosis of the pancreas was discovered in 1937. It is an inherited, genetic disease in a child. It affects the progeny of both male and female carriers. One out of four children born to these parents will inherit this pancreatic deficiency of the digestive juices amylopsin, steapsin and trypsin. Digestive function is reduced drastically due to malabsorption and the respiratory tract is hampered by thick, bronchial secretions which lead to chronic infection and progressive respiratory failure. Abnormal loss of beta pancreatic cells leads to frank diabetes Mellitus in about 15% of patients. Male infertility is present in 95%. Sweating inability causes dehydration and heat stroke. When I was interning at Ann Arbor, we did have a probable case of cystic fibrosis; and, at that time, diagnosis was extremely difficult. We learned at The Children's Hospital of Philadelphia to catherize the duodenum and collect the pancreatic juices from the ampulla of vater at the second portion of the duodenum. Then we would test it for protein digestion and if none was found, we would feel pretty certain the answer was cystic fibrosis. Another gross test was to put the stool on X-ray film to see if there was protein digestion. In the Ann Arbor case we couldn't obtain any protein digestion and the symptoms were very positive. The child was terribly malnourished and had recurrent pulmonary infections. He also had difficulty sweating and had foul, fatty stools.

Dave Dickinson, M.D. one of our instructors had specialized, more or less, in cases of poliomyelitis. He ran the iron lungs when we had cases of medullary paralysis. He was a master at teaching polio patients to talk when they had vocal paralysis of the chords. I dreaded the summer because of cases of polio. There was nothing more agonizing than a patient with bulbar paralysis due to polio, who was suffocating and couldn't breathe. The iron lung, any port in a storm, was inept and a poor solution for breathing, but it was a big help until we got CPAP (an automatic breathing device).

I did have a regrettable experience on the Pediatric Ward with a 2-year-old who had mild pneumonia. We needed blood for testing and I decided to do a deep jugular phlebotomy to obtain the blood. I had done this procedure many times in Philadelphia at Children's, but this time I unfortunately, punctured the apex of the lung, which had extended into the neck at the supraclavicular triangle. It was extremely embarrassing because the air from the lung dissected the fascial planes of the neck, arm, and chest. I was sitting on pins and needles for several days until the lung puncture leak closed and the air absorbed. Air embolism and strangulation of the trachea were ominous possibilities, but the Lord was with me and the patient made a complete and uneventful recovery. Inappropriate and untold events of this nature can lead to pulmonary emphysema, air in the mediastinum, pericardium (heart) and even inside the peritoneal (abdomen) cavity. Escaping by the skin of my teeth, I vowed never to do another deep jugular penetration. This avenue is used frequently now for nutritional and venous access by the surgeons and sometimes by emergency physicians.

Speaking of surgeons, we had a great pioneer in Fred Collier, chief surgeon at University Hospital. He was internationally known for innovative liver, intestinal, pancreatic, and thoracic surgical procedures. We pediatricians would occasionally call him in consultation for acute appendicitis dilemmas. He would respond pronto and would palpate the right lower abdominal quadrant (McBurney Point) for a few seconds and diagnose emphatically. He was a man of few words and would iterate, "Yes, and surgery," or, "No and observation." He didn't give a hoot about the lab work or history because, "They confuse me", and then he evaporated making a speedy exit.

Just before our year of toil terminated, we learned that electroencephalography had been born. Everyone including pediatrics, neurology, internal medicine, and surgical medics were quite air-born over this new revolutionary medical toy. We were exploring the waters by ordering ECG's right and left. Finally, we came down to earth and realized that there were limits to its powers and capabilities. It was really useful for neonatal seizures and especially for petit mal or absence seizures (short staring spells).

It was time to terminate my work at Ann Arbor on June 30, 1939, and move on to my third year of pediatric residency. I had applied for a Chief Resident position at Marquette General Hospital under the auspices of the James Couzens Fund for Children. My acceptance came in late May and I would have Scott Harris as my intern. Scott was a first year pediatric resident at University Hospital and desired to continue his pediatric training. Scott was a mature, honest, logical, and affable man with a big, soft heart for children. He was in his mid-thirties in age and had experienced many odd jobs before deciding full blast on a pediatric career. Doris and I had had a very exuberant and enlightening year at Traverse City and at Ann Arbor, but we were ready to take the plunge in uncharted waters and meet the challenges future life offered.

Chapter 14

Marquette's James Couzens Childrens Clinic

I had the opportunity to intern at three of the endowed James Couzens Children's Funded Hospitals, namely at University of Michigan, Traverse City and Marquette. We arrived somewhat exhausted in Marquette, the "Queen City" of the Upper Peninsula of the Wolverine State of Michigan, in the mid-afternoon of July 1, 1939. It was a travel ordeal of nearly 450 miles by land plus twelve miles by auto ferry across the Straits from Mackinac City to St. Ignace. Our trusty Plymouth made the trip without a hitch. Getting from St. Ignace to Marquette was a bit of a maze for it was definitely cross-country, zig zagish, and the muddy roads were slushy after a rainy blast.

We were introduced to my bosses and head pediatric nurse on the tennis court outside of Marquette General Hospital, quite unceremoniously to be sure. Then my chief nurse-to-be, Miss Hodge, vanquished me in a game of tennis to officially welcome me to Marquette. My bosses, medical chief and C.E.O. Moses Cooperstock, M.D. (Mo) and Miss Morse, administrative clinic head, were much more gracious and affable with their cheery welcome.

The Children's Clinic was located within the hospital and consisted of 15 beds for infants and children up to 18 years. My salary was the grand sum of $100.00 per month plus board. Scotty, my intern received room and board and a stipend of $25.00 a month. He was very capable and was unmarried and for some ungodly reason loved to work nights (the swing shift). This didn't exactly make me angry, for Doris was with fetus and she needed me for support, especially at night and in strange country. There were all new people to become familiar with here.

The clinic was located across the street from Northern Michigan College, which graduated mainly teachers at that time. We had tennis privileges there. Marquette is located smack dab on Lake Superior, where huge lake freighters ply daily. Marquette also is renowned for winter sports, like skiing, and for its coal, copper, and iron resources. It is a Mecca for Scandinavians: Norwegians, Finns and Swedes settled there in abundance. They are people who are tough, rugged and well adapted to cold climates. It is about 25 miles northeast of Ishpeming and Negaunee, the sister cities, where coal is shipped by railroad to load gigantic freighters for shipment to major Great Lakes cities.

The Upper Peninsula is preeminently known for the delicious pasties or beef and potato pies that are obtainable everywhere. Properly prepared, they are mouth watering, substantial, succulent treats.

There are many fantastic environmental attractions in this almost complete state in itself. We took a combined train and boat excursion down the Taquamenon River to see the Taquamenon Falls, the second largest falls next to Niagara, east of the mighty Mississippi River. Quaint Sault Saint Marie, at the eastern end of Lake Superior, is a major maritime shipping center, entailing passage of one of the greatest tonnage of material in the world. The ships have to be lowered by special locks from Lake Superior into the Saint Mary's River. A ride along the extensive breath-taking sandy beaches of Lake Michigan for fifty miles from Saint Ignace to Manistique is well worth while. Around 80 miles west of Marquette is Ontonagon and the Lake of the Clouds, which are truly an out-of-this-world experience. The panoramic view is indescribably beautiful from a vantage point nearly 1000 feet above the lake. The three iron cities, Iron Mountain, Ironwood, and Iron River merit visitation as well. Incidentally, there is an old iron mine and a person can descend into the bowels of the earth there. Michigan Technology Institute at Houghton and the fort at Copper Harbor pay great dividends in your travels. Escanaba, on Little Bay DeNoc is well rewarding to visitors. Munising, about fifty miles directly east of Marquette, has much to offer including the Pictured Rocks and a natural Rock Castle in Munising Bay. We took a boat excursion to the Pictured Rocks in the middle of summer and just about froze in our summer apparel.

There was one very special terrain about ten miles west of Marquette on the shores of Lake Superior named almost an island, Presque Isle. It was an island that Doris and I visited several times almost every week. It was an idyllic rendezvous if there ever was one. There were many deer and wild flowers there, especially Black-Eyed Susans. This was how our first-born derived her name for she had ebony-black eyes. All in all, we fell in love with the scenery of the Upper Peninsula and we believed that it was superior to the Traverse City environs. Our Children's Clinic was intended to cover the entire Upper Peninsula, which definitely was impossible because of distances and the scattered, poverty stricken population.

Scott Harris was a bald, gaunt, slim cavernous-cheeked individual, very mature, worldly, and knowledgeable. He was no beauty, but had amazing charm, sophistication, and a way with the ladies. His home was in Ypsilanti and his brother, Bradley, M.D., had an imposing surgical practice there. Moses Cooperstock was short, about 5' 2" and a very intelligent pediatrician, with an elegant bearing. He was full of the milk of human kindness, particularly for children. Miss Morse was a dyed in the wool spinster, wedded securely to her job. She ruled efficiently with an iron hand and would brook no foolishness or diversion. Miss Hodge was a somewhat buxom, sensuous, flaming redhead, very sprightly, energetic, and quite competent. Miss Jolene Murphy was in charge of secretarial duties for the clinic and was a master of all trades with a charisma that wouldn't quit. She could veritably sell snowballs to the Eskimos and leave them in an ecstatic mood. Jolene was the heart and soul of the clinic that really made it click.

It was a great opportunity for me to rub shoulders with all the doctors in practice at Marquette and establish close and direct relations in referrals of patients to and from them all. Dr. Lambert was the leading obstetrician and Doris's doctor. He was very personable and had a great sense of humor. Dr. Hirwas was an affable, effective general surgeon. Dr. Howe was the leading family practitioner and had a fatal, magnetism for the tender gender, first, last and always. Dr. Elzinga was the orthopedist and a dog-gone good one. Two of the general practitioners had expressive soubriquets. Doctors Bottom and Glove, who were a tad bit antiquated healers. Dr. Nicholson and Dan Hornbogen were our two reliable and old standbys for nose and throat diseases. A weird popular song was born shortly after our venue named "Old Man Mose Kicked the Bucket"'. We had a ball kidding Moses Coop (Dr. Cooperstock) and we were not too certain that he was enthralled with the guffaws. My predecessor, Dr. Cowan, moved on to his new practice in Wisconsin, just before I arrived on the scene. The information I gleaned concerning him was that he was a dedicated pediatrician, a hard worker, and possessed an almost pedophilic relationship to children, not laudable.

My duties included lectures to the nurses, performing autopsies (rare), and conducting clinics at sundry cities (which were really towns) in the U.P. (Upper Peninsula). Scotty had a particular affinity for diabetes and was delegated to take the Diabetic Clinic at Big Bay, a few furlongs west of the Queen City.

Our first priority on reaching Marquette was securing a habitat. We were housed at the Jardine Residence, two blocks from the hospital until we were able to establish a more permanent home. After a week's search, Doris was able to procure a livable apartment on 1010 North High Street, which was about a stone's throw from Coop's living quarters on Front Street. We had ideal neighbors, especially the Carlsons, Bill and Ann. They had three stalwart sons, Tom, Dick and Harry, but not in that birth order. Bill was chief train dispatcher for the Ishpeming – Marquette Railway and also chief of the winter sports program for Marquette for 1939-1940(mainly skiing). He and his wife were truly the "salt of the earth" and gave us immeasurable support. Doris became close and intimate friends with Ann and I with Bill.

One of my prime experiences on skis came early in November. Bill asked me on a beautiful Saturday to go on a ten mile cross-country ski hike, eight days hence. I demurred the invitation regretfully for I had never skied. Whereupon, persistent Carlson said, "There's nothing to it doc. I'll take you out tomorrow and teach you the basic principles and you'll be all set for next Sunday." I bought a pair of boots and Bill outfitted me with skis, gloves, poles, and jacket and we were off to the races. Manipulations on skis seemed clumsy at first, but in the wink of an eye it all seemed as easy as pie. I realized that it wasn't that complicated. With a little athleticism, all you (I) had to do was to relax and enjoy it. Just let yourself go, establish a rhythm and imagine you are (I was) dancing and swaying with the breeze. The only difficulty was in stopping (snow plowing), climbing, and making right and left 90 degree turns. However a week later I was raring to go.

We started our cross-country ski trip early Sunday morning at the Marquette Tuberculosis Sanitarium (long gone now). After skiing about five miles (half without incident), we stopped for a rest, a breakfast, and hot liquid break. It was an invigorating and stimulating exercise through the woods, hills, and valleys. We continued onward for another five miles until we reached our final end of the journey. I felt exhilarated but somewhat pooped out, for it had been many eons since I had had such a strenuous workout. When we arrived at the Carlson abode, we were greeted casually by our wives. Doris said to me, "Now that you've had your fun time, it's my turn". So, we had a hot buttered rum drink and went to the movies, where I fell asleep for the entire picture (as usual). I hesitate to relate the follow-up, but it was not exactly a bed of roses.

Bill Carlson and I took many skiing jaunts during the winter and one was particularly noteworthy. I learned to ski downhill by Bill's expert instructions. On one occasion I was sashaying down a fairly steep grade and as I hit the bottom, I heard Bill frantically shouting, "Get down, Doc. Get down on your haunches." But his advice was too late. My skis stopped abruptly and I lurched forward with gusto, turning a complete flip flop in midair and landing head first in a big snow bank. Bill breathlessly rushed over to me and helped me extricate myself from standing on my head to the normal body status of standing on my feet. Fortunately, I had disengaged myself from the skis when I became airborne, and somehow, by the grace of Jehovah, I came out of my acrobatics unscathed and smelling like a rose. Nevertheless, poor Bill was almost in shock, pale as a ghost, and almost speechless. His first words were,

"Doc, are you in pain? My God, you could have broken your neck. I've never been so scared in all my life." I tried to console Bill and assure him that I felt perfectly fine, but he couldn't believe me and kept repeating, "Are you sure, Doc?" for about a half hour more. It all happened so fast that it was just a blur and I only felt dazed, as though I was awakening from a nightmare. I've, nevertheless, never been so scared in all my life.

One choice incident is embedded in my memory from midwinter. Coop invited Doris and I over to his home one Friday evening to play a game of bridge and engage in friendly conversation. His wife, Alice, was a very lovely person and was pregnant, in common with Doris, at about the same stage of development. She had a surreptitious sense of humor and was always relating jokes with hidden meanings. Actually, all of us were far less than expert bridge players and it took us about an hour to complete one full rubber. It began to snow as we were driving to nearby Coop's residence, and we thought nothing unusual as it snowed almost daily there. But, as we were about to leave for our domicile later that night, our car was buried in a raging snowstorm with zero visibility. So, like the man who came to dinner, Coop and Alice insisted we stay overnight. Our stay, however, was prolonged on through the weekend before we could safely be ejected from Coop's place. Fortuitously, Coop was a good boy scout and had a larder full of groceries stashed away for just such an emergency. He assured us that this snow avalanche was not a rare occurrence. We made rounds at the hospital by traveling there on skis on Saturday and snowshoes on Sunday. Good thing, I knew how to ski!

One of the things that impressed me most of all was the wailing and continual repetitious cacophony of weird foghorn sounds emanating from Lake Superior during heavy fogs, which lasted an interminable time, it seemed. Believe you me, the fog would be so thick that you could really cut it with an axe. The visibility was minus zero percent. It was really eerie to the hilt and one could imagine those poor captains of the ships trying to grope their way through the pea soup fog without ramming another lost soul or vice versa. It did give me the shivers (and still does) imagining possible explosive disasters. These dense fogs occurred frequently during the winter months.

A big event for Doris was a visit in midsummer by Barbara King, her cherished girlfriend acquaintance from the Quaker City, Philadelphia. Barb flew to the Soo (Sault Saint Marie) where I met her and escorted her by the trusty Plymouth to Marquette. It was a very happy, highlight meeting for Doris as she had a few doldrums at the clinic. The food there left much to be desired for they were on a strict budget and she did not exactly see eye to eye with Miss Morse. Speaking of Doris, reminds me of my midnight excursions to a prominent "Wester" restaurant in downtown Marquette for steak sandwiches and strawberry shortcake for our Mother-to-be. She seemed to have a ravenous appetite every night at the bewitching hour for some vague reason. Of course, I enjoyed a snack at that time also, so there was double duty met to be sure.

A downright humorous event that had everyone laughing uproariously in the aisles happened at the Majestic Theater in the Queen City. Doris and I decided one evening to relieve the humdrum boredom and see a movie. It happened that "The Man in the Iron Mask" was the attraction playing at the Majestic. For once I stayed awake, because the picture was intriguing and full of suspense. About mid-film, when everyone (it was crowded) in the theater was glued with rapt attention, the silence was abruptly broken. The female usher came "waltzing mathilde" down the aisle announcing in a stentorian, repetitious voice, "Telephone call for Doctor Harry Bottom," and she pronounced the "Harry" exactly like "Hairy". The audience was immediately distracted and cracked up spontaneously with a burst of laughter. I believe Doctor Bottom completely ignored the call, as no one responded to the usher's message. We did have our lighter moments of mirth in Marquette, just good, clean fun!

We had some very unusual patients during my tour of duty in the north country, which did test my mettle. A three-year-old male came in from Germfask one day with the chief complaint of "headache" for several months and "fever". The first thing I observed when I saw him was a horrific stench of necrotic, decaying flesh. On close inspection the right scalp parietal bilateral was oozing frank pus and skull X-rays disclosed a large area of chronic osteomyelitis from where the pus was originating. His temperature was 100 degrees Fahrenheit and his vital signs were stable. Instantly, I called our ear, nose and throat person Dr. Nicholson for consult and he was shell shocked when he saw the lad. He and I were in agreement to immediately refer him to Ann Arbor Pediatric ENT. It was a no-brainer decision. The clinic afforded the transportation by a staff car.

Another patient was a twelve-year-old female from Shingleton, fifty miles distant. She had onset of menarche for two days, but had a light flow with vague, mid lower right abdominal pain. On examination there was mild muscle spasm and resistance at McBurney's Point, but very little pain to palpation. Quickly, the differential diagnosis flashed through my cerebrum and I concluded she must have appendicitis in an early stage of development or rupture. Instead of observation, I decided the best course of action was a consult with our surgeon, Dr. Hirwas. After he saw her we debated the therapeutics and finally I said, "There's a 90% chance in an adolescent girl that it is an acute appendix and if we delay, it might rupture." Dr. Hirwas didn't hesitate a split second and said, "Let's go" and alerted the O.R. (operating room). At surgery, he found an acute appendix located retrocecally (underneath the cecum). That was the reason for the vague symptoms, for it was buried and sheltered. Medical decisions are often derived from hunches and a sixth sense of telepathy, but past experience is extremely important, i.e. having seen it before.

I saw several cases of bacterial tuberculous meningitis diagnosable only by lumbar spinal puncture. With fever, especially in infants under age two, if there is the least hint of neck stiffness, irritability, or bulging of the frontanelle, a spinal tap is a positive must with no ands, ifs or buts.

One capricious incident occurred at about 2 a.m. one night. A farmer reeking with a manurish odor brought his one-month old baby to the clinic because of a scalp rash. He said, "Doc, I think my baby has_Cradle Crap." I bit my tongue and contained my internal jollity and said, "Sir, your baby has seborrhac eczema or dandruff of the scalp, and it is nothing to worry about."

We did see much diarrhea, shiga typhoid, rotavirus and pneumonia of Heinz 57 Variety. Also diphtheria and the childhood acute exanthemata were common, along with their complications. We also had a couple cases of tetanus which lived. There were no antibiotic medications with the exception of Sulfa, which was a Godsend, for meningococcal meningitis. It also worked for staphococcal infections, notably innumerable cases of impetigo, furuncles, conjunctivitis and acute joint infections. We even had a couple cases of pyloric stenosis and also a Wilm's Tumor - Medulloblastoma in an infant. All of these we shipped to pediatrics at Ann Arbor. In addition, leukemia, acute lymphoblastic leukemia, reared its ugly head, for it is probably the most common form of cancer in childhood. We also took care of newborns and had about 70/80 percent breast feeding, initiated at birth. We had two incubators for prematures and Coop was profoundly interested in preemie survival. He had a year's training under Dr. Hess at the University of Chicago regarding incubator care. Dr. Hess invented and developed the incubator in the late twenties.

Coop's first born son was birthed about February 21, 1940, perhaps 2 weeks before our first born daughter, Susan, at Marquette General Hospital. David came out with flying colors and unblemished. On the second day after his arrival, I admitted a five-year-old patient with diphtheria, diagnosed by a gram stain smear of the membrane in his nose and pharynx (throat). We gave him a shot of antitoxin and sedated him and performed an electrocardiogram because diphtheria notoriously can cause damage to the heart muscle (myocarditis). Other complications are tracheal obstruction from membranes and peripheral nerve paralysis. It is a real treacherous organism (corynebacterium) that can be utterly lethal without warning. I checked our diphtheria boy late in the afternoon and all was quiet on the western front. Apparently we didn't get the antitoxin injected in time because the nurse in Peds called me around 6 p.m. and gave me the disheartening news that she found the little fellow stone cold dead in bed. Emotionally, I felt terrible for I had visions of a much happier termination. Immediately, I called Coop to relay the disastrous news. He was eating his dinner when I reached him at a downtown restaurant. At the moment, I was oblivious to the fact that his son and wife were in the hospital. I said, "My God, Coop, something terrible has happened." Coop responded, "My God, don't tell me my son has, _____!" And I quickly realized the enormity of the situation and said, "He's perfectly OK, but the poor little diphtheria boy had been found dead in his crib." Whereupon Coop burst out, "Is that all you called about?", indescribably relieved. He indubitably had to send his jeans to the cleaners.

Another jovial incident occurred on Saturday night. Doris and I planned jubilantly to break the monotony and attend a dance. We were about to fly the kite when Susan broke out precipitously with a tempestuous and thunderous bout of crying. She was implacable and the usual ritual would not quiet her. After a bit of cogitation, with Doris in exasperated tears, I decided boldly to take the bull by the horns and administer a relaxing cocktail to Miss Suzy - 1 teaspoon of cooking whiskey (Jim Beam) in 4 oz. of water. Susan avidly gulped down this concoction and blissfully went off to slumberland. Joy pervaded the situation. This wasn't my first daring exploit of this nature to save the night/day. Whiskey is good for anesthesia and fever also!

Chapter 15

Incipient Pre-War Practice in Bay City

We reached our destination at Doctor Fern Foster's home in Bay City, Michigan, at about 4 p.m. on May 30th of 1940. We were greeted by Fern and Kate Foster, Pidge, Fernie Junior, and last but not least, Blondie, the canine female spaniel. They lived on the northeast corner of McKinley and Johnson Streets, both main arteries in the city. McKinley runs east and west and is also known as Eighth Street, while Johnson runs north and south. His homestead was a stately Cape Cod type mansion. We were royally welcomed by the Fosters, "Bill" Kendall, their dentist, and Harrison Plum, their insurance agent. Bill made a terrific fuss over Susan, as did all the Fosters.

Young Fernie Junior's entire body appeared inky blue due to his tetralogy of fallot, congenital heart disease, present since birth. Unfortunately, heart surgery for inborn anomalies hadn't developed yet in his time. Fernie did have open heart surgery when he was near age thirty but the result was fatal on the operating table. He was quite intelligent and faced his inescapable fate head on, with determined courage and intrepidation. Pidge was a gorgeous flaxen haired, blue eyed, blonde young lady of considerable magnetism. Kate Foster was a middle aged, insecure, nervous, hyperthyroid lady with bulging eyes and a fervent love for tongue sandwiches. Dr. Fern Senior was a strikingly handsome man with a magnetic, smooth charm that could docilize a pit bull. His voice was mellifluous and melodious and he embodied a personality that could sell snowballs to the Eskimos. In other words, he was the epitome of psychosocial graces and powerful positive forces. In fact, he was of fatal attraction to the fair gender.

Fern was secretary for the Michigan State Medical Society when I joined him in partnership, a position he held for about fifteen or twenty years. Also, he was Secretary of the Bay, Iosco, and Arenac Counties Medical Society for at least a similar number of years. His extra curricular medical activities demanded that he sacrifice many hours of pediatric practice and hence the necessity for a fellow medical partner to carry the load of pediatric office appointments, home and hospital calls.

Fern magnanimously offered my family, room and board until we could get grounded and find a suitable home of our own. After exploring the housing market in depth for five months, we finally discovered an appropriate residence at 221 North Lincoln Street, a neat, one floor and basement habitat. It was conveniently located within a few blocks of Mercy and General Hospitals.

My elder partner drew up the terms of our partnership which delegated a $200.00 monthly salary plus $25.00 monthly stipend to me for my car expenses. This may seem like a pittance, but actually I was overjoyed and it was substantial and plenty able to take care of all our basic needs plus. After six months, if my work was satisfactory, I would share one quarter of the profits for six months and enter into one third of the gains for a year and then become a full partner. This was the sum and substance and meltdown of our agreement. After wading through a host of fiscal terms, there was one catch in fine print at the bottom of the agreement, I couldn't practice pediatrics solo in an area within ten miles of Bay City for a period of ten years. This stipulation didn't gall me one bit for I figured my partner was trustworthy and I would never be forced to use it.

My first priority item of business was to purchase a car or proper conveyance to make all those numerous house calls and hospital emergencies. My business partner was a 100% Cadillac man who was on intimate terms with the Mitchells who had the premier Cadillac dealership in Michigan, going back thirty some years. I contacted 'Bill' Mitchell, the original owner's son, and I had my baby Cadillac in the blink of an eye. This required monthly payments, but I was exuberant, euphoric, and "in clover", so not to worry. Actually, we could purchase groceries for an entire week for less than $20.00 and they would fill eight or ten bags. Incidentally, Bill Mitchell was killed in an airplane accident many years later, along with Jimmy Wilcox, a surgeon, GP, who had a coronary heart attack in flight. I once, after WW II, engaged in an airplane flight with Jimmy to Midland to have a luncheon after a tonsillectomy with me as anesthetist. Jim was grossly overweight and loved to eat red meats, sausage, butter, cream, and chocolate. He was a tireless worker, day and night, and flew frequently to his home on Drummond Island with his wife Carmen.

Bill Gronemeyer was the other Pediatrician in Bay City in 1940, and had his office in the Allen Building on the west side of the Saginaw River. He was fortified with a multitude of "feeder" general practitioners and doctors, including Clarence Reuter, Stanley Pearson, Dwight Mosier, Walt Stenson, Hugh Cook and Arthur D Allen himself, the Physician in Chief of this group. They all had their offices in the Allen Building, owned shares of stock in the building and paid a considerable monthly stipend for rent and maintenance.

A pediatrician named McClain was the first child's doctor, immediately preceeding Dr. Foster, but there is little information concerning his practice except that he demised in 1919 with tuberculosis.

Fern established his initial practice in pediatrics in 1920 and missed WW I because he was in medical school at the University of Pennsylvania and interned at Children's Hospital of Philadelphia for three years prior to coming to Bay City. He was born in Phillipsburg, New Jersey, just across the Delaware River from Easton, PA, and two paternal uncles, for business reasons, had migrated to Bay City, the second largest city in Michigan in the early 1900's. Competition from formidable, young Gronemeyer was heating up and "Fernie" Foster realized the potency of his adversary, hence the mother of necessity to the solution was me for a counter-active force. Fern had intense magnetism and manner with mothers, especially his utterly mellifluous voice on the telephone where he could charm a lizard. But he must be out of Bay City at least 50% plus of his time for his first love involving State Medical Society's political arena. Also there was savage rivalry from the family physicians in Bay City and environs who saw at least 75% of all infants, children and adolescents. Pediatric practice here was mainly consultative.

Fern's ace in the hole was the benevolent, wonderful, Mrs. Clara Wheeler, his all American everything - secretary, guardian, counselor, telephone expert, and staunch loyal friend to her fingertips. She knew almost as much medicine and understood parents and children through many years of practical experience as many a doctor. She would "hold the fort" until Dr. Fern would return from his numerous political safaris. Clara was really a saint for Fern, covering his honest practice like a blanket, day and night, untiringly and faithful to the Nth degree.

Dr. Foster's office was set up for surgery, especially adenoids, tonsillectomies, and circumcisions. His prime ENT surgeon was Paul R Urmston, who was rough and gruff with the heart of a lamb. Fernie and I would render anesthesia and Paul would remove the tonsils with a "Schleuter" instrument. The Schleuter was a steel blade with a square, beveled window at the end that would shell out the tonsils like peas from a pod. There was practically no bleeding with this method as opposed to modern dissection. In addition, we practically never had any post-operative bleeding, the bane of the modern ENT doctor. The secret to avoiding post-operative adenoid bleeding was to remove all of them (tonsils and adenoids – T & A) in the posterior pharynx. The secret to preventing post operative bleeding from circumcisions was inserting circular sutures and excising the foreskin so that the operator could see exactly how much foreskin was being removed. The modern Gomco method is a blind operation to remove the foreskin and often results in too much or not enough foreskin being excised.

Nineteen-forty was the day and age for "kitchen table surgery" and fee-splitting. P.R.U. (Paul R.Urmston), Foster, and I would go to the homes and do our circs and T and A's, literally and figuratively, on the kitchen table after a brief scrub at the sink and application of sterile gloves. We would do three or four rounds with "good old ether" anesthesia. In all my years and virtually hundreds of ether anesthetics, with one exception, (an elderly adult), I can honestly say I've <u>never</u> had a problem with giving ether anesthesia. It is inflammable and can be lethal if not handled with the utmost, meticulous care. My excellent training in administering anesthesia at Union memorial Hospital in the "Oriole" City, armed me with life saving ability. Rendering anesthesia in surgery is a very challenging experience as the anesthetist has the patient's life in the palm of his hand. Alertness and focus is paramount. The old saying, "on pins and needles", is definitely applicable. Anesthesia has come a long way with all the gases, modern contraptions, and fees as compared to our measly ten dollar recompense for T & A, although the risk and responsibility were the same.

Fee splitting in medicine was widely practiced in Bay City in the first half of the twentieth century and undoubtedly in the nineteenth century. This practice consisted of "bribery", whereby the medical doctors would refer patients to surgeons for an appendectomy, T & A, herniorraphy, mastoidectomy, or eye surgery, and the referring physician would get a cut back or graft remuneration of 22 / 50% from the surgeon. The A.M.A. frowned on this method of wheeling and dealing in business and it finally ceased shortly after WW II when it was recognized as foul, dishonest and illegal and finally ceased.

Tonsils and adenoids were extirpated literally by the bushels in the forties until it was discovered that removing these valuable organs made children much more susceptible to poliomyelitis, especially the bulbar kind in the summer.

Our pediatric office suite was located in the Thorne Building at 919 Washington Avenue, second floor, in the center of the main business drag. Other doctors who rented there included Kent Alcorn, a premier Urologist, trained at Mayo Clinic, and my buddy Matthew R Slattery, a shanty Irishman who fought in the trenches of WWI and suffered lung damage from vile gas poisoning. Kent had a brother, Marshall who was a surgeon in Wisconsin. His father was a General Practitioner in Bloomington, Illinois, and Kent was a pilot in WWI. Matthew, a family doctor, associated with Jim Conelly, M.D.., another Irishman family doctor. They complemented each other by personality, raucous, rough, and tough but full of the milk of human kindness.

Matt had a cabin on the Au Sable River near Grayling and would often invite me to go there as his guest. His good wife, of upper class Irish, would have no part of the cottage. It was a hundred miles + as the crow flies north of Bay City, but it would take Matthew about five hours to transcend this mileage because of his proclivity to visit all the bars between here and there. He suspected rightfully that my good wife was not too enamored with far away cottages or with my absence on what miniscule free time I was tendered. Facetiously he would say, "Knobby, I'll be happy to write an excuse for you, to your spouse if you desire."

It was really a godsend for me to relinquish all the vicissitudes and demands of 24 hour on call practice. Fortunately, I could almost completely divorce and abandon my practice figuratively, when I left the office at night. As Shakespeare so rightly stated, "(it is) Sleep that knits up the raveled sleeve of care" in Macbeth. I worried, but only for a few miniseconds. My motto was "let God worry. He put them here."

We parked our autos in the alley behind the Thorne Building and my partner posted a sign which warned any interlopers against trespassing at their expense of hauling away their vehicle, although we never did. Our telephone coverage was our lifeline and it was ably managed by Jessie Slaight, who lived in the 200 block of North Jefferson Street. She was very diplomatic, soothing, and quite capable of assuaging caller's ruffled feathers.

Fern repeatedly would say, "Any mother or father who has a sick baby is crazy" and the more I delved into Pediatric care, the more I realized he wasn't just blowing smoke. After having my own children, I was aware of the tremendous, unrelenting responsibility parenthood bestows on parents. The message is loud and clear. This child normally has at least seventy plus years to live and if any damaging illness results, I am totally responsible as his guardian, for the number of years he is cut short. Most parents have little practical experience in child rearing until after their first baby.

L. Fernald Foster was also adamant about not calling him by his first name, "Louis". He would say, "A patient is your patient only as long as he or she is in your office". This brings home another truth that doctors do not own patients and bedside manner is paramount to successful practice.

The first day in practice for me was Monday, June 1st, 1940, and it was a tremendously busy one from the get go. The house calls poured in starting at 6 a.m. I was in command of the entire practice and it was a real challenge, sink or swim. I rolled up my sleeves and gave it all my might and main. Clara Wheeler would divide the house calls into the north, east, south, and west sections of Bay City and I sandwiched in both hospital visits between calls. After five hours (no breakfast) of answering calls, I went to the office at 11 a.m. to see about a dozen patients at break neck speed. Then I grabbed a sandwich next door at Ted Kant's restaurant, and was off to the races making more urgent house calls. I was back at the office at 2 p.m. seeing a horde more of patients, until I was interrupted by an emergency call on the west side of the Saginaw River at about 4 p.m. A two year old boy had fallen out of a second story window. As luck would have it, there were no broken bones, for he had fortuitously hit the limb of a tree in his descent and landed on a cushion of grass. Outside of a few bumps and bruises, he was in one whole piece. It is often remarked, "God takes care of children and drunks". I returned to the office and cranked out a few more patients and then renewed my house calls at around 6 p.m., finally terminating the most demanding ones at about 9 p.m. I quickly ate my supper on the run and made a few more house calls. Dead tired, I at last hit the sack around midnight and kissed my wife as I was dozing. A couple calls came in during the night and I was again called to duty at 6 a.m. This staggering pace continued unabated until Friday when Foster returned to his profession.

Sometimes the mother of the children will identify as wife (which she actually is in a certain sense) and establish unconsciously, an infatuation with the pediatrician as her child's father. This occurrence happens to virtually all Pediatricians, Surgeons and Family Physicians because of the close, intimate, common goal directed at intensely striving to get the child well. There is a high degree of emotional exertion involved along with the unmitigated stress of life or death emergencies, which occur frequently. It is rather easy for the mother or father to go overboard in their praise and reverence for a physician who in their mind has literally pulled the child from the jaws of death in rendering his/her usual and customary service. I'm sure this incidence has happened in my practice and it was only a temporary state of mind as it was immediately discouraged and any sparks extinguished: One such glaring example occurred when a beautiful young red headed mother became infatuated with myself after I was successful in rescuing her only son from a serious confrontation with staphylococcic pneumonia (positive blood culture). Fernie kidded me unmercifully as she came in to the office almost daily long after the boy was out of danger. All I could do was be kind, patient and non-indulgent until good old father time doused cold water on the budding enamor. They say, "Time cures all ills" and I am a staunch believer.

The medical practice continued at a hectic pace my first year as a practitioner. I remember in particular, two pediatric, unusual cases that stand out especially in those first two years. In the heat of July, Fern sent me north to Hale, MI, on an urgent call from Dr. Earl Hasty. The child, a nine year old male, had a stiff neck, severe headache, low fever, and weakness of his legs. At once I performed a lumbar spinal tap. The spinal fluid was under increased pressure with a slightly high cell count and protein mildly increased and normal sugar. The cells were lymphocytes as opposed to polymorphonuclear leukocytes, high cell count and proteins, low sugar, all seen in spinal fluid of bacterial meningitis. My diagnosis was easy, poliomyelitis for sure. But the treatment wasn't all that easy. Therapy was mainly supportive and Sister Kenny Method, <u>hot</u> packs continuous to the extremities. Around a month later Dr. Hasty reported that the lad recovered from his polio in good health with mild paralysis of the lower extremities and was in rehab physical therapy. Often there is mild continued restitution of muscle function over the period of years. I dreaded summer months because of polio, especially bulbar involvement with paralysis of the vital centers in the medulla. What a nightmare! The polio vaccine prevention was surely God's blessing, one of the greatest given to mankind!

The other unusual case that demanded an errand of mercy was one of Dr. Jardine's little girls, aged nearly two years, at West Branch, MI. She was a gorgeous little girl who had severe, croupy bronchitis and was suffocating from obstructed respirations. She was struggling to inspire oxygen but had infinite difficulty on expiration. Her chest x-ray showed severely hyperinflated lungs which were exerting supreme pressure on the heart, squeezing it to ½ it's size. I said to Dr. Jardine, "There is only one thing to do and that is to insert an intrabracheal tube to establish breathing or <u>else</u> – and I don't favor the other option." Whereby Dr. Jardine replied, "I've never done this operation, can you do it?" I retorted, "I'm in the same boat, but I'll try it because she is facing certain death." So, to the operating room we took the little girl. I said a little prayer before we started and somehow God guided me and I inserted the metal tube of life in the trachea after incision, and the child had immediate relief. Dr. Jardine was also relieved and must have done a good job on the after treatment, but I never heard any report from him. However, about twenty years later I was summoned to see a newborn at Mercy Hospital's nursery by Dr. Howard McEwan. After examining the baby and finding all parameters in order, I went in to her room to report my findings to the mother. Lo and behold,! While conversing with her, I noticed an ugly large jagged scar on her lower neck, just below the cricoid cartilage, the exact location for a tracheotomy tube. All of a sudden the message dawned loud and clear as the years and the ages coincided. I excitedly asked her if she had severe croup in early childhood, necessitating a breathing tube in the trachea, and she said, "Yes, I did." I said, "Well what do you know, my chickens have come back to roost – I was your pediatric surgeon in West Branch, working with your Dr. Jardine at that time." We were both dumbfounded but elated, and I retorted, "I believe we have made Ripley's Believe It or Not". I apologized for the nasty cervical scar, suggesting the solution of plastic surgery and she countered, "I'm proud of it and you needn't apologize for being a life saver."

I spent most of my spare hours during the 1941 summer, studying for my oral and written national board examinations in first year's pediatrics. There were four questions on the written: one pertaining to polio, one queried about calcium and phosphorus metabolism, one regarding contagious diseases, and the final question requiring a detailed dissertation on brain tumors. I took the exam in Fern's office under his supervision. The oral exams were given in Chicago at the Palmer Hotel, by four Pediatricians. I recall Doctors Parmalee, McQuarrie and Johnson, but can't remember the fourth examiner.

Before taking the orals, I visited Freddie Fehlman, my buddy fellow intern at University of Michigan, who was interning at the Chicago Contagious Hospital. It was on a Saturday following three jam packed days of CME (continuing medical education) pediatric lectures. To my astonishment, poor Freddie coincidentally was a hospital patient with severe mumps orchitis. His testicles were the size of baseballs and he was in gross agony, sitting on the bedpan when I first laid eyes on him. He exclaimed in an angry voice, "Jesus Christ, Knobloch, what in the hell brings you here at this time!" He set me back on my heels but I countered, "Awfully sorry Freddie, I know it's not a bed of roses, but I'm here to take my oral pediatric exams following the Pediatric Meeting at the Palmer House." We didn't kiss but we did make up by reminiscing about our old experiences at Ann Arbor. He managed a hearty laugh or two. After warming up a bit, Freddie said, "Howard, why don't you stay overnight in the interns quarters at Children's Hospital of Chicago on Fullerton Street, where your exam is taking place tomorrow. Most of the interns there are married and I'm certain there are some empty beds. I'll call my friend, the Chief Resident there and I'm sure he will okay your visit there." Surprisingly, the intern quarters for Children's Hospital of Chicago were located in the nurse's home in a building smack dab across the street facing the hospital. However, the bottom line was that their habitat was located on the second floor and there was a vacant space between the interns and the nurses living quarters. Also, there was a subterranean channel leading from the nurses' home building underneath the street, to the hospital. I parked my Cadillac on an avenue near the hospital and proceeded to my vacant room in the intern living quarters with high spirits. I reread Anderson Aldrich's book on "Feeding Our Old Fashioned Children" and at about 2300 the Chief Resident appeared unannounced. He asked me if I would join him on his nightly hospital rounds and I jumped at the chance. We descended to the well lighted sub-street level and crossed over to the hospital. He explained in detail the cases of several interesting sick infants to me. On returning to my designated room, I was over ready to dive into bed. I awoke bright eyed and bushy tailed, washed and dressed and made a beeline for my car. On my way, I noticed a door leading to an alley in close proximity to my car, a short cut. So, sleepily, I grabbed my suitcase and promptly threw open the door, whereupon all Hell broke loose and there was an instant, deafening alarm sounding off. My heart sank and I read on the door, "Open only in case of fire." My first reaction was to close the door, but it firmly resisted all my valiant efforts. There was a panicky feeling in my roiling stomach and I thought, if they apprehend the villain of this early Sunday morning escapade, I'll be jailed and unable to take my exam. So, "necessity is the mother of invention", I ran with my bag and beat a retreat down the steps leading to the lower level and then through the passage to my salvation, the hospital. As I exited from the hospital, I heard a tremendous commotion of fire trucks and the hustle and bustle of people in movement to the nurses' home. I asked one of the firemen, "What on earth is the trouble?" He disgustedly shouted, "Some damned fool set off the fire alarm." Enough said. I felt deeply sorry for unconsciously causing such a ruckus waking nurses at such an ungodly hour, but felt a prodigious feeling of relief and enjoyed a hearty breakfast. Needless to say, I passed all examiners with flying colors because of my euphoric, wide awake state.

I journeyed to Milwaukee, only a hundred miles north, to see my staunch friend and peer, Franklin Mellencamp. His benevolent family gave me the red carpet treatment and that night I took the overnight car ferry from Milwaukee, across Lake Michigan to Ludington, MI. When I arrived in Bay City, Monday morning, my partner asked me to delineate my experience in Chicago. After relating a vivid account of all my experiences, Fern looked up and said, "Incredulous, but it's just like a country boy lost in a big city." As a result of my labors, I was eligible and joined as a Fellow of the American Academy of Pediatrics in May 1941. L. Fernald joined the academy in 1931, when it was first formed at Harper Hospital in Detroit, by Doctors Wishropp and Martmer. Those doctors practicing pediatrics exclusively in 1931, were all exempt from examination, so I was ten years too late, but Fern Foster made fellowship by acclamation.

I joined the staffs at Mercy and General Hospitals and became a member of the Senior Pediatric Department after a proper period of probation and trainer tutelage. At Mercy Hospital doctor's lounge each day there was group of distinguished, hoary doctors aptly named "the Sages of the Wailing Wall." They reveled in all the hospital gossip and predicted all sorts of dire events and consequences such as a repeat of the 1929 financial stock catastrophe. Doctors Fred Dumond and Ed Huckins and Van Dumond were the ringleaders of doom, gloom, Armageddon, and apocalyptic future events. After a half hour of exposure to their weird proclamations and prophecies, a person would feel like the world was ending or at least going to Hades in a basket.

Our head nurse in pediatrics at Mercy, B.C., was Mrs. Etienne of French temperament. She was a steadfast friend and admirer of my fellow pediatrician,

Bill Gronemeyer. It seemed he could commit no wrong and I could accomplish no right, so it was an uphill battle all the way, for me to establish a congenial working relationship with her. I never really did get to first base. She, honestly, was quite efficient, intelligent, and maybe I was a tad paranoid.

At General Hospital, almost a mile east from Mercy, via Columbus Ave, there was a ramshackle wooden building located across Mulholland Street just westerly designated as the "Contagious" Hospital. There, there were stationed the acute infectious diseases of childhood viz, measles, meningitis, mumps, chicken pox, whooping cough and typhoid fever. Fortunately I was immune to most of these scourges by having suffered them in my youth and having had typhoid immunization in medical school. Whooping cough and scarlet fever were raging and rampant my first summer in practice. The only specific treatment at that time was good old sulfa for strep throat, pneumonia and erysipelas. I felt so compassionately sorry for the poor little toddlers and babies who contracted whooping cough. They suffered three weeks developing the disease, three weeks with intractable, harassing breath holding cough, worse at night, and three weeks recuperation complicated, usually with a bout of pneumonia. Fern Foster had a specific prescription containing creosote that we used by vaporization which did ameliorate the terrible coughing paroxysms, especially at night when it seemed to worsen. In Peds, all symptoms appear to intensify at night.

To my mind, the weather in Bay City is ideal, truly the best anywhere. It is quite capricious and changeable, "Mutable semper", but that is what makes it worthwhile. Every new day is chock full of surprises. The poor meteorologist is correct circa 50% of his /her predictions. Next to the neurosurgeon, he/she has to be the most frustrated person on the face of the earth. So many variable factors blend to control the final meteorological phenomena viz, wind, clouds, temperature, wetness, dryness, time of year, oceanic temperature, sun, moon, and location. We are strategically situated practically on the 45th parallel of latitude, or in other words, halfway between the equator, and the north pole. This means that whether northerly or southerly conditions prevail, this is your exact atmospheric result. High and low centers, and the Great Lakes effect, also are contributory to a great extent, especially when it snows. Our average rainfall and snowfall are certainly not excessive. We have practically no tornadoes, hurricanes, typhoons, tidal waves, tsunamis, earthquakes or floods to speak of. We do have occasional wind storms with winds up to 80 mph for brief periods. Our one complaint is a six month cool period, in which the only really frigid months are January and February. Over the past 25 years, our climate seems to be moderating and getting warmer. We are fortunate to be virtually in the center of the Great Lakes and they exert a temperate, moderating effect, noticeably during the winter and summer months. Our soil is very rich and conducive to farming on a super scale. Summers are ideal. We are blessed with absence of tropical insects, malarial mosquitoes, scorpions, poisonous snakes, roaches and wild animals. All in all, I would say in the final analysis, we are truly living in a near paradise.

I joined the First Presbyterian Church on Center and Jackson, in May of 1941, after surveying the ecclesiastical situation. My partner was a dyed in the wool member there and that, no doubt, influenced my decision to affiliate with Dr. Roblees' congregation. My First Reformed Church in Greensburg was not a going concern here and the First Presbyterian appeared to be in essence almost exactly a replica of the church I was connected with in my childhood. Also, I had a preponderance of Presbyterian children in my practice. I also became a member of the BPOE, Chapter #88, under Fern's guidance. Our county medical society often held their meetings there, located on Center Avenue, downtown near the First National Bank, on the second floor. They had great lunches at reasonable charges and we went there for a bite on the run. My wife attended Saint Boniface Church on Lincoln and McKinley, regularly. Our residence on Lincoln was situated next door to the Lutheran Church, so we were surrounded by churches.

Fernald Foster had a unique method for preparing his Christmas turkey. He would use a 50 ml. syringe and inject melted liquid butter in sizable quantities into the legs, arms and breast of a twenty pound bird. This operation, he claimed, enhanced the taste and moistened the turkey for a sumptuous feast. Also, he would annually, at the Yuletide Season, order a couple dozen Chincoteague oysters from southern Virginia to use in stuffing his turkey. Fernie was a gourmet eater and his paunching protuberance gave ample proof to his propensity for food. He would often motor to his favorite restaurant in Flint, Midland, Saginaw, or Fenton, after midnight to quench his craving for steaks, prime rib, porterhouse, filet mignon, or standing roasts. He also had a ravenous appetite for the ladies, but don't all males that possess their full, endowed quota of hormones at any age?!

Across the street from our dwelling, on North Lincoln, lived Elson Hood, sports director for Bay County. He invited me to go rabbit hunting with him on Sunday, December 7th, 1941, at Alpena. I hesitated for a moment, but I knew his sister, Georgia, at Marquette, so I acquiesced. I was a rank amateur with firearms and had a deep aversion to killing any animal for many reasons. But the foremost reason is that I'm sure they loved life equally as I did and I was overly well fed. Has man not advanced beyond the carnal Stone Age? Anyway, we did travel to Alpena (about 150 miles north of the crotch of Michigan's thumb) and went hare hunting. It was a bone chiller day with bright sunshine but I almost froze my toes in the deep snow and ice. Luckily, we were skunked of prey and decided after four hours to call it a day. Shortly after we left our hunting grounds, homeward bound, with the sun dipping below the horizon, the car radio ejaculated, "Standby for an important news bulletin; the Japanese have made a massive aerial strike at Pearl Harbor at 0700 and have practically wiped out our entire naval fleet stationed there." We were completely dumbfounded, distraught, and immediately knew this could only mean one thing. We were about to initiate our participation in World War II against Japan, Germany and Italy. Our allies would be Great Britain, France, and believe it or not, Soviet Russia by necessity. Germany's Hitler had organized the greatest war machine of all time for years, while the opposing countries were in a state of deep anesthesia as witnessed by Britain's "Umbrella – Peace at any Price" Man, Prime Minister Chamberlain. The Japanese sneak attack on Pearl Harbor, a real jawbreaker, crystallized our declaration of war instantaneously. We awoke from our slumber with a bang! Immediate conscription into the USA armed forces was the order of the day and for the four ensuing years.

Before describing my hitching with the army M.D.A.U.S. there are three outstanding cases of pediatric illness which are indelibly imprinted in my mind. Shortly after I began my pediatric practice, Dr. Perkins called me in consultation on a six year old boy who was very emaciated, athreptic, and a picture of absolute starvation. He was real weak, pale, had diarrhea , and had lost several pounds of weight in the past year. He had no fever and physically showed no outward signs of disease. His mother worked in the diet kitchen at old General Hospital. She was well acquainted with proper nutritional support, but in spite of her dietary expertise and vitamins, Jimmy had become about ten pounds under weight. Cystic fibrosis, an autosomal recessive inherited disease, was a prime suspect for his malady. Diagnosis of cystic fibrosis in 1940 was quite crude but necessary – frequent fatty foul stools and the cachectic clinical habitus were prominent leads to the recognition of cystic fibrosis, but definite scientific tests were required to nail it down without doubt. I had never seen a patient with cystic fibrosis, but I did know that it was a disease of the mucus-secreting glands and the pancreas, lungs, and intestines. It is a multi-system disease resulting from the production of thick dehydrated mucous and the victim is unable to sweat adequately or bring up lung secretions and this proves fatal at a very early age. To diagnose Jimmy's illness, I had to insert a gastric tube and reach the ampulla of vater through the panoreatic opening in the second portion of the duodenum. Here the pancreatic juices, steapsin, rennin, and amylopsin empty into the duodenum via the ducts of santorini.. They are the juices that digest fats, carbohydrates and proteins. The lab can determine if they are present in the extracted juices aspirated from the duodenums. In order to get the pancreatic secretions, I gave him a modest dose of alcohol to stimulate the pancreatic secretions. Our lab tests proved there was a lack of all three digestive juices and I made a correct diagnosis of cystic fibrosis - the first patient diagnosed with it, in Bay City. Now we have the specific sweat test for diagnosis. Jimmy survived until he was age 18 years, and died due to chronic pneumonia and hepatitis. Cystic fibrosis was first discovered in 1938.

Another memorable patient was Johnny Meagher, who had nephrotic syndrome, a kidney affliction. Nephrosis is characterized by heavy proteinuria resulting in low blood albumin, massive edema (anasarca), and increased blood lipids. My partner, Fern, was treating him when I appeared on the scene in Bay City, but he wasn't getting to first base, so he asked me if I would take over Johnny's case, and of course I did, enthusiastically. It fortuitously happened that Sharpe and Dome Pharmaceutical had just recently, in 1940, produced a new preparation of concentrated albumin for use in the treatment of nephrosis. I had never had any practical experience in its usage, but I figured that the conventional therapy, (steroids), wasn't cutting the mustard, so why not give it a go, for it was reasonably safe with proper directions and we had nothing to lose. So, damn the torpedoes and full speed ahead "sans icebergs". Anyhow, we did employ the concentrated albumin and had immediate positive success. Johnny lost tons of weight by diureses through his kidneys and he did make a miraculous recovery which gave my stock quite a boost.

Reluctantly, I relate the third child's sickness. Mary was a two year old, deathly ill toddler, suffering with diarrhea for several days, and was in a state of shock from severe acidosis dehydration, and depletion of all her electrolytes (sodium, potassium, magnesium, and low blood Ph). Therapy consisted mainly of drastic re-hydration, replenishing of the electrolytes, and reaching equilibrium with her blood osmotic pressure. After running the IV for about four hours, the head nurse called and excitedly said, "Mary had taken a sudden turn for the worse and is critically hanging on by a thread.'" I was at Mary's bedside in a flash and realized immediately that in addition to her moribund state from the protracted diarrhea, she had developed cerebral edema and marked increased intracranial pressure. I attempted a lumbar puncture but was unable to obtain any fluid after three tries, and she died shortly after. To say I felt terrible, is a gross understatement and I couldn't help feeling that there must have been a comorbid (complication), maybe a brain tumor, cerebral abscess or meningitis which contributed a final stroke to her death. Maybe surgical trephining and hypertonic sugar, IV could have helped. I couldn't get an autopsy permit, so we'll never know.

Chapter 16

You're in the Army Medical Corps. Now

General Hersey, in charge of conscription, organized a unique method of calling men and women (first time) to duty to defend their country. P.R.U. Urmston, a former WW I veteran, was Bay County's commander for organizing the doctors (M.D.'s only) to enter the service for Army, Navy, Air Force, and Marines. At our medical meetings, P.R.U, would say, "If you join now, as Early Birds, you may have your choice of which medical branches of the armed forces and may have a choice of duty and location of service. Besides, the sooner you enter service, the sooner you will be back to practice in Bay City." As a result of his exhortations, a great preponderance of M.D.'s here, took his advice literally, and voluntarily joined the service for war duty. Before joining, I served with Dr. Ed Huckins, to examine the civilian men of Bay County, who were enlisted. We received no remuneration, but did receive a citation award from President Franklin Roosevelt for meritorious service.

My dear friend, Doc Matthew Slattery gave me the keys to his cottage on the Au Sable River, near Grayling, and said, "Knobby, it's yours for a week, before you go into the Army. Take your beloved wife, and Susan, and wipe all your earthly cares away." Matthew had a heart of gold and I am sure he wanted to give me a glorious send off, so I called his hand and accepted his generous offer.

It was like a second honeymoon, and it was verily eventful. The day before leaving the cabin, I clumsily managed to burn my right hand on the hot tip of a kerosene lamp. I grabbed it to replace the fluid and garnered a nasty second degree burn on the palmar surface of my palm, thumb, forefinger, and middle finger. I spent the next several hours, soaking these fingers in ice water. Wisely, Matt had stocked the bathroom with bandages for fools like me. So I received my first battle wound and I hadn't even joined the Army. Also, I applied equal parts of furacin and Vaseline ointment and it immediately obliterated the pain and healing began with magic celerity.

Just before the vacation at Matt's cottage, I, along with Stan Pearson, Mike Medvezky and Dentist "Bill" Anderson went to Mount Clemens to the Air Base at Selfridge Field for the official physical and induction. Ashamedly, I almost fainted when the nurse poked my arm to draw a few c.c.'s of blood. We all passed our physicals with flying colors and I received a letter from the Army telling me to report to Barnes General Hospital, Portland, Oregon, on July 31st as Captain, Army of United States. I was overjoyed to skip basic training – heart broken.

I left Bay City on the evening of July 27th and took the "red eye" overnight, sleepless train ride on the N.Y. Central to Chicago, arriving there at 7 a.m.. From there I boarded the Union Pacific to Portland, Oregon, on a three day journey taking me over the Rockies and past Cheyenne, Wyoming, Sun Valley, Utah, and along the Columbia River to the "Flower City" (Portland). We arrived at our destination in the evening of July 30th, after a delightful and uneventful journey. I reported for duty on the appointed, fateful day, July 31, 1942, at Barnes General Hospital in Vancouver, Washington, just across the Columbia River from Portland. My first assignment after finding my living quarters in the Officer's Barracks entailed purchasing the proper army clothing and insignia befitting a naïve Captain, Army, United States, Medical Corps – Brevet.

My first assignment was to assist Med. Captain Baker on the tuberculosis ward for a brief, two week session. He was somewhat impressed with my knowledge about tuberculosis, thanks to my stint of duty at Sabillasville, Maryland State TBC Sanitarium. Baker would say, "They should spell your name, Knowblock," which I took with a big grain of salt. It was really difficult in the Army, to know who your true friends were, because everyone was desperately striving for advancement in rank, to receive a better paycheck. The Lord knows we certainly were not overpaid, and a huge portion went to our wives for family survival.

My second assignment at Barnes (Civil War Surgeon), was assistant to Major Medic William Martin Marbut, in the emergency department. Major Marbut was an almost bald, late fortyish, general practitioner, who had dove into the armed service shortly after Pearl Harbor, and had worked his way into a majority. He was a rough, tough, very capable, and efficient doctor, a very honest, sincere, committed, and conscientious person. I learned how to relieve acute, painful hemorrhoids and how to exactly describe wounds and make their closure by plastic surgery. He had an obvious affinity for the ladies and would say when someone asked him how he liked his coffee, "I like my coffee strong and my women weak." Bill had a fetish about drying between the toes to prevent athlete's foot, sometimes called epidermatophytosis.

The first Saturday I was there, my barracks roommate talked me into attending a Red Cross dance at a pavilion near the hospital. It did somewhat alleviate my home sickness and isolation being with myriads of strangers about 2500 miles from home. On my way returning to quarters, I unwisely opted to take a shortcut, and got lost in the pitch darkness. After wandering aimlessly in circles for a while, I was awakened by a stern stentorian male voice, demanding "who goes there?" I had been cautioned at headquarters that if you were challenged by an army outpost, you should answer by giving your name, rank, serial number, and station. Being a greenhorn, I nervously answered his query properly, and he replied, "advance and be recognized." I did, and was justly relieved to see the M.P.'s who directed me back to the officer's barracks.

Shortly after this incident, while conversing with my wife, I strongly urged her to come to Vancouver to join me before I would possibly be assigned to foreign duty. She acquiesced and said it would take some time to complete arrangements and preparations. My mother came to Bay City to pick up Susan and be her guardian in Greensburg, while Doris was with me.

Mother relates a tale regarding Susan, who was two years plus by this date, sharp as a razor blade, and very determined "to the last ditch", as always. She was running a sudden high fever, so Margaret (my mother) promptly took her to see the Greensburg Pediatrician. When Dr. Engel, attempted to examine Susan, she stated emphatically, "my father is a Pediatrician, and he is the only one who can see me when I am sick."

I recall an instance with Susan when she was around four years of age. She, Tom (brother), Doris, and I were dining at the Wenonah Hotel, when she and Tom got into a knock down and drag-out scuffle over some miniscule issue. Susan started to scream and wouldn't cease no matter what we did to resolve the conflict. Doris said to me, "There's only one thing you can do, take her home and that will be a lesson in proper behavior." I agreed and took Susan home to 221 N. Lincoln. She cried all the way home and never let up until Doris and Tom returned. No all out overtures would placate her.

Another instance was when Susan would have almost daily, temper tantrums. She was enjoying a real doozy, thrashing on the kitchen floor, one evening when we were alone. I became somewhat incensed, and decided to go for broke and shoot the works. My aggravation had reached the P.N.R.= the point of no return. So, I grabbed an available bucket, filled it half full with water and threw it on her. She must have been duly shocked and impressed for she deceased her tantrum and never had another. I had heard of my grandmother rendering a similar cure on my mother, and I thought, why not, it can't do any harm.

Doris finally came to Portland by train and I met her at the station there. I was all pumped up but she seemed to be deflated and singularly depressed. She's tired after such a long trip, I thought. We went to a room in a Portland hotel that I had engaged in advance. After a while, I said, "Doris, you seem to be sad, is there some problem that is bothering you?" And then all hell broke loose. I've never seen her angrier and she called me all the worst names under the sun. I was in shock and recoiled in abject humility. After catching my breath, I said, "What in earth have I done to deserve this violent outburst?" To which she angrily, in tears, responded, "You dirty dog, you made me pregnant." I said, "Why that is wonderful. Susan needs a playmate to buffer her endless energy." But Doris was inflamed with self pity to have to be pregnant alone, while I was having a ball away for the duration of the war. Nothing I could say would pacify her ill feelings and my extreme joy curdled and turned to sour milk. I don't believe either of us have ever had a more miserable night. It seems she never did totally forgive me but really I had <u>not</u> tried to impregnate her at this time. I could understand her dire consternation in this matter, but at least she could have called me a "clean dog" and a dog could not impregnate her. Apparently the only time we engaged in intercourse at Slattery's cottage in the past couple months, resulted in encyesis (pregnancy).

Ready or not, we unhappily moved in to our army apartment in the officer's barracks. We actually did not reach a healthy resolution of this pregnancy issue until three months later, during her stay with me in November of 1942. A very happy state of affairs eventuated when the Sprongs, Major David and his good wife, Eloise, moved into the vacated next door apartment about a week after we did. David was a very astute general surgeon and was built like Tarzan. Eloise was a sweet, petite, happy go lucky charming person with feline. We formed a very positive and friendly relationship with the Sprongs and the days flew by.

I was assigned to the Plasma Team of the Red Cross, Portland Blood Bank. Five days a week, Captains Edward Holstein and I, would traverse the ten mile journey to Portland and begin our venipunctures (Phlebotomies), at 9 a.m. and continue unabatedly until the 1700 curfew, except for a sandwich at noon. I don't believe I've ever witnessed such a huge number of ladies and gentlemen who were so corpulent (avoir du poise +++). It seemed like most of them gravitated to me. After our return trip to Vancouver, we would spin down all the blood we had collected and give the resulting plasma to Army Headquarters for storage. It was dispersed to the Pacific areas for usage for battle casualties at the front lines.

One Red Cross worker, Madame Irene Rowe, was assigned to assist me. She was one of the sweetest, most helpful, efficient and kind persons I have ever known – most unforgettable. In addition, she was an unexcelled cuisine artist and I was her guest at dinner on a couple of memorable occasions. In general, the people of Portland were most hospitable and welcomed us with open arms. In another instance, another Red Cross lady invited me to a college football game between Oregon State Beavers and the Washington

State Cougars. The word had gotten around that I was a sports fiend. I accepted her invitation and do recall that the Beavers were soundly trounced. She had gone to a private women's college in Chambersburg, PA, and brought along to the game a bottle of Johnny Walker Black Label. I thanked her but demurred, proclaiming that I preferred a cola. I never was, and never will be, a friend to alcohol. After the game, she invited me to a room at the Portland Athletic Club and again, I demurred and informed her I had a dinner date with my wife. She was a charming, lovely lady and I heard from reliable sources that she did "entertain" several army officers, to her husband's consternation. She must have thought I was a premier "stick in the mud".

One place Doris and I went to just about every Sunday night, was the Portland Air Base. They put on the most delectable and fancy dinner you can imagine. They had a carved ice replica of a pig in a giant punch bowl. There was a complete assortment of seafood, salads, roast beef, pork, vegetables, fruits, and desserts that have ever been invented. Being gastatory hounds, we took advantage of these heavenly offerings, (the best things in life are free).

While Doris and I were in Vancouver, we did avail ourselves of a few interesting sorties by automobile. One exceedingly memorable trip was to Mount Hood. The drive up the mountain was exceptionally scenic. We stopped at a restaurant near the pinnacle of the mountain, at about 12,000 feet. Believe me, the view from there is as magnificent as it comes. On another occasion, we toured to Salem and Eugene one Sunday in the rain and had a most enjoyable time. Also, the journey along the Columbia River, especially the Lewis and Clark route, is noteworthy for its many scenic cliffs, waterfalls and gorges.

Shortly after New Years Day, 1943, I got my orders to proceed to Seattle to the staging area for overseas duty. I was there for five weeks until my orders came through to proceed to Seward Alaska, by troop-ship, on February 3rd, 1943. While in Seattle, I went to a few lectures on hypertension and was asked to render a lecture on treatment of shock in children. One memorable event while stationed in Seattle, was a visit on a weekend, by my dear friends Irene and C.J. Rowe from Portland. We had a pleasant, memorable reunion with dinner, dancing and movies. We reviewed our alliances while in Portland.

Chapter 17

Army Medical Duty in Alaska

We embarked from Seattle for "Seward's Icebox" on the 3rd of February. It took 11 days to reach our objective at Seward, Alaska. Our "Troopship" was a converted medium-sized pleasure boat, The South American, which prior to the Second World War made summer only excursions between Los Angeles and South American ports of call. Army Headquarters (H2) had crowded 4000 soldiers on this ship and the vast majority of them were quartered in the hold, which didn't make for happy campers! I was the only doctor on board and I was assigned one poor nurse, who was the only female on board. We had sick call morning, noon, and night, practically continuously. We were warned to expect rough seas at about 0100 (1 AM) and sure enough, on target at that time in the "Inland Passage" we encountered the rolling Straits of Juan De Fuca (and the site of the unseen Killer Whales) between British Columbia and Vancouver Island, virtually tossing us out of our bunks. Our troopship was completely without lights at night because the skipper feared Japanese submarines. Woe unto the person who lit a match on the deck! We stopped over at Juneau for four days for some inexplicable reason, adding insult to injury because of out confined quarters. We did manage a couple of sightseeing trips to the Mendenhall Glacier and surrounding environs. We stayed at the Baranoff Hotel in Juneau, where the ice used in the hotel was taken from this glacier.

Most of our "sick call" patients were minor gastrointestinal problems with emesis and diarrhea prevailing due to motion sickness. There was one case of chicken pox and a couple colles wrist fractures, due to falls, to be splinted. Several mild influenza illnesses and some tracheo-bronchitis cases caught our attention. When we arrived at Seward, the port authorities tried to quarantine us. I did some tall talking and explained it was impossible to quarantine chicken pox, easier to do than isolating the ambient air. So, we did get the decision reversed, after an eon of haggling the pros and cons.

Our next adventure was to board the so-called "train" for Anchorage via the Alaskan Railway, a trip of 80 miles as the crow flies. This railroad was built in the 1880s and the locomotive and passenger cars were also constructed thereabouts. There was no heat inside the eight passenger cars and frozen water was visible on the floor. It was said that the railway had been condemned for over thirty years, but we were too sleepy to protest. Actually the railroad was reputed to be a masterpiece of engineering when it was built because it traversed tunnel wise through seven mountainous areas. Anyhow, be that as it may, we arrived at our destination in Anchorage about 3 a.m., four plus hours from our departure at Seward, half-frozen, starved, and in dire need of slumber. Outside the friendly temperature hovered around minus 20 degrees Fahrenheit and Jehovah only knows what the temperature was including the wind chill. We were saluted by the Military Police and they directed us to our living quarter barracks.

The following morning, I reported to the Alaskan Army Medical Headquarters. To my utter amazement, no one other than, Adjutant Captain William Smith greeted me. Bill, as I knew him, was a familiar sight for sore eyes. We had interned together at University Hospital in Ann Arbor, Michigan in 1938-39, he in internal medicine and I in pediatrics. He, fortunately, was in charge of physician placement in Alaska under the authorization of the Commanding General for Alaskan Troops. We exchanged courtesies and then came to the nitty gritty, the bottom-line. He asked me what and how I would like to serve. I said, "Sir, you are familiar with my capacities in pediatrics and the decision on my disposition is yours." Whereupon, he said, "Captain, how would you like to take charge of contagious diseases at the General Army Hospital here in Anchorage? Our present Infection Disease Officer is completing his tour of duty and is moving back to the States. "Of course," I said, "Yes sir, it would be right up my alley." He also told me I could have pediatric consultations and work with the local general practitioners that needed pediatric consult in their offices or hospital practices. I was assigned the Contagious Ward pronto and immediately conferred with Captain Hensley, the departing Contagion Chief.

Hensley had twenty some patients consisting of various childhood infections like mumps, German measles (rubella), measles, varicella (chicken pox), bronchitis and pneumonia. We had one mumps casualty when the patient developed hyperthermia agonally with an uncontrollable temperature of 110 degrees F. and went to see his maker in 18 hours. Hensley had devised a unique method of treating mumps patients; especially mumps orchitis (testicular swelling) which is probably the most painful affliction a man can suffer. Captain Hensley would take 20 cc's of blood from a two weeks convalescent, mumps male and inject 10 cc's in each buttock of an acutely, seriously ill patient and viola! In 24 hours the temperature would reduce to 100 degrees Fahrenheit or less, and the testicles would shrink to half their expanded size (orange or grapefruit size) and the person would feel invigorated and happy. Apparently the transfer of mumps viral antibodies from one in the stage of recovery to one at the height of illness produced a tremendous positive effect. I recall performing this exact procedure on a young man in Bay City in 1948 with similar, beneficial results and he became a principal at Handy High School several years later. Hopefully, the blood we injected to corral the mumps wasn't contaminated with the hepatitis "B" virus!

Anchorage had a thriving population of 15,000 inhabitants at the beginning of World War II. Fishing was the primary industry and the climate was temperate, influenced by the mellowing effect of the Japanese current. Alaskan land area was 570,833 square miles, more than double the size of Texas. It was a gift from Russia when purchased by Secretary of State Seward for a pittance of $40 million and was known as "Seward's Icebox" or "Seward's Folly". Alaska is surrounded by Knick and Cook's Glaciers and the Talkeetna Mountain Range on the east and north. The tides at Cook Inlet on the Bay of Alaska to the south are the second highest in the world next to the Bay of Fundy on Canada's east coast. Rainfall averages 18 inches a year as compared to Juneau's 160 inches. On a clear, sunshiny, summer day you can envision Mount McKinley, which is barely 140 miles almost directly north of Anchorage. The warriors of the Rising Sun (Japan) had invaded Attu and Kiska in the Aleutian Island chain, which were formations of defunct volcanoes. The native inhabitants were Indians, Eskimos, and Aleuts. The Russians had left their earmark of tuberculosis (phthisis) which was rife among practically all the native Alaskans. The U.S. Army inducted many native young men for a while, but under duress, these soldiers invariably developed active tuberculosis disease from quiescent lesions. If they were unfortunate enough to pick up measles, they developed raging pulmonary phthisis and inevitably succumbed within a few days. Apparently they had never had exposure to measles until the white man plagued them. Finally the Army Alaskan Command decided it was expensive and useless to draft natives into the U.S. Army.

I formed close knit, enduring friendships with several astute and congenial medical service officers during my tour of 27 month's duty in Alaska. It was a continuous Army service for this span of time, with the exception of two weeks furlough back to Michigan after one year's duty.

Lt. Colonel Conrad Earl Albrecht was a very close and valuable friend. He had practiced family medicine in Palmer for ten years before war was declared, was superintendent of a general hospital there, and had a log cabin home overlooking the Matanuska Valley and Palmer. Palmer was a small town of about 4,000 people nestled and cradled in an elongated depression surrounded by magnificent snow-capped mountains averaging ten to fourteen thousand feet in height. People who have traveled the entire earth claim that Alaska cannot be beat for sheer raw beauty.

Another close friendship developed with Major Carl Olson, our Chief of the X-ray department. We worked together on several, vital medical committees and had a close liaison with patients. Another amicable person was Major William Martin Marbut, with whom I was associated at Barnes General Hospital in Vancouver, Washington. Martin was the fatherly type, full of advice, practical common sense, and support. Captain Eveland was our lab chief and a veritable indispensable cog in the wheel for consultation and truly a real nice, affable person. Major Standiford was head of Internal Medicine, erudite with a real sense of humor. He would characterize our post Saturday night dances as "Belly Rubs" or "Navel Skirmishes". He was from Little Rock, Arkansas and was an excellent leader as well as my direct boss. We had tri-weekly conferences on all our patients with "Sandy" in charge of the discussion. Captain Wilbur's medical ward was next to my contagion ward and we had a fairly amicable relationship, although Wilbur was a bit sarcastic and hypercritical. His motto concerning patients was "rough them up now and you can always love them later". He was a lumberjack in Oregon before he entered the medical field and sort of the Paul Bunyon type. Our chaplain was 1st Lt. Thompson and we had a wee bit of humor with him regarding his "collapsible organ". He would travel to various Army installations on the post and he always carried a folding piano with him to use for singing hymns. Al Hirsch was a great friend of everyone. He was an optometrist and manufactured glasses for all medical personnel. Al's home was the "Sunshine State" and he was a dyed in the wool ambassador of Florida's virtues. He repeatedly spoke of the magnificent Orange groves and told of his happy excursions to Cuba before the strangling Castro dictatorship.

Mary Hirsch and Doris Veidt, both nurses, and I played many heated bridge games in our idle and spare hours. Bridge requires colossal concentration, memory, contemplation, intuition, and a bit of favorable luck doesn't hurt. It is not only being dealt a good hand but an innate "card sense" and ability to play the right card lead at the right time that is crucial. A person has to keep a strict vigilance to remember every card played and by whom, and every card remaining un-played in each other's hand. There is a smidgen of logic, reasoning, guesswork, and psychology that prevails. Psychology plays a prominent role. It does really wring you out after several hours of intense concentration.

We had a few games of touch football, volleyball, and frequently went skiing in the nearby mountains of 8 to 10 thousand feet on weekends. We would pile in an ambulance with equipment and sandwiches, and head for Independence Gold Mine beyond Palmer, about 60 / 70 miles. There were ski instructors from Montana and Sun Valley who would give us lessons and I honestly did learn to properly downhill ski. Carlson had taught me the rudiments of this sport in Marquette, Michigan, and I was exposed to an advanced course of instruction in Alaska. Unfortunately or fortunately, there were no ski lifts and our trusty lower extremities came in handy for climbing the mountains. It was an arduous effort, but when you scaled to the top it was well worth the struggle. Traveling down this elevation for about a mile was exhilarating and the view from the mountain peak was truly out of this world. Snow-capped, majestic mountains surrounded us on all sides. After experimenting, I discovered a neat way to fall while on skis without hurting myself. If I sensed that a loss of gravity was imminent, I would throw my body to the left side and then I would be in an ideal position to get back up. This was an important maneuver because sooner or later one must fall as the apple does from the tree. We would also get a thrill out of tobogganing down the slopes. On one of our excursions down a steep grade, poor Mary of bridge fame somehow managed to fracture a vertebra; and believe me, this is an excruciating and painful affliction with intractable abdominal griping.

We did have an officer's club with a special recreation room on the base at Elmendorf Field at Fort Richardson in Anchorage, Alaska. There also was a replica officer's club in our new 182nd hospital built in the Dispersal Containment (D.C.) area eight miles out of Anchorage on the road to Palmer, erected six months after I came on the scene at Richardson, my final destination in Alaska. Usually the Officer's Club was used on weekends and evenings where friends would gather. We also enjoyed the cinema; we would enjoy motion pictures a couple times a week. Sometimes we would take our ambulance into Anchorage from the post to the Blue Moon restaurant for a steak dinner and then top it off at the Lido Bar for a nightcap.

One special movie twists my memory, "The Song of Bernadette" with Jennifer Jones. Another picture that comes to mind was with Barbara Stanwyck, "Death of a Salesman", which I saw intermittently while attending a civilian worker who was on her deathbed with a pulmonary abscess caused by aspiration of a ruptured group A streptococci tonsillar abscess. She was being treated with a new drug, "penicillin", which had just come to us in 1943 from England. It would have saved her life had we used proper dosage. Unknowingly, I was giving her 40,000 units every four hours when I should have been administering a million units every four hours. But I was following explicit directions as presented on the instructions. She was the most beautiful young 18 year-old lady you can imagine, like the famous drawings in Esquire by Vargas.

Occasionally I would go to the Methodist Church in Anchorage with Colonel Albrecht. Two of my buddies were Captains Bill Bishop from Tallahassee and Larry Reck from San Diego. Both were pediatricians my age. We would lament, commiserate and sympathize with each other, especially during the holidays at the end of the year. At these times family nostalgia was too great to sweep under the carpet, especially when the air was dripping so dulcetly with those sugary World War II songs. "Long Ago and Far Away", "Don't Sit Under The Apple Tree", "Till the End of Time", "Lovely to Look At", "A White Christmas", "Embraceable You", "Some Enchanted Evening", and "Till We Meet Again" were a few choice ones. There were also "In the Mood", "One O'clock Jump", "Celery Stalks At Midnight", and "You'd Be So Nice To Come Home To" to stir up smoldering cardiac fires and the romantic hormones.

We had several cases of acute meningococcal meningitis during my 27 months of duty in Denali, Alaska. The enlisted men that developed this disease would be perfectly well and then all of a sudden they would be slugged with a devastating headache, high fever, stiff neck, and atrocious projectile vomiting. My good friend Sulfa did a real workman's job to eradicate this gram-negative diplococcus in short order. The spinal fluid was usually a smidgen cloudy and it would spurt out under pressure. When doing a spinal tap, the operator must be extremely careful to prevent herniation of the cerebellar tonsils and vital medullary centers into the foramen magnum causing instant death. Extracting the stylus from the needle and being extremely cautious to have the spinal fluid drip slowly into a blood agar plate for culture obviated this event (slow decompression).

Major Bernes, our chief of Psychiatry, called me one day and said, "Howard, one of my patients is acting very peculiarly. He is screaming violently, complaining of an awful headache and banging his head against the bathroom toilet tank while vomiting." I said, "Bob, does he have a fever and possibly a stiff neck?" Bernes replied, "I'll check and call you right back. Don't go away." Shortly after, Bob called me excitedly, saying, "His temperature is 105 degrees and I can't bend his head." I immediately answered, "That clinches the diagnosis; it has to be meningitis for sure. Send him to my ward stat and I'll call you pronto." After my examination, there was no doubt about it and the lumbar puncture confirmed unequivocally a diagnosis of bacterial meningitis, probably a meningococcus, which occurs mainly in young, adolescents and infants. It is acquired infrequently through contact with a carrier in a nonimmune, compromised individual but really is not epidemic or contagious except by intimate contact. This coccus, named for its founder Weichselbaum in the late eighteen hundreds, is invasive where teenagers congregate in close quarters, notably in dorms. About 1 in 20 people are "innocent" throat carriers.

A dramatic incident involving the meningococcus organism happened shortly after Bernes' case. I received an emergency call from an enlisted soldier in the barracks one afternoon. He was extremely agitated and stammered that his buddy was unconscious and convulsing. I took an ambulance and arrived at his bedside on the run. I found him in a comatose state of deep shock. Upon reaching my ward, we performed a spinal tap, which showed normal fluid and a complete physical was otherwise negative. We learned that he woke up perfectly well and happy that morning and complained of a mild headache about two hours before he lapsed into a stupor progressing to la-la land. Apparently, he had an adrenal hemorrhage, otherwise known as Waterhouse-Friedrichsen Syndrome, which is almost invariably fatal. This young man did die about an hour after the lumbar tap. Just before death he developed a pinkish, voracious rash on his chest and abdomen, which is usually due to septicemia and our friend the meningococcus. We shipped his body to the Army lab in Seattle for a post-mortem autopsy and burial by his parents. I must have taken care of a dozen cases of meningococcal meningitis during my medical career in Alaska, with only this one mortality as proven by report from the lab in Seattle.

I recall two red-letter pediatric consults. One was a male two-year old who was brought in to the hospital with chief complaint of a painless abdominal swelling. The mother had inadvertently discovered a smooth, round, large swelling over the right side of his belly while giving him a bath. This history was a familiar narrative as it was a dead ringer for a couple identical cases I had experienced during my internship and brief stab at practice. The child was perfectly healthy in every other way. A diagnosis of Wilm's Tumor hit me smack dab in the face like a lightening bolt out of the blue. It's like Dr. Arthur G. Shipley, my surgical mentor in medical school, stated "How do I know what this malady is? It is because I've <u>seen</u> it before." Usually the history of a child's illness is much more enlightening in nailing down a diagnosis than the physical examination. After informing the mother of my tentative diagnosis, we made arrangements to transport this young lad to the University of Washington Hospital in Seattle and a month later received the good news that his Wilm's Tumor was totally removable and he was recovering completely. Early diagnosis is the sine qua non to complete cure because this tumor is highly malignant and metastasizes to opposite kidney, lungs, liver, bones, testis, brain, and peripheral lymph nodes. Treatment consists of preoperative chemotherapy and radiation, with extensive exploration of abdominal organs, surgery, and postoperative radiation and chemotherapy for several weeks, depending on metastasizes and size of tumor. Biopsy of the tumor before removal must be avoided due to possible leakage of tumor cells into the abdominal cavity. A doctor feels especially exuberant when he knows that he has rescued his patient from the jaws of death and I am no exception to this heavenly feeling.

The second memorable consultation was another two-year old boy in Seward, which my boss, Conrad Albrecht, allocated to me. I traveled by train down to Seward. It is a gorgeous, scenic ride from Anchorage through tunnels, over mountains and waterways. It takes about four hours on a clear day. Upon arriving at the station in Seward, I was greeted by Doctor Francis Foreman. He was a large, handsome, middle-ages country practitioner, very affable and down to earth. I could sense worry and concern in the lines of his face. Immediately, he escorted me to the patient's bed without fanfare and in a few pertinent words described the little boy's symptoms. He was a native Alaskan child and had been ill for over a month with low-grade fever, gradual weight loss, weakness, anorexia and a severe, deep cough with expectoration and night sweats. It was evident that he was cachecnic, stuporous, and recently had complained of headache and explosive vomiting. His temperature was now 103 degree plus. His skin was hot and dry and his pulse was weak and thready. Noonak was moaning and groaning ,and his neck was as stiff as a board. When I raised his head, the entire body rose as a unit and he screamed with pain. His chest X-ray showed a tuberculous hilar nodal pattern. I did a spinal tap and it was under pressure, cloudy, with high protein cell count of a couple thousand, and low sugar. The conclusion was acute tuberculosis meningitis with Mister Brinks (death) staring us belligerently in the eyes.

Dr. Foreman said, "I was afraid of TBC but didn't want to be realistic because my son, who lives across the street, plays with him like a brother." We had no anti TBC antibiotics except penicillin and a new one, streptomycin, which had recently been discovered. Penicillin never fazed the tubercle bacillus, which was encapsulated and very resistant. However, I had recently read in the American Medical Association Journal that at the University of Minnesota they were using streptomycin for injection into the spinal fluid pathway as successful therapy for TBC meningitis. I relayed this information to Dr. Foreman and told him to watch his son closely for signs and symptoms of the dreaded childhood TBC in his own son. The patient certainly required surveillance, but there were no pulmonary cavities and children with lung tuberculosis usually are not contagious as they seldom have cavities, unless in a far advanced stage. This fact relieved the Doctor's mind somewhat. The crucial question was how and where did this little guy acquire the disease with which the Doctor and local health department could wrestle? I was graciously invited by the Doctor to be his guest overnight at his home and I accepted. The next morning I caught the train back to Anchorage, but before

I left, the Doctor asked me for my charge. I told him that the Army paid me a livable wage and there was no charge for my services. After about an hour on the train I reached into my right coat pocket, lo and behold, I did find a plum! Surprise! It was a check for $75.00, which in those days was a bonanza. It seemed to me that I'd done him a big favor by maybe salvaging his son's life. Before I left, I did advise Dr. Foreman to do a tuberculin test on his entire family. If any positives arose, he was to examine early morning gastric contents for tubercle bacilli and to contact the University of Minnesota regarding use of streptomycin and consider injection of BCG (bacillus calmette guerin) as a possible immune booster. Also, I reminded the Doctor of the essential importance of calcium (all forms of milk) in the diet to wall off any tubercle microbes.

My living quarters in Anchorage were about four blocks from the hospital. I was assigned to a house with Major Robert Bernes as my roommate. Bob and I were compatible, he being a psychiatrist and myself a pediatrician. Bob was a congenial, astute, soft-spoken, somewhat effeminate, single, and Jewish young man. It was obvious that he was male oriented, for almost daily, young service men were his guests at our humble habitat. We roomed together for several months and then I was transferred to the newly built 182nd Station Hospital. My relations with Bob were strictly above board and non argumentative. He had a stereo music system devoted to purely classical music. His favorites were Wagner, Rachmaninoff, Brahms, Beethoven, and Mozart. For the first time I was exposed in depth to the great romantic classic composers and when I returned to the States, the first thing on my agenda was to purchase a stereo and to obtain the symphonies and piano concerts. I remember the first 78 records. Doris and I bought Rachmaninoff's Piano Concerto #3, for me, and Beethoven's Emperor 5th Symphony, for her. To conclude Major Bernes' saga, he was returned to the States because of his male sex relations. I felt quite sorry for Bob Bernes, for he was really a talented and personable man, rendering an excellent service to the Army. However, the Army would not tolerate this disposition of hormones and I can understand where they are coming from.

A sometime humorous event occurred at Elmendorf Field before I was transferred to the 182nd Station Hospital. It so happens that a native Eskimo, Klutch, while cogitating in his tent one night became agitated and went stark berserk. He pulled out his revolver and went on a rampage, spraying bullets all over the tent, fortunately not hitting any of his fellowmen. He loudly exclaimed, "This give Alaska back to Indians must cease," several times until someone could restrain him and extinguish the fire. Apparently, he was supersaturated with the continual razzing and teasing he had absorbed over a lengthy period of time.

In moving to my quarters in the brand, spanking new D.C. area 182nd

Station Hospital, I acquired a new chief, Lt. Colonel Conrad Earl Albrecht, who roomed just across the hall from me. On the room to the right of me was my good friend Major William Martin Marbut. Our location there was really rustic, on the side of a mountain inhabited by neighborly black bears. They were harmless usually, unless there was a mother with cubbies. We were taught if suddenly confronted by one to clap hands or shout loudly, and if they became angry and charged us, to lie down and play dead. They are near sighted (presbyopic) but they are fast, agile, and can climb trees. Intense noise seems to frighten them. One of our corpsmen shot a bear that was frequently searching for food in the hospital cuisine, enabling me to taste bear steak. It was very tasty and succulent, just like prime rib beef.

Another bear incident tweaks my memory. It involved the night Charge of Quarters. While making rounds at around 0200 one drowsy a.m., the on duty sergeant heard a vague clicking sound behind him. After searching a couple halls, he aroused to full consciousness and peered behind him. To his consternation there was a big black bear following his footsteps. He took off with celerity and headed for the kitchen. Upon reaching the kitchen, he hastily grabbed a large piece of meat and enticed the bear outside. Then he faded out of the picture and reentered the hospital after tossing the raw steak to the bear. This really is a true story, cross my heart.

I really loved my surroundings at the new hospital location. It was a breath of fresh air and gave me a feeling of freedom from the rigid army life on the main post. We would take daily hikes up the mountainside. We also would ski often on the road in front of the hospital, for there was fresh snow from October until May. Surprisingly, there was a little theater about 1 1/2 miles down the road towards Anchorage, and it afforded us recreational advantages three nights a week. We relished in the extended light period in the summer, when there was almost blinding light from 2 a.m. to 11 p.m. daily. In fact, sleeping was difficult, as the light penetrated our window shades (no curtains). However, in winter the environment was opposite, very depressing and conducive to cabin fever. So-called daylight or semidarkness prevailed from about 10 a.m. until 2 p.m. if we were lucky. The dark side was especially depressing for the female gender. Be that as it may, the nurses had one explicit advantage. If conditions became too harsh and unbearable, they had a natural easy escape that we men were negated. All they had to do was to let nature take its course and succumb to pregnancy (<u>accidental</u> of course). The servicemen did try valiantly to get back to the States, but to no avail. They would frequently go on sick call for unmitigated disabling backache. I was on a medical board that functioned to evaluate the chronic backaches, and we would meet at least twice a week. They were a scourge, for X-rays and physical exams were invariably negative and non-productive, like searching for a needle in a haystack. Others would taunt us with a chief complaint of polyuria and feign diabetic symptoms. They surely deserved an "A" for trying and for concocting dramatic schemes to return to family and loved ones, for Alaska in war times is no beach party.

One feature that intrigued and delighted me in Alaska was the northern lights, known as the Aurora Borealis. It was an electrifying, fascinating display of bright, shimmering, shuddering, darting fingers and spears of various shades of blue, green, gray, and yellow lights overhead in the sky. They would occur at least twice weekly in the winter sky.

When we arrived on the scene in Alaska, we were told repeatedly to hang a white paper on the wall and when it turned brown we were ready to disembark for home. I believe one of the main ways to keep our equilibrium during the time in Alaska was to keep up a good sense of humor. Another attribute was to think positively at all times and to keep smiling, keep running, and never look back. Fortunately, I kept extremely busy and developed many worthwhile friendships. I became integrated thoroughly to the black race and to the realization that color was the only difference between them and anyone else. I'm sure their intelligence is on an equal footing with any race, barring none, but generally speaking it just isn't as developed. They are arduous workers, quite affable, loyal, consistent, and persistent in their work habits. Man originated from Africa, so we should be kind and respectful to our Black brothers and sisters.

The Eskimos love dried salmon and it is known as "squaw" candy.

One of the native matrons approached me one day and asked me to get her some aspirin to combat her arthritic, painful fingers. Luckily, we just happened to be loaded to the gill slits with aspirin. In fact we had a trunk, full of this drug left over from World War I and honestly, it was still functional, although as hard as a rock. It would dissolve if softened with a hammer. I gave her a generous supply of our "modern" version of aspirin and she promised to make an Eskimo outfit from hat to mukluks for my darling 3 year-old daughter, Susan. I had really become oblivious to this promise, but, lo and behold, in about six weeks this native lady presented me with a really beautiful, complete little girl's ensemble from stem to stern. There was quite an odor to the rabbit fur and I learned that the Eskimos cure the furs with human urine. After thoroughly airing out this furry clothing, I boxed it and mailed it to my wife at 221 N. Lincoln in Bay City. I thought, Doris and Susan will love this regal outfit, but, alas! They had the opposite reaction and discarded it with disdain because of unrelenting olfactory odor.

During my entire Alaskan duty of 27 months, I had only one furlough of 10 days for a home visit. It came a year after my entrance to Alaska, on February 10th 1943. I clearly remember when our plane took off from Elmendorf Field in Anchorage. We were over loaded with passengers and equipment, and our C-47 just barely escaped upwards at the very end of the runway. What a thrill! We all had bucket seats (metal only) and our first stop was Edmonton, Alberta Province, about a five hour run. We flew north to Fairbanks, then south along the Alaskan Highway. Edmonton is a thriving, bustling, large city teeming with intense activity as the hub and capital of central Alberta, almost 500 miles directly east of Calgary. Our next flight took us to Minneapolis, and thence to Detroit and the Tri-Cities Airport. Doris was reaching the 35th week of her gravid state with number one son, Tom. My visit served as a picker-upper, but a drastic let down when I returned to Anchorage. Tom was born on April 21st 1943, about 2 months after my home furlough. My contagion nurse, Hester Stilabauer, Lt. Colonel Albrecht, Captain Olson, and I broke out a bottle of champagne (bubbly) and lit up "It's a Boy" cigars in celebration. Little did I know it would be 13 long months (centuries) before I would see my first son in the flesh, head to head, and then I would be a total stranger to him, as Doris had to assume double parentage.

During my first year in "Seward's Icebox" Lt. Colonel Albrecht flew to Seattle on two occasions and was rewarded with an adopted baby on each sortie. My close friendship with the colonel designated me as the pediatrician to render medical care for his babies. He and I would journey to Palmer, 50 miles northeast, each weekend to check out the little critters. Apparently, there was some cogent reason that he and wife, Lucy, were barren and unable to bear children. Albrecht had an old Packard and usually turned over the driving duties to me. I didn't mind these trips one iota for the drive was really picturesque, over narrow, mountainous dirt and macadam roads. In the spring and summer we would pass through miles of gorgeous yellow and red flowers. Lucy Albrecht was a large; happy go lucky, intelligent mother to the babies and carried out instructions to the letter. The infants thrived under her tutelage and were immensely healthy for they never came in contact with the outside world.

Mrs. Albrecht told me about her multiple experiences with black bears while she was hanging clothes, planting flowers, or working in the garden. Vegetables and fruit had a short growing season over a 2 1/2 months period with temperatures usually around 60 to 70 degrees Fahrenheit and seldom as high as 80 degrees, tops. One time I had a picture taken while holding a thirty-five pound cabbage and it was somewhat of a task for me. The strawberries, raspberries and tundra berries were huge, one would fill a cup, but they were pretty much all water. Actually, you could practically see them grow in July under the "midnight sun". Major Marbut was an excellent photographer with much artistic talent. He enlarged three pictures I had of Doris, colored, and framed them. They turned out spectacularly realistic. They enhanced her natural beauty to the nth degree.

It was a production which would put a professional photographer to shame. He enlarged two other pictures, one of the surrounding snow-covered mountain peaks and the other of Palmer in the Matanuska Valley. His talent truly was explicitly outstanding and verily incredible. Major Marbut was a prime coffee klatcher. When asked "How do you like your java?", he would respond "I like my coffee strong and my women weak."

Christmas was the loneliest, longest day of the year, but our Christmas packages were a Godsend of enlightenment. We would all cheer each other and commiserate with one another. We just had to tighten our belts, keep a stiff upper lip, and bite the bullet. We did have three U.S.O. visits from Hollywood actors and actresses. Two special actresses that came our way were Olivia DeHaviland and Ingrid Bergman. One renowned actor, who found us was the "lady killer" Errol Flynn. Olivia DeHaviland was fresh from her appearance in "Gone with the Wind" along with her leading gentleman, Leslie Howard. She shared a noon luncheon with all the M.D.'s. After our repast Colonel Albrecht said, "Captain Knobloch, would you kindly give Miss DeHaviland the cook's tour of our Station Hospital?" I replied, "Colonel, if that's an order, I will gladly acquiesce with the utmost pleasure, immediately"; whereupon I promptly escorted Miss Olivia to every nook and cranny of our hospital and it's environs. During our tour she told me she was born in Tokyo, Japan, as her father was the U.S.A. envoy to the empire of the "Rising Sun" at that time. She didn't reveal her year of birth, and I was shrewd enough to beg the question. Also, she related that after the big picture of "Gone With The Wind," was shown in Tokyo, headlines appeared in the Tokyo newspaper, "Local Girl Makes Good in the Movies". Olivia's tour covered the South Pacific, England, and Africa to entertain the GIs. I was impressed with her charming, down to earth, humble conversation and innate beauty. She indubitably embodied the "lady fatale"; and I believe her charisma could charm a cobra. Poor me!

Ingrid Bergman gave us a classic acting performance. She seemed to be very intelligent and was a basic, what you see is what you get, high-class lady. The Colonel did not ask me to escort Ingrid around the hospital, but decided to fulfill this gracious duty himself. Errol Flynn came with a bevy of beautiful ladies and put in a flamboyant, swashbuckling appearance. I don't believe I have ever seen a more handsome man without makeup and a personality which would mesmerize a toad. Intellectually, he was an airhead and gave the semblance of life was just a bowl of cherries. Indubitably, his social genes predominated to a high degree with hedonic pursuits his forte. Surely, he would never succumb to depression.

There was one gorgeous nurse who worked on the officers' ward and who was given a sobriquet of "The Blonde Bomber". Maybe we had been in the wilds too long, but she was a reasonable facsimile of Marilyn Monroe.

She had all of the male hearts, especially the older officers, beating in triple rhythms. However, it was useless for she had a sweetheart (a private soldier) in Whittier, about 60 miles southeast of Anchorage and she would go there every weekend. Jenny loved the younger, more virile type men. It was like that song, "Go Away Old Man, Go Away". She really was devastatingly lovely, but she was well aware of her attributes including a <u>sound</u> mind.

We really did have one special battle in late 1944 at the chain island of Attu, in which the entire 10,000 Japanese retinue was annihilated for we didn't take any prisoners. The men in combat swear that the "streams ran red" as the Japanese were herded to the extreme eastern part of the island. We had a superior force and weapons, and it was just like shooting fish in a barrel. Few of our men were killed, but we did have large, severe casualties (1300) with Immersion Foot Disease because of improper, faulty footgear. Instead of having shoe pack boots like Colonel Castner advised the San Francisco Headquarters, the big shot Army generals decided our soldiers should wear regular, old-fashioned, cheaper Army leather high-top boots. The temperatures during the battle were in the twenties Fahrenheit and the terrain (tundra and rivers) was almost knee deep with freezing water. Therefore, the water went through the leather boots like a sieve. The combat lasted three days and after immersing feet and legs for long-time intervals, the circulation in the lower extremities became frozen with little or no movement or oxygen. This caused necrosis and gangrene (death) of these tissues. All 1300 of these wet, hypothermal injury cases came through out station hospital. The more serious, almost gangrenous feet and lower leg cases were sent packing to Seattle. Less injured cases remained for physical therapy rehab. They responded very slowly to heat, massage, whirlpool and graduated exercises. After weeks and months of gradual recovery, they were sent back to the States for reassignment and further medical care.

Our second debacle with the Japanese occurred on the Island of Kiska about four months after the Attu skirmish. Colonel Castner was in charge of this pseudo battle and was slated for Brigadier General if the outcome was successful. Castner was a champion of survival in the wilderness and was a "Buffalo Bill" type of caveman, existing against primitive nature with only his own ability to survive. Unfortunately, the Japanese personnel on Kiska realized our attack there was imminent. They weren't enthused about suffering the same fate as the Japanese garrison on Attu, so they evacuated the island by submarine on the night before our invasion and we were left holding an empty bag the next day. The strain of this lost battle and loss of promotion to general was too much for Colonel Castner to bear, and he developed a sudden coronary embolic heart attack. He was routed as an emergency to the officer's ward in our hospital, where I was in charge. Colonel Castner was literally heart broken mentally after the build up in preparation for several months and then the sudden let down, like pulling the rug out from under your feet with a sudden jerk. His wild anticipation had been dashed on the rocks and reduced to ashes in the wink of an eye. He had a consult with the chief of internal medicine and it was decided to rehab him with morphine, aspirin, and complete rest and relaxation, as near as possible, for six weeks. After about two weeks, he regained his sense of humor, mental composure, and reasoning. He reasoned, "Life is like a squirrel cage and a guy has to take the bitter with the sweet while working for the ultimate goals". After stabilization, Colonel Castner was transferred to Seattle for evaluation and reassignment.

After the non-battle of Kiska, we received a psychiatrist directly from that battlefield. His name was Captain Imperatrice and he truly lived up to his epithet. He was a real hard-boiled, weird, middle-aged man in whom the milk of human kindness had congealed. Actually, Imperatrice was deep in the doldrums and could see only the dark side of life. He had very little empathy with his patients and was harsh and unfeeling in relations with them. His room was only 2 doors away from mine and he always kept it locked day and night. Finally, after approximately two months, we noticed several marks on his right forearm. Colonel Albrecht sensed there was something rotten in Denmark and he confronted Imperatrice one night in his room, which was forcibly opened by the M.P.'s. Imperatrice was in a daze and had just shot himself intravenously with morphine. A cache of a trunk full of morphine was found in his room. It was taken from the Japanese on Kiska by our psychiatrist and brought to Anchorage somehow. He was arrested on the spot and sent packing to a psychedelic drug rehab center in the States. At last we gleaned an insight into his peculiar psychopathic behavior.

It seemed like every psychiatrist we received had unusual character and personality traits. The psychiatrist who replaced hard-nosed Imperatrice was strictly asocial with his fellow officers. He appeared to have a chip (plank) on his shoulder against the world and an attitude of persecution. Maybe it could be explained by his isolation in Alaska from family and constant exposure to the crazy behavior of his patients without any cushion to counteract this stress. I tried assuming the duties of psychiatrist while pinch-hitting for that position when Imperatrice left us. But, after one month, I gave up because of undue psychic pressure.

Two public health personnel were admitted to our hospital in July of 1943, with severe pain in all extremities. They had a history of killing a black bear and eating insufficiently cooked muscles. My diagnosis, at once, was trichinosis spiralis, a parasitic disease the bear had innocently acquired by eating infected pigs. There was no curative treatment available, but a biopsy of their gluteus maximus did confirm this disease. Supportive treatment was mainly ablation of pain, rest, and physical rehabilitation. I learned of this illness in medical school, but to my utter amazement, the 1998 Authoritative Textbook on Pediatric Practice, by Saunders Publications makes absolutely no mention, total blank, regarding trichinosis spiralis in its book of 1024 pages. Apparently it is quite rare now.

Another unusual occurrence was admission of a patient with toadstool poisoning. Apparently he thought he knew the difference between mushrooms and the poisonous variety of amanita, the muscatine group. The prime symptom is vomiting, dehydration, alkalosis, and electrolyte imbalance. Pumping out or evacuation of stomach contents is number one if the ingestion has been within 12 hours. Also IV normal saline or lactate ringers can be started as soon as possible if the patient is in or near extremis exchange transfusion or intraperitoneal dialysis may be considered. Our patient made an uneventful, complete recovery in 48 hours.

Another uncanny experience occurred on a wintry night when an army private entered the dispensary complaining of heavy, purulent, penile discharge. A quick gram stain slide of the emission revealed the gram negative diploid intracellular gonococcus to be the guilty offender. History was that he had intercourse with a native, Alaskan female in the street at 20 degrees below zero Fahrenheit. Apparently, Mother Nature conquered the weather, impossible, as it seems. A big penicillin shot was curative and restorative to instant active duty.

I remember a case of epiglottitis that hit me with a bang one morning while I was making routine daily rounds on the contagion ward. Casually I examined this young GI's throat and suddenly on visualization there appeared a cherry red swelling, filling the space between the tongue root and the pharynx. There was an electrifying realization. This was the epiglottitis, the lid that covers your trachea (tube to the lungs) when you swallow. Any inflammation or tumescence of the epiglottis can impede swallowing, breathing, or speech and contribute to aspiration of food in the lungs. Mainly, it can shut off the airway and prevent exchange of air to and from the pulmonary organs. This can lead to cessation of breathing and finally death. I noticed that his speech was soft, slurred, and barely audible or understandable. A feeling of dire urgency swept over me and I took him stat to the treatment room to start an IV of sulfa, our only reliable antibiotic at the time. I held my breath (figuratively) for a few hours, giving him one on one care. By evening the swelling was lessening, the color was receding to pink, and his signs and symptoms were ameliorating. Heaving a sigh of relief, I said a prayer of thanks to our Creator for pulling him out of the woods.

A humorous incident to arouse our consciousness happened one spring fever day when the Military Police reported a lost locomotive. It was last seen near Portage, about forty miles from Anchorage. This must be a joke, we surmised, but a week went by and after intensive searching night and day, no locomotive! Our commanding general, Emmons, in desperation said, "A watched kettle never boils so let's abandon the search." Sure enough, a month later, the "lost locomotive" turned up in Anchorage as big as life. No one ever came forward and we were left in the dark as to the whereabouts and adventures of the missing locomotive.

One of my missions was to investigate a so-called epidemic of hepatitis at a small Army medical installment at Homer on Cook Inlet, sixty miles south of Seward by railroad. It turned out to be a false alarm as the signs, symptoms, and blood tests for antigens were all imaginary. The doctors and nurses believed each other had jaundiced (yellow) sclerae, abdominal cramping, dark urine, and pale stools. They were injecting each other with 4,000 units of penicillin every four hours A.T.C. (around the clock). I checked their bilirubin, ALT and AST (liver enzymes), blood counts, LDH, and alkaline phosphates and found them all to be normal. I disillusioned them and exposed their fake "epidemic" to Colonel Albrecht. This situation mimicked medical students who contracted every disease they studied.

Our contagion ward patients were the only ones who received whole liquid cow's milk because of our tuberculosis cases. Every other patient and hospital personnel received powdered milk, which really was not too bad once you got inured to it.

There was a huge lottery concerning the exact time in day, minute and second that the Tenana River Ice Cap in Fairbanks would begin to melt and liquefy. Just about every person in Alaska would feverishly bet on this proposition because the winner would get a fabulous sum of money, well over a million dollars. This lottery had been in vogue for eons, since the Russians had invaded Alaska. We all bought tickets with about as much chance of winning as a snowball surviving at the equator, maybe more. Anyhow, "What fools these mortals are!" We all defied the odds and entered the contest hook line and sinker. No one I knew won.

I studied the state of vitamin C in our soldiers in Alaska by checking their blood levels to determine if any deficiency existed. Symptoms and signs of scurvy were also minutely investigated. As expected, our results were practically 100% negative. Colonel Albrecht, who asked me to make the study, and all the "top brass" felt reassured that out dietary fare, especially vitamin C, was definitely in order.

Col. Albrecht, ordered me to make several trips during my 27 months duty. My most memorable excursion was the trip to McGrath, Bethel, and Goodnews

Bay, all on the Kuskokwim River, which parallels the mighty Yukon southerly and empties into the Bering Sea. McGrath was merely a "whistle stop" for a few hours, but at Bethel there was a medium large army installation on an island in the middle of the Kuskokwim River, about ten miles up river by motorboat from Bethel. At Bethel, there was a Lutheran Church and a U.S. Government Hospital of 20 beds. There were two medical officers, Captain William Jackson (a distant descendant of Stonewall), and a surgeon. Captain Hoyle. The purpose of my visit there was to assess the quality of medical care in the army unit and the hospital. The care rendered at the hospital was adequate and consisted mainly of acute and chronic ear, nose, throat, and sinus infections with viral pneumonia and suspected pulmonary thithis ever present. I worked in the dispensary with Jackson each day of my week there and on one occasion removed a foreign body imbedded in the cornea – very gently.

Capt. Jackson related an unusual occurrence that happened to him one night at a dance being held on the post. Music was furnished by phonograph and the ladies were Aleuts, Eskimos, and Indians from nearby villages, transported by canoes. Jackson was dancing with one of the girls and tried to strike up a conversation but she was mysteriously silent and aphonic the entire dance. After the dance ended, he saw her older sister and queried why her sibling wouldn't return his speech. She replied in a loud voice, "Well, Captain, she hasn't been f-----much." Bill confided to me that his face turned scarlet and he wished to hide under the floor. But this was normal behavior for the native; candid, honest explanations and Marquis of Queensbury rules.

After four days of inspection, I flew on to Goodnews Bay, located at the beginning of the volcanic Aleutian Chain. The army personnel there were engaged in extracting and purifying several minerals from ore surface mined locally. These included iron, lead, zinc, tin, and silver in moderate quantities, which were transported back to the states. I spent two days there and returned to my home base at the 182 Station Hospital.

There were two overnight fishing trips. One by myself and my sergeant to the Susitna River, twenty miles by car, northwest of Anchorage and the other to Krechbak Bay, 500 miles southwest, with Albrecht, Hirsch and Eveland. We caught about fifty sizable trout at the Bay and I have a photograph to prove this statement. The fish were real battlers, caught by flies. Fishing here was practically primeval as the fish were heavily stocked and hungry. All a fisherman had to do was throw in the bait and in no time there was a 25-30 inch fish on the line. It was virtually a fisherman's paradise where finesse and piscatorial art were not required. We also would reserve wintry Sundays for ice fishing. The ice on nearby lakes would be 1 to 2 feet thick and we would all take turns at cracking the ice with spuds (long poles with a chipper on the end). We did have some lighter moments.

There were also air journeys to Juneau, Annette Island, Yakastat, and Prince Rupert, to check the health and dismissal of their units. The Juneau junket was a three day affair. I did meet a charming young lady, my age, at a dance in Juneau. Douglas and she invited me to dinner the following day. But we were both married and her partner was a fisherman away on a fishing expedition. After considerable cogitation, I got cold feet and called her the next afternoon and told her a little white lie, that I was sorry to cancel our dinner date because of a sudden, immediate recall back to Anchorage. My old fashioned religion kicked in, and apparently judgment was victorious.

In Juneau, Victor Pluvius, the rain god, holds full sway as there is an average rainfall of 148 inches yearly, which leads to vitamin deficiency diseases, i.e.: rickets, pellagra, and scurvy among its inhabitants.

The trip to Annette Island near Ketchikan was really special. There I met Captain Jim Nelson and we had a ball touring the island and visiting Ketchikan, a fairly populous and thriving city (for Alaska) located on the panhandle in the southern Inland Passage, near Wrangell and Petersburg. Landing a plane at the Annette Island Airfield is a breeze compared to landing and taking off at the Juneau Airbase. The Annette runway approach is flat as a pancake, whereas the Juneau approach is perilous because the airfield is situated at the bottom of a cup of surrounding mountains. The plane must fly into this air runway, making several circles while gradually descending until it hits bottom. Captain Nelson and I did some fishing and it was the strategic time of the Humpback Salmon run upstream. Watching literally for hours, I was amazed at how the Humpies would take several runs at the falls until exhausted or successful in going upstream to lay their eggs.

The ride to Yakutat comprised about 400 miles directly east of Anchorage. I visited Captain Zelvin and his first aid station. Phil had been on the post with me at the Elmendorf field hospital for several months and he was in charge of a medical ward there. Yakutat was strictly a fishing village and I visited a large fishing company engaged in packing, freezing, and transporting the caught fish to the U.S.A. Zelvin was a very nice, middle aged gentleman, of Jewish heritage, from Brooklyn stateside. He was a born optimist, happy go lucky man, who knew how to roll with the punches and was reconciled to not swimming upstream.

The Prince Rupert junket was a brief trip by air and boat to the southernmost city of the Alaskan panhandle. It has a moderately wet climate, warmed by the Japanese pacific current and borders on Midwestern British Columbia. It is built high on a steep hill just off the coast of the Pacific Ocean. The time was near the end of April 1945, so I put in a telephone call to Bay City as we were not permitted to call from Alaska previously. After an interminable time, I finally got connected to my wife, Doris, (if I still had one!) and all hell broke loose. I was so filled with ecstasy and euphoria at hearing Doris's voice that several soldiers came rushing into my room, thinking that I was delirious and had gone off the deep end. It was really quite a thrill for me to talk with my spouse, after two years' separation, and my son whom I had never seen and was one year old!

I forgot to mention a highlight which occurred when I toured Bethel at the government hospital. Captain Hoyle was the medical officer in charge of the patients there. One morning when I visited the hospital to make rounds, Captain Hoyle, M.C. greeted me excitedly, as though I was his long lost brother. He blurted, "Boy, am I glad to see you! We just admitted a fresh newborn, pre-term baby boy weighing 5 ½ lbs, delivered in the early morning hours today in a canoe on the Kuskokwim River." Amazed, I said, "Is my hearing correct? Did you say delivered by the father in a canoe while on the way down the Kuskokwim River to the hospital?" Being knee deep in pediatrics until before the army, I embraced this distinct opportunity with gusto, right up my alley. The baby was in an incubator for a warm up, rest, and to preserve hydration. After learning from the father that there was no unusual blood loss and he had securely tied the baby's cord with a shoelace and cut the umbilical cord with his teeth, I performed a microscopic quick exam on the baby. The vital signs were stable, his peripheral pulses were in order, and his cry would arouse the deaf. The external body and facial features were intact, but lo and behold there was no anus present! It was an imperforate anus! I related the presence of this congenital anomaly to Dr. Hoyle. After a lengthy detailed consideration of all options, we decided to promptly institute intravenous normal saline solution and wait 24 hours for equilibration of vitals and adjustment of the circulatory system to the outside world. Imperforate anus is a malformation of the rectum consisting of complete absence of an anal opening, sometimes a dimple where the anus should be, whereby bowel movement elimination is totally obstructed. The incidence is slightly higher in boys, but overall is in the neighborhood of 1 in 4000 or 5000, according to pediatric surgeon, Edward Austin of Saginaw, MI. There are three main types of Imperforate Anus, 43% low (trans elevator) 18% intermediate, less common, and 13% high (supralevator) The risk for accompanying genital or upper urinary tract or spinal abnormalities is increased the higher the level of imperforation and is also increased for boys. This little man's anorectal malformation was high, as evidenced by a small dimple in the approximate location where the anus should have been. The only thing we could do for our patient was to perform a colostomy or create an artificial opening on the right abdomen at the site of the cecum. This would allow passage of intestinal contents which is quite essential to life. He withstood the operation, which required one hour under very light anesthesia. I did the anesthesia with drop ether, with nary a problem. Abdominal flat plate x-ray gave us a hint of the whereabouts of the bowel end location. He was dispatched by plane to Children's Hospital at University of Washington, in Seattle, along with a nurse on the second post-operative day with IV running and frequent small formula feedings. When the baby was grown to about 25 lbs heft, he would have a definite rectal pull through and repair of any rectourethral fistula. This event made my trip to Bethel worthwhile.

Before my departure to return to the states from Alaska, I was visited by two notable Army Medical Corps Physicians. Captain Larry Reck came to Fort Richardson on his way back to San Diego, California, and civilian life. He had served two years in the army installations at Kotzbue and Nome as a medical officer. He was, and is, a pediatrician around my age and had many interesting stories to relate concerning the natives and army personnel. He got his hands wet in pediatrics and obstetrics by delivering, as emergencies, a few local mothers and caring for their newborns.

My second guest was 1st Lt M.C. Mike Medvezky who came to Anchorage via Cold Bay Army Medical post, with a diagnosis of rheumatoid arthritis on his way to an army hospital in Chicago. Mike was one of my prime buddies as a fellow family medical practitioner in Bay City. We had worked together for two years in Bay City, he as a general surgeon and I as anesthetist and consultant for his pediatric medical and surgical patients. Cold Bay weather was probably one of the worst posts in the Fox Islands in the Aleutian chain. Mike had been in service there for two years and gradually became seriously incapacitated due to swelling and pain in his hands, ankles and knees. He did some hunting and fishing as he was a true sportsman. Mike claimed it rained every day and bragged that it had to be the only place on earth where the wind blew from all four directions simultaneously. If you were voiding, he said the wind would switch 180 degrees suddenly and your urine would blow back in your face. Also, if you were leaning forward into the wind for balance, it would instantly reverse itself and you would fall forward, flat on your face. Every time I heard these weird tales, I got down on my knees and thanked my creator. Shemnya, the furthermost western army post in the Rat Islands of the chain, was probably the most rigorous and hardy of all. There were no trees in the Aleutians and on Adak, a G.I. made a wooden tree, calling it the National Forrest Reservation.

I went hunting for Ptarmigan in the winter but they were too elusive for me. Their ghost-like camouflage was beyond my reach as they are similar to pheasants, except that they turn white in winter. The mosquitoes around our station D.C. hospital would hatch out in late spring and early summer. They were about ten times the average in size and you could hit them with a baseball bat. The worst pesky flying insects were swarms of tiny black no-seeum flies, in June, which had a really painful sting. The standing humorous saying was that the mosquitoes would check your dog tags to see what blood type you were before stinging you. Actually, they were slow movers, probably because of their immense heft.

Shortly before I departed from my Alaskan stay, one of my patients was an affable and spirited nurse who was afflicted by pulmonary TBC. She had an unusually cheerful perspective for having such a dire illness with unknown prognosis. Gretchen was waiting exportation back to stateside for further testing and management. One morning, during my daily rounds, I examined her and passed the time of day to elevate her spirits. Apparently I was the one who really needed an up-lift because she turned sharply to me and said, "Captain Knobloch, you look mighty depressed today. What on earth is going on?" I said, "I'm sorry if it shows for our roles should be reversed. To be honest, I haven't had a letter from my wife for a couple weeks and frankly, I am worried that something untoward may have happened to her or our daughter, Susan." Gretchen looked me straight in the eye and replied unflinchingly, "Sir, if I may be so bold as to analyze your situation with a word to the wise. When I'm in a quandary or presented with a disturbing unchangeable event, you know what I say? Yes, I say 'Piss on it' as my solution and go about my business." Changing the subject, my answer was, "I feel much better already, thank you very much for putting me back on track. I feel like a new man and realize how stupid of me to let this miniscule matter get under my skin." Gretchen stated, "Now you are talking and you are like your normal self. Don't ever forget my homespun solution to clear the air."

There were a couple bits of humor, which helped us to lighten our burden of service while sweating out our plight before returning home. They gave us a superficial cushion to mask our unctuous feelings of homesickness and to tide us over a period of stress. We would query one another with the question, '"What is the first thing you will do when you get home?" and the illogical answer was, "I'll take off my skis." Another conundrum was "What is the first thing you will say to your wife when your ship reaches Seattle?" Answer, I will shout, "Hello honey, let's F.F." But what if a verbal battle develops and she replies, "No, honey, let's E.F." Well, this friendly differential could ensue back and forth indefinitely, your stand "Honey lets F.F." and hers, "No honey, let's E.F." Finally you disgustedly agree "Okay, honey, you win let's eat first." There was absolutely nothing as important or supportive as our precious letters from home. They were undoubtedly worth their weight in platinum and the glue, which preserved our sanity and buoyed our spirits to make life worthwhile.

Chapter 18

Terminal Discharge from the U.S. Army

My 27 months duty as a medic in the army in Alaska ended, mercifully , the middle of May 1945. Before I departed I received a highly prized Certificate of Commendation from General Emmons, General of Alaskan Forces, and Colonel Albrecht, my commanding C.O. We retraced our flight path through Alaska and Canada to Minneapolis and thence to Detroit where I was greeted by my loving wife and her sprightly companion, Florence Moore. I was never so excited and happy in my life. We toured to Bay City and I was utterly oblivious to our ride home while Florence took the wheel. Florence was orthopedist Dr. Neal Moore's wife, and he was doing Army duty in the European theater at this time. Neal called Doris a name of endearment, "Mama Do-Do", to her consternation.

I received orders to proceed at once to Miami Florida for a ten day recuperation furlough. I at last got a chance to see and hold my infant son, for the first time, after 14 months of agonizing overseas duties. John Howard Thomas Knobloch and I, as expected, were total strangers to each other. It was understandable and logical since Doris fulfilled both of his needs in the double personage as mother and father for over one year, and I was merely an interloper without a mission. Actually, it took about six years before we could establish a definite bondage and true identity relationship. "Tom", as he was called, to my utter amazement, couldn't walk without support and couldn't speak words understandably – just babbles. Apparently, he had been sheltered and smothered by mother love and devotion. We gradually broke the ice and gradually nurtured an ironclad friendship.

Doris and I entrained for Miami Beach, Florida, in June via Cincinnati and the Atlantic Coast Railroad. I thought I would be incinerated by the intense heat when we hit the orange country. It was quite a switch of climates from the thirty degree Arctic Circle to the one hundred degree torrid, near equator country with only a two weeks adjustment period. The enormity of the raw heat was overwhelming, and the only relief was the cool Atlantic Ocean breezes at night. We stayed at the Grosvenour Hotel, smack dab on the beach, and enjoyed our second honeymoon. We were duly impressed by the gigantic cockroaches when we would enter our room at night after a stroll on the beach or sumptuous dinner and movie. When the light was flicked on, myriads of these creatures would fly from the walls to the shower or sink. They were about the size of a tarantula spider and exceedingly acrobatic. We did swim afternoons, but it was literally impossible to enjoy walking outdoors until late evening when the sun submerged beneath the horizon. We did see my cousin, Dorothy Haynes, and her husband and enjoyed an evening of southern hospitality at their home in Miami. Our rendezvous in Miami was extremely enjoyable but we were ecstatic to escape from the unbearable heat when we left for heavenly Bay City, incomparable mild tundra and polar bear country.

Shortly after arriving back home, I received orders to proceed to Fort Sheridan, Chicago. There, I was engaged in the process of mustering out and discharging G.I.'s from army service. While at Sheridan, I met my roommate Captain M.C. Hugh Cook, and we formed a close knit, permanent Damien and Pythias type friendship. Hugh was a gracious, euphoric, positive and erudite young man with intense desire to succeed in medicine. He had had excellent training for several years under the tutelage of famous chevalier, Jackson, number one in the profession of ololaryngologist and ENT. Dr. Jackson was especially renowned for his expertise in endoscopy. Quite often the army hierarchy would put square pegs in round holes and vice versa. To bear this travesty out, I was in charge of Ear, Nose and Throat, and Hugh was in charge of chest examinations when we gave the enlisted men their discharge physicals at Sheridan. Coincidentally, Hugh had decided to go to Bay City to set up his practice in the Allen Building when he received his army discharge.

I would often go home on weekends to socialize with my family via the New York Central Railway. Returning to Chicago was a seven to seven hour overnighter, cat napping or dozing on the rocky passenger train seat. While at Fort Sheridan, Hugh and I discussed our future plans for practice in Bay City. Also we did take in some ball games in our leisure hours. We saw the White Sox and Chicago Cubbies in baseball contests, and Northwestern football in the big-ten football league. I recall one game in particular between the Cubs and the Brooklyn Dodgers where Cub, Hack Wilson, hit a grand slam home run over the ivy covered right field wall to win the game in Hollywood style in the ninth inning.

I was in Alaska when we got the news of Franklin Delano Roosevelt's demise, in Warm Springs, Georgia, at 4p.m. on a sunny afternoon in the D.C.

station Hospital. Colonel Albrecht dispersed the news, which really was not a shocker as we knew he was gravely ill. Everyone seemed to have extreme confidence that Harry Truman could carry on ably in the presidency, to put the finishing touches to a war which was winding down. When World War II did finally end, August 14th 1945, in Europe, we celebrated with delirious happiness for we realized that our heartsick suffering away from home was showing a light at the end of the tunnel. My official honorable discharge culminated in January 1946, although I was separated from the army for all practical purposes at the end of October '45. It was a mighty grand and glorious feeling of rank liberation to be extricated from all army rules and regulations. As my final reward just before discharge, I was promoted from captain to major and given an honorable discharge. I had thought I would get my majority before I left Alaska, but the table of organization had room for only one Major M.C. promotion there. I was told Captain Carl Olson, our x-ray chief, had seniority and he was elevated to that major ahead of me.

Chapter 19

Initiation of Solo Practice in Bay City, MI.

My first priority of business was a settlement of my relationship in practice with L.Fernald Foster, my prewar partner. We decided upon mutual dissolution of our partnership after due consideration of all options. Fern and I were on excellent, friendly terms socially and mentally by sharing the same wavelength of thought. He was immensely involved with Blue Cross and Blue Shield insurance and eventually became their president in 1950. After a month living at home, I established my office practice temporarily in my pal Dr. Mike Medvezky's office in a building on the southwest corner of Farragut and Kosciusko streets. Mike kindly invited me to share his office space at no reimbursement until I established financial competence. We had always meshed gears and we would refer patients of mutual interest to each other. I would often give pediatric anesthesia to his children's surgical cases.

Mike had a huge Polish clientele in south end Bay City and we shared pediatric practice, he surgically and I medically. Our wives were staunch friends and we often would have an evening of bridge. He was a doughty business man and would always collect cash on his 40-50 daily house calls. The money for the call was often stowed away under the bedroom mattresses. Mike was born with a silver spoon in his mouth and was a real perennial winner and shark at poker games. He related winning fabulous sums of money in army poker games, while stationed at Cold Bay in the Aleutians. The soldiers had no place to spend their money and gambling was the only form of entertainment and way to spend the time. His story unravels that in one all night session, he won several thousand dollars and the following day bought one of every item in the Post Exchange. Also, Michael claims royal heritage from the Crown Duke of Austria.

After conducting pediatric practice, for three or four months in Medvezky's office, I found one of my own in a new edifice downtown on the northeast corner of Madison and Fifth Avenues, dubbed the Professional Building. It was on the second floor and there was a laundry underneath. By a stroke of good fortune, Clara Wheeler became disenchanted with her relationship binding her to Dr. Foster and became my secretary, and the chief cook and bottle washer in my office - my right arm. I was further favored by the Gods in obtaining for my nurse Betty Zacharko, a recent nursing graduate of Mercy Hospital School of Nursing. We formed a solid triumvirate and my practice in pediatrics took off like a jet plane with smooth sailing.

I reconnected to the senior pediatric staffs at Mercy and General Hospitals and joined with fellow pediatricians, Fern Foster, Bill Gronenmeyer, and Fred Chapin. Gronenmeyer also was returning from army services in WW II. Chapin had joined the Allen group of doctors in 1944 on completion of his internship at University Hospital in Ann Arbor. Coincidentally, he was rejected by the army because of a fractured right leg (tibia). The fracture resulted from a fall when he was inebriated while celebrating his entry into the army on the night before. Fred swears this is gospel truth and the fall was not perpetrated purposely. He was later joined in practice partnership by fellow pediatricians, Thomas Benjamin Wright, Albert Ellison, and Richard E. Bickham.. Chapin's first love really was psychiatry, his wife was a psychologist and after 24 years in pediatrics, he left Bay City to become a psychiatrist. This transformation was accomplished by a three year course of psychiatric training at the Mental Hospital in Traverse City.

During the war years 1943 to 1945, Bay City experienced a profound lethal epidemic of diarrhea in babies and children which was attributed to enteroinvasive escherichia (E. coli bacilli). It was very widespread and intensive and I am told the mortality rate was at least in the fifties plus. It invaded the nursery at Mercy Hospital and apparently Fred Chapin, M.D. was swamped day and night with critically ill infants and newborns. Many families described horrid, gory details of this ravishing diarrheal epidemic to me when I returned to practice.

Realistically, my pre-war pediatric families welcomed me with open arms in toto and I hardly missed a beat when I returned to reestablish my pediatric practice. My old, true blue patients welcomed me back. When we returned from service the doctors who were left holding the bag in Bay City while we were cavorting in the armed services, related gruesome tales. Apparently, P.R.U. Urmston, the medical procurement officer for the Army, had medically castrated over 50% of the local practitioners of medicine here (Bay City) in one fell swoop. There was a real dearth and shortage of M.D. physicians left for Bay County medical care. They were swamped with office patients and demands for house calls. Each doctor would alternate taking all calls all night, one at Mercy and another at General, regardless of his/her specialty. We did have one female physician, Dr Saba Kessler, in general family practice. She was the wife of Dr. Mana Kessler who specialized in Ear Nose and Throat diseases. I remember her poignantly, when she was president of our county medical society and I was its secretary. My arms were almost paralyzed at the termination of her term in office because I had to carry her for the entire year.

I believe the doctors who pinch hit for us during the war period exhibited more than the usual wear and tear aging process. Our return was like a transfusion and they welcomed us back like the "flowers in May". It was interesting that the army command wouldn't take doctors of osteopathy in the service. They made hay while the sun shone while we were absent and now the D.O.'s were on an entirely equal footing with the M.D.'s. There is no difference between the two branches academically now, except that the D.O.'s are much more congenial and affable personality wise. They have the identical training now in medical school with an addition of chiropractic manipulative skills as advocated by originator, Dr. Still, in the Civil War days. Competition is the spice of life and maybe it is best that the Osteopaths maintain their individual heritage and ideology.

My number one priority after my reconnection and allegiance with my family, was to obtain a car for transportation and making house calls. Not being too flush money wise, I settled for a 1936 Buick sedan with 140,000 miles on the speedometer and very scarce tread on the tires. Our first excursion in July '46, was to Baltimore to visit Doris' relatives and show off our two wonderful children. We hadn't traveled more than fifteen miles, on the Lincoln Highway, when to our abject consternation, a right front tire blew out. Fortunately, I was able to control the car's thrust and stop on the right side of the highway. After changing the exploded tire with a shaky spare tire and wheel, our next stop was a tire shop in Ligonier, Pennsylvania, about ten miles from Greensburg, our travel intervention. Following the purchase of four safe, rideable, second hand Goodyear's, we proceeded uneventfully to the Gibson residence in the suburb of Hamilton in Baltimore, where we repaired our frayed nerves. Aunt Nettie Gibson welcomed us with open arms like a mother hen finding her lost chicks. Johnny beamed with boastful pride when he saw our darling Susan and J.H. Thomas. Of course, he was ecstatic to see daughter Doris, the apple of his eye. Nettie was a cook par excellence and she whipped up our culinary favorites, including those scrumptious, unbeatable brownies.

A cold spell enveloped Bay City from our "friendly" neighbor to the north, Canada, on, of all times, the 4th of July '46, with temperatures in the twenties Fahrenheit. Fortunately there was some bituminous coal in the basement of 221 N Lincoln and I actually built a fire in the furnace on July 4! The following day we got lucky and had a torrid blast from our "friendly" neighboring country to the south, Mexico, and our temperature escalated to the nineties Fahrenheit. This is a sample of how capricious and flighty our Michigan weather can be. The meteorologists with all their toys are correct about 50% of the time and cannot be blamed for committing suicide if worse comes to worse. There is never a dull moment weather wise in Michigan, with constant change and surprises from the every day to day variation. It's thrilling once you become acclimated.

Clara Wheeler separated a long lasting association with Dr. Foster mainly because of his inordinate and exorbitant love for the female gender of the species. Apparently, his Don Juan characteristics earned him this reputation statewide, for I was warned about it several times before I left Marquette. A large proportion of the doctors and nurses, locally, would query me about his proclivity and weakness for feminine charms. In fact, doctor dalliance relationships were not uncommon here, and there was a tale concerning a prominent doctor who was murdered in his office by a jealous husband who pushed him through a large second story window on Center Avenue. Medical duties and affairs of the heart are incompatible, similar to oil and water.

Chapter 20

Pediatric Practice - 1946 to 1951

It is a well known fact that many lonesome women do fall in love with their doctors. My Grandfather Haines often would sagely advise his male grandchildren, "Don't let your pecker go overboard with your brains". I believe this paramour behavior of Fern's was a paramount reason I wanted to dissolve our partnership.

A mysterious incident developed shortly after we returned home from our Miami, Florida vacation. I was invited to a stag, card party by my friendly neighbor, Elson Hood, who lived directly across the street from our Lincoln Street residence. I consented to Elson, for it was a welcoming celebration for my return home from the army. Elson was sports director for Bay County and I knew his older sister, Georgia, who taught sports activities at Northern Michigan College, in Marquette. She would play tennis with Scott Harris and I, as this institution was just across the street from my children's clinic at Marquette General Hospital. An incident involving my daughter, Susan, (age 5 years), and Elson occurred one day when he was visiting me and he was holding Susie on his lap. Suddenly, while we were deeply engaged in conversation, and out of a clear blue sky, without any warning, Susan clobbered Elson on his forehead with a toy engine, bringing a gush of blood. She got our undivided attention stat, if that was her purpose. I apologized profusely and put in a suture to stop the bleeding. Susan was noted for her pranks and did an identical repeat job on my father while he was asleep in the arms of Morpheus one afternoon. When I told my wife that I was going out to a card party at Elson's that evening, she blushed and angrily, in a vehement voice said, "No you're not." I couldn't comprehend the reason for this dynamic negative response and said, "Elson Hood is my friend and I promised him I would be there." She replied, "If you go, don't come home." Doris wouldn't divulge her specific reason for her attitude and stormed out of the room. The only explanation I could conceive for her behavior was that some untoward confrontation had occurred between Doris and Elson in my absence. I believe I can imagine what this happening was, so I decided to let sleeping dogs lie, dropped the issue, and remained home that night. However, I did telephone his home and spoke to his wife, Sylvia, stating, "I am very sorry, but it is impossible for me to consummate my invitation to Elson's card party tonight, but I'll take a rain check." I never did ascertain why my spouse reacted positively so negatively, except possibly he made some unwanted romantic advances toward her.

I would be sorely remiss if I didn't extol Mrs. Laura Boelte's superlative qualities as caretaker for our children. She was a venerable bulwark of strength and benevolence for all four of our progeny. Laura lived in a cute little domicile diagonally across the street from us. Mr. Boelte was afflicted with coronary heart disease and succumbed to it shortly after coming to Bay City from Monotowoc, Wisconsin. Laura was an eternally happy, optimistic, benign elderly woman who had a positive way with our children. She was afflicted with severe allergic dermatitis which baffled her physician, Dr. Sam Horowitz. He was very adept at ameliorating her frequent flare ups of eczema in all flexures of her body skin. Scratch skin testing for multiple allergens was ineffectual. Cortico-steroidal ointments, along with benadryl did render her a measure of relief from the intense desire to scratch all itchy, inflamed flexures of arms and legs. Cool wet compresses and mineral oil were also a boon for survival and insomnia.

When I came to Bay City, my membership in the First Reformed Church in Greensburg, Pennsylvania, was extinguished for there were no Reformed Churches here. My pediatric partner, Dr. Foster, was a staunch pillar of the First Presbyterian Church on Center Avenue and Jackson. After attending a few sessions of this Presbyterian church, and being introduced to the Reverend, Dr. Roblee and some congenial parishioners, I decided to join in May 1941. The First Presbyterians here resembled almost exactly our Reformed Church services back home, so I transferred my church membership. When I was interning at the University of Michigan Hospital in Ann Arbor, I often attended Sunday services at the First Presbyterian services there and found them quite favorable. Doris joined the Catholic church at Saint Boniface on McKinley and Lincoln, just a hop skip and jump from the Foster residence on McKinley and Johnson Streets. I later shared several pleasant years with the deacons and elders of the Presbyterian Church. I assisted Fern in the care of the Roblee children when the boss was away.

My father and I went on a happy, most memorable fishing trip in August of 1946, with Dr. Clyde Tarter and his son, Jimmy, to Batchawanna Bay in Ontario Canada, just a wee bit north of Lake Huron. I'm no shakes as a fisherman, but it was by far the best outing I ever had with my Dad. It contained about a week in golden moments. We went out in the bay with a professional navigator in his ship and caught trout, whitefish, and walleyes. There is no delicacy superior to freshly pan fried catch of the day. What a juicy, succulent, ultimate delicacy and gastronomic delight! Our breakfasts were loaded with the most wonderful fresh eggs, direct from the hen house, homemade, grade A sausages, homemade butter and bread and buttermilk flapjacks were also incomparable. We did go fishing in the Blind River but the current was a bit turbulent from recent rain and wind storms. My Dad and I enjoyed several games of catch baseball with the ball he caught from a foul ball struck by Gus Suhr of the Pittsburgh Pirates at Forbes Field in Pittsburgh, circa June 1932. We basked in the warm rays of sun in pure relaxation without any worry. I've never, ever enjoyed such a delightful vacation with no telephone dictating and commanding me to interrupt my sleep saying "Go to the ER, stat".

Alas, unbeknownst to my father and I, it would be our last big hurrah together because he died from a stroke in May of 1950 at the age of 64. Even in death he looked like a younger man of around the late forties with nary a grey hair. To me, my father was a saint. Never did I hear him ever say an evil word about anyone regardless of their provocation. Rarely did he lose his temper, not even once a year, and he was most adamant about the usage of alcohol. Once yearly, at midnight on December 31st, he would imbibe one ounce of scotch in celebration of the New Year. He lived and breathed sports and loved children and animals. He always carried a smile and a song in his heart. He took me to church faithfully every Sunday and took engineering courses continually at Penn State University. He encouraged me to the hilt in my schoolwork and was profoundly happy when I finished with high honors in all my elementary grades and ranked tenth in my Greensburg High School graduating class of 245. It seemed as though he was living his life through me for he was rudely jerked out of 8th grade to help support his family of seven children, when John (his Father) died from alcoholism. Apparently John was a master of newspaper printing, shortened by his untimely death.

In December, 1945 I reentered the private practice of pediatrics going bare and alone entirely on my own merits. Up until now, I was nurtured, protected and supported, under the wing of my mentors, hospitals and the U.S. Army. It was now or never, and with a stout heart and a bit of trepidation I decided that with all my experience under fire and with expert tutelage I was ripe for solo practice.

There were six doctors with me in the Professional Building when I reestablished my practice. To my east was Dr. Neal Moore, orthopedic surgeon, and his father, Dr. George Moore, family physician who practiced a lifetime in Munger, Michigan. Dr. Neal was not boarded in orthopedics, but there were <u>none</u> better in this medical specialty. He also persuaded Dr.

John S. Campbell to join him in orthopedic practice. John had trained at Duke University and Ashville, North Carolina, and had just taken his orthopedic board exams. To my west were Dr. Jim Connelly and Dr. Michael Dardas. Jim was a general family practitioner and was closely aligned with Dr.'s Matt Slattery and Mike Medvezky, professionally and socially. Mike Dardas was a benevolent, happy go lucky obstetrician, and a true friend of mine with unlimited empathy for his patients. To the west and north of me, was Dr. S. Franklin Horowitz, a premier general family practitioner of Napoleonic habitués with a profound interest in surgery. Frank did tonsil and adenoidectomies and I would administer the anesthetics. His office was a virtual pharmacy and he dispensed practically all medications to his patients. Frank had several associate nurses and would administer to two hundred plus patients through his office each day. His nurses would see at least ½ to ¾ of his patients. They would run his office traffic on days when he was away, which were far and few between. There were occasional instances when a patient would have a serious allergic reaction to a shot of penicillin or other I.M. medication and his office staff would face the dire predicament of an emergency with possible demise. His buddy, surgical partner Clyde Tarter, might or might not be available at the time to help them resolve this sticky problem.

I resumed my hectic schedule of a five day week, morning, afternoon and evening office appointments and Saturdays 9a.m. until noon or whenever as needed. I also made every day hospital rounds and responded to house calls and the emergency room at Mercy and General Hospitals when necessary. House calls were dwindling in number because auto transportation was freely available to almost everybody and time was precious and of the essence. Doctors could do much improved examinations and treatments in the office where they had adequate equipment. I frequently had to chase the patients from under the beds and off the ceiling with a mite more than gentle persuasion. I've always been truly amazed at the innate strength of the "terrible twos" and even the strength of 6 to 12 month old infants. Sometimes it would take three adults to restrain one poor "helpless" little one. I had a special hold for those life and immortal struggles whereby the mother would, in a sitting position, hold the child in a sitting position on her lap with both the child's lower extremities firmly held between the mother's legs, the mothers left arm wrapped firmly around the child's chest and holding both arms against the body and using the right arm and hand to support the head in the upright position. It was a trick I had learned during internship and it really worked to perfection. Sometimes with a particularly stubborn and resistant child, I would employ a mild Mickey Finn sedation to spare the timid mother's musculature. The strong nurses would also render a helping hand to corral the toddlers and preschoolers.

These were the penicillin intramuscular days and most children had a rigid aversion to "shots". No amount of verbiage could or would convince them otherwise. It comes to mind on two specific occasions while the mothers were holding the little ones for an injection, that the syringe holding the penicillin became disengaged from the needle hub "accidentally" during the struggle and the penicillin sprayed all over the mother's clothing, arms, and face. It was a most embarrassing moment and I had much explaining to do to keep peace in the family.

One of the benevolent tricks I learned in the army was sharing "on call" nights and weekends with my peer pediatricians. In this way, we could enjoy family life and share home duties and nights out with our wives. In addition, we could give prime time to our children and help our harassed partners with discipline and setting limits for our children. We also had time to referee the children's battles among themselves. The fathers usually have better control and command over the kinder mothers. It's probably due to being with the moms for 24 hours a day and familiarity will breed contempt. Whereas the fathers are usually away for at least half a day at work and usually there is a love fest when he arrives home. When he speaks with a deep stentorian voice, with a few well chosen words, the kids "listen up". The father is the behavior moderator and means business and no foolishness when he admonishes the children. Whereas the mothers, with their tender hearts, can't say no; and if they do say no, the off springs know they really mean maybe and they can usually twist mother's arm and get their ends accomplished. We never used physical punishment with our little ones, but we drew a line and their punishment was time outs for cooling off periods in their bedrooms.

I talked with Dr's Foster and Chapin about drawing up an on call schedule for weekends at first, from Saturday noon until Monday, 7 a.m. Fred Chapin and I remained in Bay City the entire call weekend, but Fernie had a cottage on Lake Huron near AuGres and he retreated there every weekend. When he had the call duty, he would take calls from his AuGres abode. Apparently, the parents calling him, accepted the space between them as being perfectly okay, for everyone was used to this behavior. Fern's mellifluous voice and persuasive logic could pacify a raging bull and sell snowballs to Eskimos. I don't believe I have ever seen a person with more hypnotic magnetism. Many times I have seen a client enter his office with sheer blood in his/her eyes and after a few seconds melt with loving kindness under his magic spell. One incident strikes my memory forcefully. A healthy, one year old that I treated with a DPT (diphtheria, pertusses and tetanus) shot, had a violent adverse anaphylactoid reaction. The mother erupted with blood and thunder and Fern entered the picture pronto and quelled her anger before you could say Jack

Robinson. He saved my bacon one other time when a diarrheic child, died suddenly and unexpectedly for no apparent reason even with an autopsy. The grandfather erupted in anger and Dr. Foster went into his dance and extricated me with his soothing gentle persuasion. Later on, when Doctors Ellison, Wright, and Bickham joined Dr Chapin in his pediatric group practice, we established a true, weekend alternating call system which was unparalleled. Still later, we acquired Dr's. Sundara and Devonagondi, both of Indian (India) extraction as fellow pediatricians. Finally, Dr. Felick and Dr. Hendrickson broke the female pediatric barrier and joined our ranks as a fellow pediatric peer.

Anesthesia fascinated me to no end and I devoted a large share of my work time to rendering ether anesthesia to children and infants undergoing pediatric surgery. Initially, for a couple years, Foster, Urmston, and I teamed up for "kitchen" and office tonsil and adenoidectomies (T & A's). Then we became "modernized" to hospital performance of anesthesia. However, to my knowledge, we never, (never say never) had any problem with home operations and postoperative bleeding was rare as hens' teeth. I also did T & A's with Clyde Tarter, S Franklin Horowitz, Robert Criswell, Knute Sherman, and Hugh Cook. Actually, I averaged 10 to 20 T & A's a week at my heyday. I also gave anesthetics for family surgeons, Mike Medvezky, Ed Miller, Pit Husted, Bob Gunn, Dick Scrafford, Mike Dardas, Orlen Johnson, Bob Crissey, Jimmy Wilcox, and Ed Taheri. I believe that my intense anesthetic training at Union Memorial Hospital lit a fire under me for I really enjoyed being an anesthetist, despite its life and death responsibilities and very dangerous propensities. My only death on the operating table came with ether anesthesia, rendered to eminent surgeon Ed Miller's patient. An 80 year old "young" lady was pronounced "safe" for surgery by pro "Bo" Mosier, a generalist family physician. I gave her practically no anesthetic and the operation was "only" a cyst removal from the neck that Ed said would just take 5 to 10 minutes to extract. Realistically, it took over 2 1/2 hours to remove with all of its roots, and she did leave the operating room alive, but expired in recovery. A post mortem revealed a lady with extensive myocardial infarction and coronary thrombosis. She may have survived with tracheal intubation but this is very doubtful. After that one fatality, I decided to irrevocably stop doing adult anesthesia. Up until then, I had given many, many adult sodium pentathol IV anesthetics for M.D.'s Horowitz and Tarter, and had never run into any trouble. Other than T & A children's surgery, I anesthetized for pyloric stenosis (youngest was a week old, 4 lb preemie), eye muscle surgery, hernia, intussusceptions, burn grafts, myringotomies (ear drums) fractures, and even brain tumors for Taheri. Our first bona-fide anesthesiologist was Walt Pelczar, who did family practice in Unionville for a few years before taking a course in anesthesia at the University of Michigan. Then we had anesthesiologist doctors, Leo McSherry, Nick Tsonka, and

John T. Genesco. I remember John T. G. vividly as my golf partner when we were invited to a golf outing in Kalamazoo by Upjohn. In fact, we were bunkmates one night and we hitched a night airplane ride back to Bay City with Jim Cooper sans flying instruments. John T. G. was a premier, astute anesthetist who contracted pulmonary TBC and had a lethal coronary attack in the late sixties.

Speaking of golf, my prime favorite sport and pastime for all seasons, I joined the Bay City Country Club in 1947. It was my first serious experience with the links, although I had slugged a few balls at Mountain Inn while a senior in high school in Greensburg. Also, I had played a couple rounds at Marquette with "Mo" Cooperstock as a rank novice sans any lessons. Dr. Robert E. Criswell, prime E.E.N.T specialist, (my T & A surgical buddy), convened with me concerning a golf issue. We met while he was ill in Mercy Hospital with bilateral varicose venous vessels in his lower legs. A bright idea dawned and I said, "Bob, why don't we reserve a special golf day each year where the doctors get together with the dentists and pharmacists for a real donnybrook filled with a C.M.E., golf, dinner and prizes. We can call the blowout "DDD Day". He concurred vigorously to this idea, and thus a historic frolicking joyful day was born, enabling all these conjoined medics to let down their hair and make whoopee. This event originated in 1948 and we have had 56 successive outings following this date.

Beginning in 1958, we also celebrated a super special gold day meeting at Dr. William (Bill) Follis' cabin on the famous Au Sable River, 15 miles east of Grayling, on the fourth Wednesday in July each year. It was designated as the "Follis Open" and a group of 20-25 doctors would join forces for a caravan leaving the doctors parking space behind the hospital at 7 a.m. Bill's rustic cabin was a dream come true in an ideal setting nestled among the pines above the crisp clear Au Sable. This river touted an 8+ mph current and was a haven for canoeists and trout fishermen. Actually, this excursion was probably the pinnacle of happiness for the year and was anticipated with glee all year long. We would reach this ideal rendezvous around 10a.m., have a round of doughnuts and coffee and relaxing libations while enjoying blissful camaraderie and relating Paul Bunyan yarns. At noon promptly, we would proceed leisurely to the Garland Golf course about 3 miles east of Lewiston. Garland is just about the most beautiful course you can imagine. It was a diamond in the rough and its natural setting made you think you had gone to heaven. After 18 holes of challenging golf, (about 25+ for me), we would all convene at the bar and really let our hair down with a couple beers or tall ones (my favorite was a Bloody Mary). After a verbal exchange and peals of laughter we would proceed back to Bill's abode and live it up with a vigorous dice game of "folly-folly". Stan Cousins and Joe Loree were the life of the party. Bill VanDenbelt and I would play cribbage, and John Ley would go fishing. Dick Bickham would compute all the score cards and handicaps and award all the monetary prizes for close to the pin, long ball, and high score. We would each have partners matching the "good" and "poor" golfers for balance, giving everyone a chance to win. I usually had a handicap of 40 to 50, and one year I won for Low Score counting my handicap. After the prizes were doled out, we would have a dinner of lasagna fit for the gods. Bill had a lady chef that could conjure up the world's best, tasty lasagna. Before dinner, we would have a picture with everyone taken by Farrel LeVasseur or Marc E. Mulholland, our oral surgeons. After reluctant, parting farewells, we were homeward bound and believe me, we didn't need anyone to rock us to sleep that night. Bill Follis gradually lost his ability to ambulate and we were forced to relinquish our yearly golf sortie to the Au Sable.

On one of my golfing escapades at the B.C. Country Club, I reluctantly remember wildly shanking a golf shot away to my left. I yelled, "Fore!" but unfortunately it struck Connie Cook on the left thigh, where there was fortunately ample padding. Also, I struck Larry LaPorte in the rump with one of my wayward balls, but he was a good sport and laughed it off. Joe Loree was a WW II bomber pilot in the Canadian Air Force based in England. He was a general surgeon and he had a cottage on the Au Sable near Bill's place. Charley Rogers, also a good surgeon, commented on one of my poorer golf tee shots at Garland, "Knobby, why don't you use your putter, it will go further?!" My best score for 9 holes was 40 and for 18 holes, 92. My problem in playing golf was lack of focus and inability to relax. I had plenty of muscle but would smother the ball and hack it. Putting was my forte, probably because of my pool table ability and a good eye for depth perception.

Regretfully, I gave up my membership at the old B.C.C.C. due to financial burdens, when I separated in 1964 from Doris, my first wife. Pediatricians have big hearts for kiddies but also flat pocketbooks for recompense. It is a labor of love and our payback is the thrill of helping tiny little ones get over the hurdles of illness. The more serious the sickness and higher the stakes, the more satisfaction. Monetarily, we are the bottom rung on the totem pole, but as someone wisely remarked, "You can't take it with you." If you can live comfortably in the middle of the pack, you've got it made.

Respiratory diseases head the list of infants and children's sufferings in the Saginaw Valley. Pneumonia is preeminent in all seasons, but predominant in the winter months. I believe the main factor of causation is the drastic fluctuations of weather changes. As I previously mentioned, here, we are amazingly unstable with meteorological conditions varying ungodly from day to day and often hour to hour. It is my firm conviction that these severe climatic switches don't allow the body time for adjustment or re-adjustment. It probably would be a sage idea to carry clothes for weather adjustment in a backpack wherever you go. Almost every child in this area has at least one bout of some kind of pneumonia during childhood. This pitfall is almost unavoidable regardless of the most meticulous health care. However, we are gaining on this malady by leaps and bounds with our vaccines, hygienic measures, and antibiotics.

Speaking of antibacterial rings a bell about a little three year old boy I was treating for strep pneumonia in Mercy Hospital. While making rounds one morning, Danny was about to be on the other end of a penicillin injection. He was raising a mighty fuss, yelling, "I don't want it. I don't want it. I don't want it, but I need it." Another instance that pricks my memory concerns a two month old infant male with chest disease. I was summoned out of a cozy warm bed at 3 a.m., in the middle of February, our coldest month, by a frantic, crying mother, claiming her baby was dying. I responded ASAP dressed in pajamas, bathrobe, and overcoat. They lived near the Kawkawlin River and I instructed the mom to hang a white bed sheet over her mailbox, for it was pitch black outdoors. I traversed the five or so miles in a hop, skip, and jump and entered the abode. The baby was cradled in her arms and she had tears streaming down her cheeks. The baby had a real thick mustard and onion poultice wrapped around her chest. The odor was stifling, especially with a kerosene stove for heating. After unwrapping the poultice, a quick examination revealed and corroborated my first impression, the baby was lifeless. One of the most difficult duties in my practice confronted me, telling a mother her child had died. Death of a young one, near the termination of my practice was quite rare, but in 1950 it was not uncommon. Thank God for all the many cataclysmic advances and discoveries medicine has harvested from 1936 to 2000. And it has been my exquisite privilege and pleasure to have survived them all. Now we have hospice and most parents are better acclimated to death, especially for the chronic diseases.

Death of children can occur with Sudden Death Syndrome, mainly in your infants, and with adolescent's sports resulting from heat stroke and cardiac auricular and ventricular arrhythmic disorders, anatomic anomalies of the heart prolonged Q-T. Syndrome, Brady Arrhythmia and cardiac shock. Sudden Infant Death contributes to sudden demise without apparent cause. Prolonged Q-T disorder is usually congenital and can only be detected by electrocardiograms and electrophysiological study. The etiology of sudden infant death is unknown, but the supine (back) positioning of babies has cut this event at least in half. Theory points a finger at medullary vital centers and sleeping disorders, especially two to four month olds. Until recently, babies slept prone in America. With the face turned sideways, the carotid arteries to the brain were restricted, the baby was re-breathing carbon dioxide and there was danger of the nose being buried in a soft surface, (especially a pillow). United States' pediatricians learned a lesson from their European counterparts who placed their infants on their backs, and they reaped much better success against this scourge. Boys, preemies, and adverse weather are also risk factors. Sleeping with adults is extremely hazardous with possible crushing and low oxygen accessibility.

Asthma is another extremely common affliction in our neck of the woods. Probably our capricious weather variations are, again, a tremendous factor in causation. Almost every family is doused with a generous touch of asthma and there is a strong inheritance proclivity. Another contributing element is the stark prevalence of upper respiratory infections, which are profound triggers of asthma. Sometimes it seems like every person in the pediatric age group has asthma at some period in their life. It appears that this malady is becoming more prevalent by leaps and bounds yearly and, unfortunately, the morbidity and mortality rate is increasing every year, possibly due to rank pollution of air, water, and soil by chemicals, pollens, gases, smoke, and automobile exhausts. To medicine's credit, there are a host of effective medications to relieve this bronchial constriction. The corticosteroids are number one, anti-inflammatory drugs are number two, and the bronchodilators which are antispasmodic and open up the bronchi for oxygenation are third. Theophyllines were originally our chief standby for symptomatic relief but they are very dangerous, for the margin of safety and error is miniscule and the dosage is different for everyone. Cromolyn sodium is a preventative mediator and the leukotrienes are the latest development to ameliorate severity and decrease the necessary dosage of the rescue medications, (steroids, oxygen, and beta agonists). Treatment is divided into management of chronic asthma and acute exacerbations (episodes). Usually, if a child is going to become asthmatic, before five years of age he/she will develop chronic night cough, wheezing, or manifest allergic signs when exposed to cold air, cats, tobacco, colds, strenuous exercise and pollens. Boys show a higher prevalence by a 2 to 1 ratio and there are early and late phase reactions in each asthmatic episode.

Tobacco is a real number one scourge to an asthmatic child. My elder son, Tom, suffered severe asthmatic episodes as a preschooler, but as expected, the disease ameliorated to a high degree by his adolescence. He volunteered for the Army Air Corps and passed his written examination in San Antonio, Texas, but developed asthma when he ran the two mile test. Otherwise, he was as healthy as Tarzan, but the wheezing killed his chances for an army air corps career.

Many incidents involving asthma cases jog my memory. The first indelible imprint, concerns a little two year old boy from Pinconning whom I treated at

Mercy Hospital several times for severe, unrelenting, asthmatic attacks. On admission, we would usually give Billy a stat injection of adrenalin to supply immediate relief. Epinephrine (adrenaline) is a very powerful bronchial muscle relaxant and is employed only as an emergency measure. The dose by PDR is stated as 0.01 millimeters per pound. His weight was about 28 lbs. and I usually gave him 0.1 ml. subcutaneously per shot and this was my order. However, the pinch hit nurse did not see the decimal point and administered 01.0 ml to Billy sub-q. He had a humongous reaction , stat, consisting of violent shaking and generalized flushing. His blood pressure was increased immeasurably and heart action pulse 250/300 rate was extremely intense. I saw him on the double, probably within two minutes, as I fortuitously was in the hospital. I was scared to death that he would have a cerebrovascular hemorrhage due to the sudden tremendous blood pressure elevation or that pulmonary edema would develop with the pulmonary arterial constriction. We applied cool packs and gave Billy a big dose of vistaril, (a relaxant). Valerie, the head nurse, reported stat to Sister Thomasine and after the reaction subsided uneventfully, I reported it to the parents. If ever I said an emergency prayer, this was the occasion. It is amazing how well nature compensates for medication errors. This is one instance where the metric system can really cause serious compound trouble. One misplaced decimal point can magnify or decrease an error by a multiple of ten, and that can be lethal for an infant or young child. I'll stick with the cumbersome avoirdupois system for safety sake. In fact, we're stuck with it in the USA, but it is sagacious to be familiar with both systems.

Another one of my challenging asthmatic patients was Jan Fettig, who lived on Nurmi Drive in Bay City. I made so many house calls there to bail out Jan's almost deadly, asthmatic spells that it was just about my second home. My favorite rescue medicine would be a hefty , don't spare the horses, dose of a corticosteroid viz decadronby l.m. injection. Amazingly, Jan would usually be converted to her normal state within about four hours. If this miracle, ace in the hole drug did not do the trick, she would have to be admitted for a huge shot of IV steroids plus aminophylline and beta two agonists by inhalation. Recovery ordinarily ensued in 24-48 hours.

Additionally, Dr. Smelzer called me in consult, in the middle of the night for a hospitalized two year old male who was recalcitrant to the usual rescue therapy for asthma. I administered aminophylline IV, as I had done successfully in Marquette, and it broke the critical spell of his gasping for air. You have often heard the expression of "sweating blood" under duress and I must have been close to this state figuratively and literally before the little boy came around and broke the spell.

Another severe asthmatic patient was a girl, aged three years at first acquaintance, whom I doctored for over ten years. She would present at least monthly, with extreme wheezing, coughing, and dyspnea,(difficult respirations). Her hospital courses were usually protracted, more so than any of my scores of other patients with asthma. Nothing in my armaments of meds seemed to work. After a few years of this recalcitrant behavior, I sent her to Ann Arbor for consultation with their allergy gurus, to map out a beneficial program to control her disastrous, frequent exacerbations of asthma. They, after many trials and tribulations, didn't appear to accomplish much more success than poor little me. I thought that puberty might have an ameliorating, favorable effect for her, but she continued on the edge and her episodes were morbid but less numerous. Immunotherapy (shots) do help dramatically in an occasional severe, recurrent asthmatic, but benefits with this mode of treatment in my experience are few and far between. I believe father time and natural exposure immunization to sensitizing allergic antigens are the bread and butter helpers. My second daughter, Melissa, did have intense allergic rhinitis and had non striking benefits from allergy vaccine shots by Dr. Meryl Fenton, of Detroit, over a period of five years.

I recall another patient, an infant male from Clare, Michigan, who had recurrent asthmatic events combined with pneumonia and cerebral palsy requiring repeated hospitalizations. The mother was quite intelligent and could almost smell a bout of asthma occurring in its infant stage. She would phone me and say "Charles is going into his dance and having another one of his attacks and I'm on my way over to see you." I would reply "Fare thee well and full speed ahead." His symptoms would worsen with amazing alacrity on the 50 mile jaunt from Clare, and he would just about always require hospitalization for recovery. I am convinced that his periodic, recurrent pneumonia and asthma were in large part due to aspiration and reflux regurgitation syndrome.

Shortly after returning from the recuperation furlough to Miami, Florida, Doris and I decided to have a mini honeymoon trip to beautiful Mackinaw Island in the summer of 1947. We had to cross the straits by ferry from Mackinaw City to the island tourist haven, about 9 or 10 miles by water. No cars are allowed on this idyllic piece of terra firma and transportation is by bicycle, shoe leather, or horse drawn carriage. There is a scintillating journey by carriage around the outer rim of the island. It skirts the governors' mansion, a British Revolutionary War fortification, and many scenic outposts. Downtown is a lovely park and a Mecca of fatal tourist traps, shops for the unwary. Several stores dispense the heavenly Mackinaw fudge which is famous worldwide. We did a one night stand at the Grand Hotel, which is no inexpensive venture. Our room was in the middle of the second floor and I spent a somewhat sleepless night conjuring up thoughts of fire, as the hotel was a 150 year old plus wooden building without a fire department. The highlight of our stay there was a Sunday dinner in the grand ballroom. The waiters were all men dressed to the gills in flashy, red British colonial uniforms. The silverware was probably 24 carat gold and proper etiquette ruled the roost. We had eight courses of the most delectable food you can imagine served with flawless decorum. It was well worth the price of admission. I almost forgot a three piece string ensemble that played classical gems of Mozart and Beethoven.

The pre-vaccine polio epidemic would strike abject fear and horror in all parents' hearts when it progressed from the southern United States in May to Michigan in July. Paralysis of extremity muscles was an anathema per se, but paralysis of the vital centers in the medulla oblongata was pure hell. Apparently the polio virus is in love with <u>heat</u>. To see a child dying from suffocation and unable to breathe was about the zenith of nightmares. To see a child struggling for air and choking helplessly, before mechanical breathing evolved, was the worst possible scenario. The Iron Lung, an invention of the devil, did help a smidgeon but of itself was a woefully weak substitute for the real McCoy. The only benefit from the polio disease was an abolition of the tonsil and adenoidectomy operation in children because surgery opened up the avenue of entrance of the polio virus into the throat and blood stream directly.

One of the most pitiful events during our battle with this virus involved Dr. Jim Connelly's 8 year old daughter, Jennie. She was virtually, completely paralyzed - arms, legs, larynx, diaphragm, and respiratory muscles. Dr. Chapin and I labored and suffered exquisitely as her doctors for several months while she fought tooth and nail in an Iron Lung until death forced her to abandon this planet. Jim Connelly was a great apple pie baker but with his buddy Mike Medvezky had a fatal penchant for gin (not gin rummy) unfortunately.

Another episode of polio involves my flesh and blood son, Greg, at the age of five years. Our family was enjoying a hearty picnic in Carroll Park one evening in July 1953, when I noticed Greg red faced and asleep on the ground, quite out of character for him. Upon feeling his forehead I was instantly aware that he was burning up with fever. With trepidation we hustled home and put him to bed. His temperature was 105+ degrees and he complained of tenderness and shooting pains in his legs. The lower extremity calf and thigh muscles were very sensitive to touch, weak, and hurt when moved. An explicit diagnosis of polio was confronting me head on. I at once gave him two hefty shots of penicillin and gamma globulin in each buttock and then prayed with all my might and main. The Sister Kenny treatment with continuous <u>hot</u>, wet packs to the affected muscles was in vogue at that time so I called my good nurse friend Evelyn Lewicki . "Evie" had nursed hundreds of my patients at

Mercy Hospital for years but now was working for Bay County Public Health. She was truly "Old Faithful" and responded at once to my call, bringing with her the proper equipment to effectively administer the steaming packs to Greg's legs twice daily. I was consumed, emotionally overboard with Greg's polio, so I decided for his sake to call in Fred Chapin, a peer pediatrician, to care for him and discharged myself. By the grace of God our combined efforts did help and Greg made a miraculous, probable complete recovery within a week. I had always previously been my children's pediatrician through all of their illnesses and injuries, but this one affliction of Greg's was just too hot to handle, threw me for a loop, and I capitulated.

One tidbit strikes my memory regarding Greg, I used to sing him to sleep with my favorite hymn, "The Battle Hymn of the Republic." He queried me one night, "Dad, what war were you a doctor in?" Connecting my song with the appropriate war, I glibly and dreamily answered him, "Why the Civil War." About a month later during parents' night at McKinley School, we lived at 1911 Center Avenue, Greg's teacher quizzed me out of a clear blue sky, "Doctor, I was totally unaware that you were a physician in the Great War between the states." She caught me off guard and I was dumbfounded; and after a pause I stammered back, "Why, don't I wish I were." We had a hearty laugh and she revealed the explanation. The teacher related, that one day in class, they were discussing the invasion of Normandy in June of 1945, in WWII, and Greg, with fire in his eyes, spoke up emotionally and proudly announced, "My father was a doctor in the Civil War." Molly tried to correct his thinking process but Greg was adamant and would only accede to my correction. Doris would never let me live my faux pas down. I was always secretly hoping, strongly in my mind, that Greg would sometime emulate me and become a pediatrician, but I made up my mind that I would never try to sway my children's choice of a vocation. Their decision for their life's work would be 100% their very own. Greg was brilliant and possessed all the basic qualifications to succeed in this profession. Manufacturers of Cool Cigarettes, gave me a first aid kit and cap with the caption of 'Dr. Cool' printed on the bill. Greg would wear the cap and he was known as 'Dr. Cool'. The first aid kit was his "house call" bag.

Little did we know at that time, what a horrendous anathema on the human race, that tobacco was, in disguise. More addictive than morphine, more poisonous than arsenic, and more cancerous than radium, it was. A wolf in sheep's clothing, lethal to the lungs, heart, brain, and all organs, it promoted the four horses of the Apocalypse. I smoked cigarettes for over twenty five years, but didn't inhale much because of the bitter taste. I did not like having my teeth turn yellow and my clothes smell like the bottom of a birdcage. Besides, I had a constant cough and was beginning to develop emphysema and asthmatic wheezing. In the army, cigarettes were dirt cheap at $1.00 per carton and just about <u>every</u> male smoked. The female gender slowly caught on to the odious habit but when they did, they bit, hook line and sinker. By 1959, I realized how vile and morbid the ill effects of tobacco were and I said to myself, "Howard, common horse sense dictates that this addiction is gradually killing you." Actually, I never became inescapably addicted and I abruptly told myself, "You have absolutely smoked your <u>last</u> cigarette", (Chesterfields and Camels), and I did irrevocably stop, cold turkey, thank Jehovah. I did try a cigar and pipe substitute for a year, off and on, but found it equally distasteful, uncouth, and unfulfilling, so I finally gave up the ghost entirely.

Being a total inveterate sports lover, when I came to Michigan in 1938, I turned my full attention and focus on the Wolverines, Spartans, Tigers, Wings, Pistons, and Lions. I had two season football tickets at the Big House in Ann Arbor, from 1947 to 2000 and attended the vast majority of those games with misses far and few between. I fortunately witnessed World Series baseball games in Detroit in 1940, 1945 and 1968. Also, I was present for several Lion football games when they had some <u>real</u>, bona fide All-Stars, such as Bobby Layne, Joe Schmidt, and "Night Train" Lane. In addition, I was fortuitously in Detroit for a pediatric meeting and saw a Stanley Cup playoff game between the Red Wings and the Montreal Habs. I was delegated as ringside physician at the annual amateur boxing matches at the Bay City Armory for several years. Also, I was team physician for many high school football games for Handy and B.C. Central and did many of those team examinations gratis. My most favorite sports were college football, Big League baseball, and college basketball, in that order. My least favorite sport, if you can call it that, was boxing, which is "caveman" and should be banned forever. It usually attracts the dregs of society and consists of two people trying to kill each other by bashing their brains out.

There was one football game to end all football games, November 22nd, 1950, the Snowball Bowl Game between Michigan and Ohio State in Columbus, Ohio to determine the Big Ten Championship. I possessed a ticket and was raring to go as a frenzy of hype was whipped up by the media, as it was always the "<u>Big</u> Game" with the most intense (crazy) rivalry. The train to Columbus left from Saginaw Station on Washington Avenue in Saginaw, at 6:30 a.m. <u>sharp</u>. I had worked like a beaver 'til midnight for 16+ hours that Friday, November 21st. I decided to take a little catnap at the witching hour and use my mental alarm clock to awaken at 4 a.m. and proceed leisurely to Saginaw, which I always could do from my army training. I went to sleep with all my clothes on, on the downstairs couch, and I awakened at 6:15a.m.! I shuddered and muttered, "Oh brother, I've got 15 minutes to catch that train and I'll never make it! But I have to make it, or miss the game of my life!" I kept thinking what my father would say, "Howard, are you a man or a mouse? Go for it, full speed ahead". So I did, with a wing and a prayer to the Almighty. I had my boots on and I grabbed my alpaca, ran and jumped into my trusty new blue Ford and was off to the races. There was snow and ice on the ground, but that didn't deter fearless me, as I was flying low through red lights, uninhibited by almost no traffic. I proceeded down the River Road at break neck pace (75-90mph), and when I pulled up anxiously to the train station, lo and behold, the diesel train was still there! I jumped out of my car in a flash and started my dash for the train which was approximately 100 yards away. After I was ¾ of the way to "Shangri La", it started to slowly pull out. So, alpaca in arm, I increased my pace and began running down the tracks. A railroad car workman looked up at me in disbelief, his mandible dropped several inches, and he was speechless. I was a track luminary in high school, so I poured the coal on the fire, and finally caught up to the rear coach. But, the diesel was picking up speed so I desperately flung my coat over the railing and made an impossible phantom leap to luckily grab the post of the observation car. Fortunately, at that precise instant, a man came out of the rear door and upon glimpsing me shrieked in disbelief,. "Jesus Christ, where did you come from?" I had grabbed the post with my left hand and he grabbed my right arm and pulled me on to the platform. I'll never know his name, but my savior said, "Come on in and get some breakfast." I was completely winded and could barely whisper a thank you. The porter served me a hearty breakfast but I could hardly relish it because I was breathing about 100+ per minute and my heart was racing to the maximum rate of over 180 per minute, I'm sure.

I no sooner was in my seat when a sports reporter from the Saginaw News appeared and began to grill me for the story regarding my miraculous adventure in catching the train. It must have been a couple hours before I could relax and really catch my breath. I literally ran into my favorite friends, Oscar and Jimmy Baker, two renowned lawyers from a famous Bay City black family of attorneys. I was invited to join them in a friendly game of poker to pass the time. This must have been my day in the sun, for I couldn't lose and must have accumulated about fifty green ones. We made a stop at Toledo, Ohio, in time to board the University of Michigan football team and I noticed it was snowing lightly. As we sped on to Columbus, the snow gradually increased to a raging snowstorm and I became a wee bit apprehensive about whether the game would be staged, but they <u>never</u> cancel a football game. Our train pulled into the Ohio State University campus. We parked about 75 yards to the left of the stadium. Believe it or not, the snow blizzard prevented entirely the visualization of the stadium.

We had lunch at a bistro on the campus, High Street, and immediately, at noon, I decided to leisurely wade through the snow, over a foot deep, to find my seat for the game if it were to be played. When I reached the playing field, I started fumbling through my stack of clothes to find my ticket. The ticket collector said, "Don't bother, I know any damn fool coming here today has to have a ticket." With consternation I replied, "But where will I sit?" He said, "Pick out a seat" in a stentorian voice. So, with my ticket pocketed, I proceeded to enter the stadium and found the seats to be covered with about 14" of snow. Blindly, I picked a high bleacher spot, one quarter way from the south end zone, being, I think, the first person to be seated. Pretty soon the bleachers began to fill up all around the bowl with an open end. Lo and behold, I was stationed right in the middle of the Ohio State student rooting section. They must have thought I was a fellow Buckeye student, because the young man next to me kindly offered to share his blanket with me. I snapped at the offer because the temperature had plummeted to near zero F. One student in the next row down, derisively remarked, "When does Purdue come on the field?" and I thought silently, "Anything's possible today!" and truer words were never spoken.

The snow kept falling and you couldn't see the yard stripes. The stadium workers kept sweeping the goal lines. The announcer on the loud speaker said the people in charge of both teams were debating whether the game would be played or cancelled. After a half hour's deliberation, the officials announced, "The game, because of it's importance for the Big Ten championship Rose Bowl selections and a full house of 75,000 spectators, will be played today in it's entirety." The two combatant teams and referees appeared on stage (tundra) for warm-ups and after a few moments, it was well nigh impossible to distinguish either team by their color uniforms or letters. Michigan's white shirts blended perfectly with the snow, which was densely swirling with reckless abandon. Ohio's scarlet and grey uniforms were resplendent for a brief period and then were about as clear as mud as the dark sky resembled semi-darkness. In spite of all the adversities, the contest began in earnest. The statistics were most unique. Michigan did not register one first down and Ohio State ground out three first downs. Michigan punted 22 times and Ohio kicked 20 times, bearing out the 'foot' in football. All punts were delivered on third downs for both teams because of the treacherous footing, (ice skates for cleats would have been much more appropriate). Every time Michigan would make a good play, I would cheer lustily and my blanket buddy would loudly say, "That wasn't Ohio State, that was Michigan." And I would reply, "Oh gosh darn it, I thought it was Ohio State. You really can't distinguish who's who." In spite of the slithery field, Vic Janowicz, their All American Halfback, kicked a 40 yard field goal at the north end to my left circa the middle of the first quarter. Both teams fumbled several times but recovered their own fumbles. Only two short forward passes were completed by the

Buckeyes. Michigan's only scores came on two blocked kicks. The first one occurred at the beginning of the second quarter, at the Ohio State 20 yard line, in the south end, to my right, by the Olentangy River. The ball rolled through the end zone for a big two pointer touchback. The second one was a critically obstructed punt occurring at the end of the second quarter with one minute to play on the Ohio 3 yard line. This one was at the north end of the field to my left side. The kick was blocked by our own Ben Pederson playing left tackle when he burst through the defensive Buckeye line. The precious pigskin was recovered by Michigan in the end zone for six points and we miraculously kicked the point after touchdown, going ahead in the score 9 to 3. (Ben later graduated from Michigan Medical School and went on to become a renowned obstetrician practicing in Bay City, Michigan.) The entire second half of this impossible game was very boring and a monotonous scenario of three downs and a kick repetitively. I stayed until the bitter end and was just about frozen in all extremities. The only beneficial reward was that we won; and because the northwestern Wildcats beat the fighting Illinois in Evanston that same afternoon, we were big ten champions. We had won the right to engage southern California in the New Year's Rose bowl in Pasadena, California – which was won by the indomitable fighting Wolverines!.

I went onto the field after the game concluded and, believe it or not, it was covered with at least four plus inches of ice, just like a skating rink. The crowd had dissipated to probably a thousand when the referee blew the final whistle. With my numb feet and the exuberant feeling of victory, I was flying high and could not feel the ground on the trip back to the train. It had almost stopped snowing and there was impending darkness, but in the twilight we could actually see the train. It was a joyful, uneventful, somnolent trip back to Saginaw, but I was a bit worried whether I had turned off the car lights and ignition in my mad dash to make the train. I had done, and all's well that ends well.

Upon returning from the armed services, I ran into a disagreement with our hospital pathologist, William G. Gamble, Jr., regarding my administration of transfusions to my pediatric patients. The tiff was finally settled in my favor by the executive committee at both hospitals, to Bill's dismay. I figured this operation was rightfully mine as I had been doing all my own patients' transfusions in all the hospitals where I had interned four years in the army and in the Bay City Hospitals before WWII. My prior two years in practice, I had never had any serious reactions or complications. Poor "spitting" Bill G. didn't have a leg to stand on.

Gamble was quite the character! His sartorial garb was a sloppy shambles, with gravy and jelly stains all over his shirt, tie, and trousers, buttons missing on his shirt, hair unkempt, and occasionally fly unzippered. When he conversed, he would be right in your face and he unconsciously would be spitting all over you. He was ungodly penurious and would squeeze the buffalo on a nickel until it howled. When he opened his pocketbook, a moth would fall out, dead. With all his slovenly faults, he was a kind and gracious host of many parties for his staff and all the physicians he served. His laboratory staff was constantly turning over because of starvation wages. He became alcoholic after his wife and son drowned in a tragic boat accident in Saginaw Bay due to a sudden storm one summer Sunday. Bill owned vast acreage in his home state of South Carolina.

I had numerous babies in the 9-12 month category, who became quite anemic because of iron deficiency in their diet plus acute infections. They were typically "milk babies" or, in other words, the vast composition of their diet was milk, which contains an infinitesimal quantity of iron. It was much easier for mother and babies for them to drink their meals. I would use 50 and 100 ml. syringes to pump the blood, usually a scalp vein, but any port in a storm. There was an art to cannulating those tiny, collapsed rivulet veins and giving the blood was a slow, laborious, tedious process requiring steady hands to keep the needle in the vein. We (Peds) gave all our own intravenous fluids.

On one desperate occasion, I recall giving lactate ringers, 1000ml intraperitoneally, to John Meyer's 18 month old daughter. I was called out of the Washington theater at approximately 10:30 one Sunday night, while Doris and I were enjoying a leisurely moment watching Humphrey Bogart and Lauren Bacall, in "As Time Goes By". Before I could catch my breath, John shouted over the phone, "Doc, come quick, I think my little baby is dying. I'm at 400 Pine Street in Essexville", and clicked the receiver. My wife and I made a hasty exit from the drama and high tailed it to John's abode. He was waiting for me and had the door open. On entering the living room, my gaze revealed a little girl lying on the couch in athreptic shock. She had had a week of devastating diarrhea and was as dry as a bone in the desert. She was limp, lifeless, pale, and hardly breathing. I picked up the skin on her abdomen and it remained stationery and inelastic, tented in a fold, two inches high. I said, "Oh brother! She is really flirting with the Grim Reaper. Our only hope of saving her is a fire engine run to the hospital." I grabbed her up in my arms and as I was getting into my car, I transferred her to Doris and John said, "Make it Mercy." We were off in a flash and John and his wife followed closely. I hit the pediatric 3rd floor running and summoned a nurse on the double. "Bring a quart of lactate ringers into the treatment room and I will give it intrapertoneally. We don't have a minute to waste." Recognizing the gravity of the situation, the nurse, Evelyn Lewicki, exclaimed, "Oh dear! I'll be right with you." Mary Lou's pulse was barely perceptible and she had Cheyne-Stokes breathing signifying dire organic acidosis with comatose state. After infusing a liter of life saving lactate ringers solution intraperitoneally by gravity the color began to return to her skin and she began to regain consciousness. Her veins were completely collapsed and a rapid flickering pulse was barely discernible. External and internal jugular veins were an alternative but they too were collapsed and speed was the essence of the moment. I had used intraperitoneal fluids in an emergency situation many times when interning at CHOP, so now it was a piece of cake. Almost instantaneously, my patient began to show signs of reviving, eyes opened, pulse slowed and became stronger, breathing improved, arm and legs begin to thrash, and tissue turgor pinked up. Hallelujah! The sweetest sounds this side of heaven – not even Guy Lombardo - cries burst forth in full bloom. Needless to say, her parents, and all those people in attendance, heaved a tremendous sigh of relief and smiles pervaded.

In the fall of 1947, diphtheria organisms invaded Bay City in the guise of a mild epidemic, creating rank panic in the minds of its citizens. Everyone rushed to catch up to date on their D.T. immunization. I sometimes had a couple hundred patients daily coming to the office for diphtheria vaccine shots. It requires a magnum of toughness for an adult to volunteer and submit to a shot, but the corynebacterium organism is a most powerful persuader. In fact, the pharmacies and hospitals plum ran out of syringes and needles after the first week of the scare. Indeed there were only three proven cases of the real "McCoy" of this culprit. They were concentrated in the south end, around Broadway and Fremont Avenues. I treated one patient with diphtheria antitoxin and they all survived the ravages of the disease. The most dreaded complication of diphtheria is complete heart block from paralysis of the electric bundle of HIS which controls heart beats and rhythm. Of course all out blockage of the nose, throat, and trachea is an agonizing killer also.

I remember several severe critical burn cases and hundreds of mild burn patients I have treated during my medical career. One devastating third degree burned family with one infant and three boys, ages 4, 7, and 8 occurred at 208 South Lincoln Ave. when there was a huge gas explosion in their home while they were sleeping around 2 a.m. on a Sunday in 1948. I received a distressed phone call from Dr. Norris Asline asking me to come quickly to meet him at the "Old" General Hospital to attend this ravaged family. If ever I have witnessed a horrendous tragedy, this was number one in red letters. Both parents were burned beyond recognition, like two overgrown lobsters covered with smoke and soot. They were in an extreme morbid state, on the very edge, and staring death in the face. Their demise occurred about two hours after I arrived at the hospital. Their severely burned children were my prime assignments for immediate attention. The one year old girl was moribund gasping her last breath and did go to see her maker shortly after being hospitalized. She was third degree burned from head to toe and didn't have a ghost of a chance. The three sons were all gravely burned, arms, legs, chest, abdomen, and face. We covered the burns with cool, wet normal saline compresses, administered large amounts of intravenous lactate ringers solution, corticosteroids, and penicillin. Infection, vital organ injury, dehydration, and chemical imbalance of electrolytes were out worst enemies. As soon as stabilization was secured, several days later, skin grafting of third degree burned areas was begun. Dr. Orlen Johnson, a general surgeon, did grafting with skin from unburned skin sites while I gave them light ether anesthesia. Miraculously, all three brothers were salvaged, thanks to the Grace of God and abundant prayers. It was a most intense and stressful daily struggle all the way, but the happy end result was well worth it. Doris and I knew the mother by first name as she did our wash and cleaning and I was pediatrician for the children. In addition to the gruesome repercussions of the ghostly morbid and mortal injuries, they were additionally compounded and complicated by the emotional factors involved in losing parental ties. Two parents lives were snuffed out and three beautiful children were atrociously maimed for life, and one child died in one lightning stroke.

Another unforgettable burn patient strikes me between the eyes. Leo's twenty month old daughter, Mary, pulled a boiling hot pot full of coffee off the table down upon herself one night while the parents were hosting guests. Again, Doris and I were enjoying a movie with Barbara Stanwyck in "Death of a Salesman" at the Regent theatre, beside Trahan's Pharmacy. Upon answering the phone I heard Leo's deafening, stammering voice imploring me to rush ASAP to his home to see Mary because of severe coffee burns. Doris and I hastily put the pedal to the medal and reached our destination in "Banks" on Bay City's west side in record time. I knew by the urgent tone of Leo's voice that this incident was a true emergency, and it was. Poor Mary had deep second degree burns on her neck, chest, and abdomen. Over the telephone I had instructed Leo to immerse the burned areas in clean, cold water, and emphasized not to put anything (salve or ointment) whatsoever on the scalded body parts until I arrived. I also admonished him to give her half of a five grain aspirin tablet stat. Upon arrival, I plastered her burns with a heavy coat of my burn life saver – equal parts furacin and vaseline. Furacin ointment diluted ½ is indubitably the unchallenged best healer and immediate pain squelcher on the market. The ointment did the trick and within the brief span of two weeks, Mary's third degree burns were healing famously and she required no grafting. It was incredible. All I did was daily dressings and liberal applications of the ointment. That, and Father Time, who also is a great healer and solves may medical problems sooner or later, did the trick.

To save my soul, I could never convince my obstinate fellow practioners of the furacin/vaseline ointment's miraculous and magical properties for burns and for most skin infections. I had innumerable wonderful results using it with happy parents, happy children, and happy me. It is entirely my own concoction which I stumbled upon by experimentation in the early fifties.

Chapter 21

Our Postwar Children Duo

Doris and I were the proud parents of two wonderful children after my emancipation from the Army as a Major in WWII. Our first newborn was a male named Gregory Haines (my mothers maiden name) born at 11:30 p.m. on Saturday night September 14, 1948. I don't believe I've ever been more excited and euphoric in my life as on this blessed occasion. He was birthed by my staunch friend and superb obstetrician Mike Dardas at Mercy Hospital in Bay City. Vividly, I remember that night with a passion of pent up emotion and exuberance. I called just about every doctor in the Bay County Medical society from midnight to dawn announcing his birth in saturated terms of pure joy. The doctors were all very tolerant with my interruption of their somnolence and expressed their feelings of empathy and goodwill. The delivery was smooth and uneventful, without any hitches. Mother and baby came through with flying colors. Greg came into the world with a loud fit of crying and did not need the proverbial slap on the buttocks. He had a touch of "Cole Porter Colic" (day and night) for several months. However, it was not in the same league as Susan's year long bout with indigestion. Gregory was a well behaved baby and grew by leaps and bounds, but he was quite demanding of attention and service. He was a very handsome and happy baby and was bonded intensely with his father. He accomplished all the physical attainments of walking and speech in shorter than average time periods.

We had moved from 221 North Lincoln to 2112 6th Street just a few months before his arrival. I had a chance to buy our little home on Lincoln and should have grabbed this option with the gusto of a snapping turtle, sale price $7,500. We needed more room for expansion and our finances were quite meager at this time. We did purchase the house on 6th street and lived there until 1951.

We became intimately acquainted with a venerable elderly lady who lived across the street on Lincoln, Mrs. Laura Boelte. She became a veritable "mammy" to our children. She was a widow due to the sudden death of her husband, stricken by a massive coronary arterial blockage occurring in 1946. We had implicit faith in Laura Boelte, originally from Three Rivers, Wisconsin on Lake Michigan. She had a passionate, innate love for children which was unquenchable. Her culinary abilities centered on baking cakes, cookies, and muffins, all prime requisites and delights for kids. She suffered the agonies of severe eczema due to manifold allergies to milk, eggs, wheat, berries, fish, beef, and you name it food stuff. Laura was bedeviled with constant, exquisitely itchy rashes over all the flexure skin surfaces which were well nigh uncontrollable except mildly by corticosteroids.

Speaking of infant colic, the medics have been completely baffled as to its etiology. The dictionary (Webster's) defines colic (Greek derivative colon) as a paroxysmal abdominal pain due to spasm, obstruction, or distention of any of the hollow viscera. Apparently milk allergy plays a prominent part, but I believe it is multifactorial in causation. It occurs in certain babies who have a typical behavior pattern of spastic crying for over 3 hours a day and over 3 days a week for 3 to 5 months. They are very sensitive, easily provoked to anger, very irritable, and restless. It has been proven conclusively that mother anxiety and mother stimulus overload do not cause colic. Fern Foster used morphine in miniscule doses to control intense colicky babies and it did a superb job. Addiction <u>never</u> seemed to be a problem. There was one mother who used morphine in marked overdose and the baby did develop marked somnolence. If used in prescribed dosage, it is harmless. Personally, my innocuous but effective therapy for colic was cooking whiskey, 1 tsp to 6oz of water, given in a bottle. The baby would guzzle until he/she dozed off and it <u>really</u> worked like a charm and never caused a problem. Dicyclomine is also used and its purpose is reduction of pain which is certainly the humane thing to do. Parents must understand from the beginning that the normal period of infant crying is actually 2 to 3 hours per day. It varies depending on the child's temperament. Vast instances of colic are easily managed by measures of relaxation, comfort, and resignation to nature's designs.

Gregory was quite determined and demanding in his wishes and desires. Every time I left the home on 1911 Center Avenue, he would point me in an easterly direction. If I failed to obey his explicit directions he would jump up and down and scream vociferously to middle C and cry crocodile tears. His mild colic was quite tolerable and in general he was a good natured, well behaved, non belligerent, male child.

Melissa Mary was our fourth and last newborn on November 25th of 1951. She, like I, never did see her paternal grandfather because he succumbed to strokes and cardiovascular disease in the fall of 1950, at the young age of 64. Her birthplace was Mercy Hospital, birthed by proficient physician, Robert R. Crissey. Melissa first saw the night lights at about 10:30 p.m., on a Saturday, during football season. In fact, I had tickets for the Michigan - Ohio State game at Ann Arbor and I could have returned in time to observe her emancipation from the womb. But the mother to be, dear wife, put her foot down and like a stern staff sergeant, gave me stentorian orders to remain in Bay City that day if I valued my life.

I had asked Ken Barker, a close friend, who is nuts about nuts, to accompany me to this game. We became acquainted with the Barkers when we moved from Lincoln Avenue to 2012 Center Avenue, into a garage apartment across the hall from Ken, Lisa, and Libby Barker's abode. Ken was school psychologist for Bay City Central High and we would attend all the Wolves' home games. Lisa met a horrendous fate in 1968 when she burned to death in her car one night upon returning from her Akron school teaching duties. Her demise is shrouded in mysterious circumstances and was never solved. Ken's wife also met an untimely death from lung cancer due to our cobra cigarette tobacco enemy. Ken must have warned Libby a thousand times to banish her addicted smoking habit, but to no avail. Ken eventually moved to Akron, Ohio, and worked his way up to become Men's Dean at Akron University. We're still very good friends and exchange Christmas greetings yearly. Kenneth B. will eternally have a soft spot in his heart for the Wolverine State.

There was an especially humorous happening between my son, Greg, and my staunch friend, Ken, when my number two son was three years old. The Barker family was visiting us and we had to double up on sleeping quarters. Ken was slumbering with me in a twin bed in my bedroom. Along about 0700, Greg entered our room and confronted Barker saying in an austere tone, "Mista Barka, I'se gonna give you a shot." To which Ken replied sleepily, "Okay Greg, go ahead" thinking it was just a childish prank to get attention. At that juncture, Greg really and truly did plunge a syringe, with hypodermic needle attached, into our guest's thigh. Barker jumped two feet straight into the stratosphere and screamed, "Oh my God, that was a real needle!" This explosion awakened everyone in both families. I apologized to Barker profusely and had a heart to heart conversation with my young son. It appears that Mr. Gregory was jealous and resentful that my friend was sleeping in a bed beside me. He found my "Black" medical bag and extracted a 2cc syringe and sterile hypodermic #26 needle and put one and one together. I took Greg on many house calls with me and he had seen me use this apparatus often for penicillin shots. He knew exactly the modus operandi into the lateral thigh. Before Ken Barker left Bay City for Ypsilanti and a position as school psychologist, he gave Gregory an IQ test. He was duly impressed with his above normal 120 score at age three years.

Melissa was as welcome to our household as the flowers in May. For some mysterious reason, she was an unhappy baby and cried vociferously and inconsolably for interminable periods daily, until she was almost a year old. As far as I could fathom, she seemed like a fish out of water and couldn't accept our way of life. She seemed to have her own specific ideas of living and they just didn't coincide with ours. Finally she seemed to find her niche in the family constellation and she did elicit a sunny smile. She was mighty pretty and seemed to reek intelligence to a high degree. Melissa was born near the end of November, and when she matriculated for kindergarten, I was logically apprehensive because she was only four years old. Her teacher consoled me and said, "Let's give it a try and test her readiness. She surely is not the first four year old child who has made the grade with honors." I acquiesced with confidence and lo and behold, our four year old daughter passed the test of fire as one of the best pupils. From then on I had high, positive expectations for our "poor little" Melissa Mary. She was my "LOVE" child, conceived on Valentines Day, 1951, I'm indubitably sure.

Melissa's bodyguard was Susan, who assumed the role of little mother to all her siblings. I believe Susan inherently embodied and reflected her grandmother's DNA preeminently. Also Susan was physically a facsimile of my mother in toto. Our other children appeared to absorb a heavy dose of the Knobloch and Haines genes equally in their makeup. I'm positive that my mother's chromosomes were quite dominated by her father, J.T. Haines. His strong genes were passed along to yours truly, as J.T. lived 89 years and worked as a laboring millwright until 8 ½ decades.

Chapter 22

True Blue Friends

The Cogans, Howard and Norine, were special friends we cultivated following my honorable discharge in October, 1945, - officially January 31st, 1946. Doris and I saw them frequently on home to home visits until they moved to Atlanta, Georgia. Their son, Sonny Cogan, graduated in Journalism, from Michigan State and we attended football games at Spartan Stadium in East Lansing and The Big House in Ann Arbor for inter-rivalry games in the late forties. Howard was a shrewd engineer and worked for a welding company in Bay City. We visited the Cogans in Atlanta when Howard was practically on his death bed from the ravages of cancer. Sonny met an unfortunate, untimely demise in an automobile accident near Sebewaing, MI.

In the fifties, we bonded with three other families to have social get togethers including dinners at alternating homes once monthly. Our circle embraced the Dardases, Mike and Katie, the Blumenaus, Roz and Jerry, and the Englehardts, Carl and Connie. Our meetings embodied conviviality and good fellowship. Each wife endeavored to out do the others with gourmet meals and culinary expertise. I believe Katie Dardas was the champion. Her standing beef rib roast was to die for.

Mike Dardas was an outstanding Obstetrician, with a heart of gold and a perpetual smile. He also served in a surgical capacity in World War II and was a participant in the death march on the road to Mandaly, which utterly destroyed his feet. Katie and Mike were parents to a deaf mute child, Karen. Katie was a graduate nurse and was extremely active in the field of audiology. She tried valiantly to tutor Karen to learn speech and language and had a large measure of success for her intense efforts.

The Blumenaus' were a happy go lucky couple, quite the fun lovers. They had a handicapped child – a boy with cerebral palsy and reduced intelligence. I would often watch the Detroit Lions play football Sunday afternoons with Jerry at his house on 7th Street. Jerry had a rendezvous with death from a massive gastric hemorrhage in circa 1970, caused by aspirin uncontrolled over dosage, taken for arthritic pain. He required 20+ pints of blood to staunch the flow of blood while hospitalized for an interminable time. He eventually won the battle with the Grim Reaper, barely by the skin of his teeth.

I have always been on friendly terms with pharmacists and drug representatives (Reps). They are quite intelligent, college graduates and are extremely informative and helpful. Their expert counsel is especially helpful in preventing adverse drug reactions, especially related to incompatible medicinal combinations. Bud Frantz was a Rep for Mead Johnson Pharmaceutical Company and was a real friend of the physicians. I was doctor for his infant son, Chuckie, who had excruciating "Cole Porter" Colic, almost without letup, for three months. I must have made at least twenty house calls to their second story apartment above a drug store on 3rd Street, at all hours of the day and night. Chuckie was the healthiest unhappy baby you ever saw. Thriving like a million dollars in spite of his gut ache. Bud was as nervous as a cat on a tin roof in a hail storm. He constantly complained of chest pain over the procordium (anginal). Poor Doctor Hal Shafer, an excellent internist, examined Bud weekly/monthly for many years, but always came up empty, heart disease wise. His multiple EKG's always were perfectly normal. Finally, after the umpteenth EKG impelled Hal to pronounce Bud's heart perfectly normal, Bud dropped dead about an hour later. Unfortunately, medical technology was in its infancy and there were no available cardiac imaging studies. EKG's are about as useless as the iron orchids (testicles) on Lafayette's horse when it comes to diagnosing heart disease.

Another true pharmacy friend was Linda Leach, a Ross Laboratories district manager Rep. Linda was 100% dedicated to her job and her all out enthusiasm endeared her to all the pediatricians. Her intelligent and forceful salesmanship branded her as one of a kind. Dick Bickham, pediatrician, and wife, Dottie, made up a foursome at a round of golf with Linda and myself before the N.E.M.P.S. meetings twice a year – usually at Frankenmuth's Bavarian Inn third floor restaurant, with myriads of stuffed reindeer heads. Linda, Dottie, and I were rank duffers, but Dick was a true pro who had a suave, perfect swing as smooth as glass.

The N.E.M.P.S., "nymphs", included pediatricians from Bay City, Saginaw, Flint, and Midland and was designated as the Northeastern Michigan Pediatric Society. It was sponsored socially by Ross Co. Inc. Ross Co. furnished Mullsoy, Enfamil, and non-allergenic artificial milk to the newly born infants. Thus, there was a skin tight marriage between the pediatricians and Ross. We were compatible bedfellows. Our society originated circa, September 1949, and Wolfe Zuelzer, Peds Professor at Detroit Children's Hospital, was our initial speaker on "RH Babies".

Robert Drew, an Eli Lilly Rep, became one of my most inseparable friends. We became inveterate golf buddies right off the bat, in the late forties, shortly after I joined the old Bay City Country Club on Fisher and Euclid. Bob was a hulk of a man, a rugged individual with a definite mission, perfectly coinciding with a drug salesman. He was from Traverse City and his father was a sea captain on a Great Lakes freighter hauling iron from Duluth MI to Cleveland. Bob had a nifty wife, Cleo, who was quite the culinary artist. She wrote the book on fried chicken and also was a golfer. Somehow she developed a shoulder separation which rained on her golf game. You know, “it never rains on a golf course or football field”.

Robert constantly fought the battle of name brand vs. generic drugs. He was utterly convinced that the name brand species had some mystic properties that rendered them above the generics quality wise. However, actually there is practically no difference except cost because of strict, rigid regulations imposed upon the drug industry.

Bob and I golfed weekly at the Bay County golf course, until his osteoarthritis incapacitated him in the eighties and he finally succumbed to septicemia on Thanksgiving day in 1990. We played a foursome with Varin Kule, a gastroenterologist, and Vince Haroon, a pulmonologist – both elite craftsmen. They were just raw beginners at the golf game, and very appreciative of our teaching efforts in fathering them under our wings. Our so called “pupils” mastered the game in amazingly short order and soon were showing up their teachers. Haroon became a long-ball hitter while Kule was more of a finesse and placement whacker. Vince had a catastrophic occurrence while on vacation to view the luscious and gorgeous fall leaf color changes in the Upper Peninsula. While he was passing a truck at high speed, that vehicle, unaware, turned abruptly left into his Cadillac, causing it to catapult and roll over several times. Unfortunately, his car was equipped with only one air bag on the driver's side. His wife, Mutosh, was killed outright and his daughter sustained a serious head injury necessitating surgery. Vince survived this accident physically, but went into a mental fugue, blaming himself for his spouse's death.

When I began practice practically all the pharmacy Reps were men, similar to the same situation with reference to the doctors. Now, thank God, this disparity has completely reversed itself so that the tender gender has practically equilibrated to equal representation in both fields.

Red Blaise was a venerable, long standing Rep for Lederle and was an outstanding favorite of all the physicians. Red was an expert raconteur of tall tales and was always good for a hearty laugh. His pharmaceutical company was primarily engaged in the production of disease prevention vaccines. Namely, they comprised pertussis, polio, influenza, tetanus, mumps, and measles and were cultivated on animal embryos. They are active or passive in their initiation of immunity from disease and generally were effective at an 80 to 90 percent rate. The active mode means the causative organisms were alive, but attenuated by heat. The germs are known as antigens that stimulate the production of protective antibodies to fight off actual disease. They may completely obliterate the disease process, or at the least grossly lessen the severity if disease breaks through the barrier.

Passive immunization, on the other hand, is the process whereby the antibodies are already present in the vaccine to challenge the invading microorganisms. Unfortunately, needles and syringes have to be employed to inject these life savers to activate them. I daresay almost 100% of humans have an astounding aversion to pain. It is veritably impossible to penetrate the skin without causing some degree of trauma, physically or mentally. Other avenues of entry inside the body embody the nose, mouth, and possibly the eye, but they are not really practical. The acid gastric juice is a big deterrent. The "gun", as used in the army, causes very little agony, but is time consuming, messy, and of doubtful efficacy. Local anesthesia of the integument has been pursued but is not pragmatic due to pain with infants and young children. Diversions such as infant nursing and music do help to ameliorate and distract the acute impact. There is a misconception that babies do not feel much pain, but there is nothing more fallacious. At least they do not build up a psychological aura and the pain centers are supposedly immature.

In active immunization, where the antigen is not dead, there is a precarious situation in which a person could develop the real disease instead of building up protection against that specific disease entity. As I previously mentioned, with the Sabin oral polio vaccine, where the virus is attenuated but alive, about 3+ people will develop the real McCoy (polio) each year. Apparently this occurrence is caused by a natural individual immune deficiency. For this exact reason, live vaccine is not administered to anyone whose resistance is compromised or to those people suffering with cancer, ulcerative colitis, organ transplantation, post splenectomy, leukemia, and acute illnesses such as pneumonia. Pregnancy is a contraindication for giving virtually all vaccines, active or passive, because of the direct danger of injurious effects to the fetus. Because of the risk of developing the disease, we now employ the Salk vaccine exclusively for polio immunization, in spite of having to use the injection method. Actually, the Sabin oral polio vaccine is more effective than the Salk vaccine, because it endows intestinal immunity and there is the supreme advantage of giving it orally. Due to the benevolent influence of the vaccines and the antibiotics to fight disease, the human race has profited immensely. Now we are much taller, robust and healthier than ever and our age has soared infinitely. Who knows but what the utopian age of 150 years for the human race is not attainable? Medicine has emerged from the dark ages to unbelievable enlightenment, from the seeming impossible to the possible. But really, we have been discovering what has been here from time immemorial. The vaccine future is limitless and combinations are the order of the day. We have been able to conjure up vaccines for practically all but the HIV virus, which has thwarted and stymied all efforts to lasso it.

One other beloved drug Rep deserves meritorious mention. John Cosgrove, the Mead Johnson man, was with us, body and soul, since the termination of the greatest war, (WW II), ever fought. John Cosgrove was a very honest, reliable, obliging man of few words. He was erudite, pleasant and non pressuring in contradistinction to most of the other salespersons, especially the tender gender. His motto was, "Try it, you'll like it."

John's company was in heated competition with Ross Labs, manned by our buddy, Linda Leach, while striving desperately to win the battle of infant formulas. His company manufactured Similac, Isomil, and Alimentum, all substitute formulas for breast milk for baby's nutrition until solid food stuffs can be introduced at six months of age. Mother's milk has multiple advantages over these artificial formulas. Mainly, it has protective antibodies to combat the common infant illnesses, especially the colostrum. Other incomparable advantages include: convenience, intimate bonding relationship with mother, absence of allergic food sensitizations, essential proteins, hormones, and enzymes, and much better weight control for the infant. The mother also benefits from uterine involution and some protection from becoming pregnant. Nursing babies eat much more frequently in smaller amounts and experience increased satiety. It is more like one continuous 24 hour meal daily.

Chapter 23

Friends Galore

We became acquainted with Doctor Robert Fisher and his lovely wife, Sally. Robert was an astute internist who was awarded a citation for his research on insulin in 1975. Poor Sally was cursed with frequent bouts of renal calculi which caused excruciating pain in her side. During these attacks, it seemed to help her to grab hold of another person for support. Frequently I was the target. We often went dancing at the Elks Club in the late forties. Bob left Sally for a femme fatale in Battle Creek, Michigan, and settled there. Sally had a less auspicious ending, as she succumbed to uterine cancer at University Hospital in Ann Arbor.

Dr. Neal and Florence Moore lived across Lincoln Avenue from us when we moved to 221 North Lincoln, in 1940. Doris regarded Florence as a close buddy, along with Dr. Medvezky's wife, Jean, and Dr. Mike Dardas' wife, Katie, during the long, lonesome, stressful years of the war. They were temporary "War Widows", keeping the home fires burning.

After WWII, Doris and I formed endearing, lasting friendships with numerous families. The following were the paramount true friends: Bid and Mary Cranage, George and Alice Ward, Kent and Belle Alcorn, Orlen and Dottie Johnson, Bill and Joy Reed, Frank and Regina Bearsh, Mike and Jean Medvezky, Carl and Linda Olson, Harry and Cora McGee, Jim and Judy Connelly, Tom and Althea Tupper, and Tom and Florie Wright.

We perpetuated our social ties with Bid and Mary Cranage, whom we knew rather intimately in Baltimore during medical school days. As I previously mentioned, Bidwell had conducted a boarding home on Park Avenue our sophomore year in medical school at Maryland and Mary was a nurse at Women's Hospital nearby.

Another lasting and binding friendship was established with Alice and George Ward just after the war. I made frequent house calls to render pediatric service to their five progeny, Ashley, Mary Ann, Katy, Georgie, and Nicholas.

We were often dinner guests for grilled steaks by master chef, George. There were two very memorable trips we engaged with the Wards. In July, 1954, both entire families rented cottages at a resort about three miles from Oscoda for two weeks. We all had rollicking, frolicking, enjoyable times and parted the best of friends. Greg and Nicholas went fishing on a raft at the mouth of the Au Sable River one day, and drifted unconsciously, out into the lake, a ways from shore. Fortunately, they were rescued by an obliging yacht. While there, I was destined to return to Bay City for a monthly, General Hospital Staff Medical Meeting, to fulfill my duty as President.

On another occasion, we joined the Wards and the DeFoes on an unforgettable excursion to South Bend, Indiana, to witness the Notre Dame versus Oklahoma football game. The only time George Ward and I crossed swords was when Michigan played the Irish in football, and then, for only a few hours. Notre Dame was soundly trounced by the Oklahomans on that occasion. Our surprise came after the game, when we returned to our rented home. The madam in charge declared war with us because of "rowdiness" and evicted us from her domicile. We weren't crying in our beers as she was such a rigid sourpuss. However, rooms were at a premium due the "big game" with Oklahoma. To make a long story short, we found the last three available rooms at a moth eaten South Bend Hotel on the top floor. We all were guests at an elaborate, elegant dinner dance blowout on the campus following a disastrous Notre Dame defeat. We bedded at around 3:00a.m. and our home bound Grand Trunk train, left at 8:00 a.m. The only incident that occurred there after the dance was a real donnybrook of a battle of loud words between Bill and Mary Jo Defoe, in the room next to my wife and I. The wall between us must have been plywood, so we gleaned a few explicit choice words before peaceful sleep overtook us all.

I recall one memorable event which happened perennially on March 17th of each year viz Saint Patrick's day for the Irish. In the fifties, dear George Ward became the erstwhile, self appointed band leader of the Notre Dame University Band, which led the "Big Parade" gaily, down Center Avenue in Bay City.

I am compelled to relate one other unctuous matter concerning precious, lovable, Alice Ward. She improperly developed the dreaded lady killer named breast cancer in the nineties and died at Bay Medical Center. But before succumbing on her deathbed, during one of my consoling visits, she made a soulful hearty request as I was parting. "Kiss me goodbye Howard." I complied with a buss on the right cheek and she reacted negatively, stating, "No, my darling" and pointing to her mouth, said, "Here, my dear." I believe a pediatrician's relation with a mother and her child has deep roots, almost like a father and pseudo husband.

Doris and I had happy, friendly relationships with the Alcorn Doctors and their wives. Kent Alcorn was a super urological nephrologist and practiced his skills in the Thorne Building on Washington Avenue, along with me, for two years before I entered the service to fight the "War to end all wars." Marshall Alcorn was a general surgeon practicing in Wisconsin and after several years there, decided to establish a joint practice in Urology with brother Kent. The brother doctors were sons of a family physician who practiced in Urbana Illinois. The wives, Kent's Belle and Marshall's Lilly, were affable lovely and dignified ladies who welcomed us into their homes. Kent was an aviator in the first WW, and related tales about his harrowing experiences as a flyer. I made a flight with both brothers to witness a football game at Champaigne, IL, between the Wolverines and the Fighting Illini. Lucky me! Michigan won both games, and Kent and Marshall were quite chagrined. On the way back to Bay City with Kent Alcorn, we ran into a violent rain storm and dense, low fog. Our plane made a pass at the runway at Tri-City MBS and Kent shouted excitedly, "Go back up, go back up!" The pilot must have heard him for we zoomed at breakneck speed back into the stratosphere and touched down finally at Bishop Airport, in Flint. From there we bussed to our home destination.

We also formed a close friendship with Orlen and Dorothy Johnson. Orlen was a general surgeon of exceptional ability. He performed a vasectomy on me after we decided our family was intact, and Doris was admonished by Bob Crissey to desist regarding further pregnancy. Dorothy was from my home city of Pittsburgh and was reared in a charged social elite atmosphere. A beautiful lady, with personality to burn, but prone to carry tales out of school with weird delusional tones of prevarication - probably due to her alcoholic habitués. For instance, it was reliably reported that Dorothy J. was seen cavorting on the first hole of the Bay City Country Club on Euclid in her birthday suit at 5 a.m. on a Saturday in July. On another occasion, while we were attending a party at Dr. Charters' (DDS) home, she accused me angrily of saying disparaging remarks about her while on the stage at Washington School. This accusation was purely a delusional figment of her imagination for I was never near any school on this date. I'm sure Orlen was soundly embarrassed and harassed many times by her uncanny and nasty provocative behavior. He was totally one of my true friends.

Orlen and I were golf buddies at the Bay County Golf Course on many occasions, for many years. On one happening, he accompanied me to Detroit Children's Hospital to consult an internist pediatrician at Detroit's Children's Hospital. The consultation concerned a litigation case of a ten month old baby girl who had a complete right lung atalectosis with a very low hemoglobin of six grams, breathing her last when I first saw her in consult for ENT Dr. and lawyer, John Grigg. (Also, I was anesthetist for John's pediatric surgical cases.)

Orlen was also a staunch booster for General Hospital and was a real life saver for their campaign to raise operative funds in circa 1950. He was an intimate associate of Hoyt Hayes, President of the Hospital Board and lived in a home on Hoyt's estate on Center Avenue.

Orlen's relationship with the Dafoe's ship building operation enabled me to become ship doctor on an Australian destroyer bound for Boston via the Great Lakes. We proceeded from the shipyards on the morning after Thanksgiving in 1968, with Bill Dafoe at the wheel. Son, Greg, accompanied me as we circled the Michigan thumb and passed the Detroit skyline at about the witching hour. As we were passing into Lake Erie, a cruiser came out of nowhere and cut across our bow just missing us by the skin of its teeth – a harrowing experience. We enjoyed immensely, our passage through the majestic locks connecting Lakes Erie and Ontario, while skirting Niagara Falls, Saturday a.m., on a gorgeous autumn day. On Saturday night we had much needed help from an expert lake pilot, to guide us through the beautiful Thousand Islands light signals. Saturday was also my daughter Melissa's birthday and I called her by phone from our ship, via Kingston, Ontario, to wish her a happy birthday. Saturday also encompassed the OSU – Michigan annual showdown for the Big Ten title. We heard this game on radio, but were not pleased with the result. On Sunday, we voyaged the mighty St. Lawrence River, passing Montreal and reaching Quebec by midnight. When we hit the Atlantic after passing around the Gaspe Peninsula, the ocean became exceedingly choppy. While visualizing the numerous whales, I experienced a sudden sinking feeling of nausea and vertigo. I made tracks to my bunk and assumed the total horizontal position until my fugue evaporated. We entered Boston Harbor at 10 a.m., Monday, moored, and turned our destroyer over to the Australian sailors for their disposition. Greg and I bolted to see my cousin Mary Eisamon and her husband Lewis in Arlington, a suburb of Boston. Mary has always been my favorite cousin, for we were like brother and sister for several years during childhood. Mary even taught me to dance to "I'm Looking Over, a Four Leaf Clover" and "Roll Them Girls, Roll Them". Mary had gained weight and was having arthritic pangs, but she cooked us a delicious roast beef dinner. We then caught the plane at Logan Airport and flew back to Bay City.

Tom and Florie Wright were two of our most staunch pediatric doctor friends. The pediatric triumvirate of Al Ellison, Fred Chapin, and Tom Wright was formed in the early fifties, in the A.D. Allen Building on Jane Street on the west side of Bay City. Ellison was always oppositional and contrary in arguments relative to all medical issues at all times. He was a true iconoclast and would convincingly debate that "water runs up hill," against the established phenomenon of gravity. Fred Chapin joined the Allen Clinic in '43, fresh from his internship at Mott Children's Hospital in Ann Arbor. He was celebrating his joining the U.S. Army, on the night before reporting for duty when fate intervened and he fell (alcohol induced), and fractured his right lower extremity (tibia). This resulted in his abject rejection from army service and necessitated the option of private practice. Bay City was ripe for a pediatrician. Tom Wright came here from his Mott Hospital residency in partnership with Ellison and Chapin. Tom was the epitome of devotion and conscientiousness to his patients, and was an immediate, huge success. A pediatrician in a group practice has the tremendous advantage of capturing all the referrals from all the doctors in the group; and at Allen Medical there were about 50 doctors - one half of the Bay City medics. In solo practice such as mine, we knew that our patients were entirely loyal and there was a more binding relationship known universally as LOVE.

Tom B. Wright was inducted into the U.S. Navy during the Korean War. He served in the capacity of a pediatrician, even giving exchange transfusions to erythroblastic RH babies. Tom and I were, and are, definitely on the same wave length in our devotion to total service for every patient, regardless of social or monetary affluence. He was an accomplished pianist and we would share our profound love of classical music when we would gallivant to the annual American Academy of Pediatric Meetings, usually held at the Grand Traverse City Resort or by Torch Lake, MI. While en route by automobile, we would listen to our favorite piano concertos and symphonies on CD recordings. One time, in 1998, we were ably chauffeured to the meeting at Shanty Creek by my Grandson, Jon Prengel, who was visiting from his home base in Frankfurt, Germany.

Tom and I had an intimate friendship, socially and professionally, with Aaron Stern and his good wife, Nel, who lived in Ann Arbor. Aaron was professor of Pediatric Cardiology at the University of MI. Mott Hospital for many years. He would come to Bay City General and Mercy Hospital to conduct cardiac clinics on our congenital heart cases. Aaron had an inherited spinal deformity which caused a handicap in ambulation for him. He was a very affable and intelligent person, down to earth, humble, and honest to a tenth of a penny. He was a real gentleman. All our heart problem children were referred to Aaron in consultation. His diagnosis and therapies were exact, practical, and had excellent results. On a couple occasions, we all were together at pediatric meetings held in New Orleans, which was Nel's birthplace. Also, we all ended up several times at Zehnders famous chicken dinners restaurant in Frankenmouth.

Florie and Tom Wright had five children and there were never more devoted parents. The children all metamorphosed into superb human beings, excelled in their professional pursuits but, like my progeny, none pursued

M.D. degrees, probably due to the grueling and arduous work. Apparently, our examples of rigorous devotion to medical practice dissuaded them that a happy home life was possible. I've often entertained the thought that pediatricians should mimic chaste priests and sacrifice all personal pleasures and ties to their patients' welfare. But this is selfish and impractical in nature's schematics and the big picture.

Benjamin, one of the Wright boys, at age 14 years accompanied me to a Michigan-OSU football game in Ann Arbor on a Saturday in late November of 1963 - incidentally which we lost. I had arranged to meet Ken Barker at the gate of "The Big House" after the game, but was unable to do so because of the 107,000 attending consumers. When we reached our car, I told Benji to remain car-bound en garde, while I endeavored to contact Barker by phone. After a fruitless mission, I returned to the car to discover Benji in a state of heated agitation, saying, "Boy am I glad to see you! About a dozen car owners have been hassling me to move this vehicle for the past fifteen minutes, and I've fought them off by tooth and nail." There was a massive car jam and snarl and I know these car ragers did not display their Sunday manners when they accosted poor Benji. I apologized to him profusely for being such an immovable person and letting him hold the bag alone for me.

Florie Wright was a nutritional expert extraordinaire and held a degree in food preparation from study at Central Michigan University in Mount Pleasant. Also, she was a graduate R.N. (registered nurse) from Crawford W. Long Hospital, in Atlanta, GA. I've been the recipient of some of her culinary masterpieces over the years. Her specialty is standing beef or pork roasts, which are also my favorites. My taste buds had a liberal education from my wonderful mother who was known all over Pennsylvania for her unique cuisine. Her granddaughter, Susan, is a chip off the old block and is developing rapidly into an outstanding chef persona.

Tom and Florie had a harrowing experience one summer while on vacation in Caseville. They were rudely interrupted on the second day of their stay by the dear telephone informing them that their house on Handy Drive was on fire and their immediate presence was requested (if not sooner). Their offspring had been left in charge and some secretive hanky panky had prevailed during an impromptu teen party. One question you never, ever asked Tom, unless you had time to kill, was "How are you feeling, Thomas?" It seems as though brother Tom has had almost every physical human infirmity discussed in the textbook of medicine and he would liberally describe them in infinitesimal detail when queried.

The telephone has literally and figuratively been the necessary bane of my existence in medical practice. On a busy day, we would receive over one hundred calls. I would interrupt my interview with the patient to respond to all important "must" calls, such as hospitals, doctors, and emergencies. On a few occasions, at the height of heated frustration, I was known to vehemently slam the phone receiver down, sometimes injuring it severely. I would get calls all hours of the night and mostly they were of the frivolous gender. Often I would state that "I pray fervently that no one inserts a telephone in my casket." God bless the telephone, it has its benevolences and its iniquities, a double edged sword. In my case, it is my blessed lifeline with my children and their spouses, who are all globally positioned.

Shortly after the holocaust (WWII), Doris and I became familiar with Frank and Regina Bearsch. Frank was a very proficient orthodontist, and he and I made a trade-off pact. He would use his expertise for correcting any orthodontic problems our children confronted and I, in turn, would use my pediatric knowledge to care for any problems his daughter encountered. This arrangement was a concoction perpetrated by the "great" '29 stock crash, because money became scarce as "hens teeth". The doctors would trade their services for chickens, vegetables, and fruits because no one had any expendable cash. You can imagine my chagrin and frustration during my college days, '29 to '36, trying to scrimp and scrape to meet deadlines in tuition payment especially. Even though my father had an excellent job as foreman of forty five pattern makers, my poor parents had to "sweat it" with the money for my education. I made a solemn promise to my mother that I would repay every cent. But she, in reply, said "You may have a free ride on your schooling, if you promise me that you will give all your children a college education for their life occupations." This promise I actuated to the letter (and then some). Tom and Greg hung on for a couple extra years of didactics. I told my kids there were only two stipulations I would promulgate regarding their college education. First, you will not marry before graduation, and second you will attend a college in Michigan. They each adhered strictly by these rules and they all graduated from respectable colleges with respectable grades. I believe sincerely, that a post high school education now for every adolescent is a definite "must" for him/her to succeed in life and develop their complete potential for health and happiness. It gives them a fighting chance to earn an honest living.

Frank Bearsch was a golfer par excellence even though he was a mighty mite about five feet four and weighing 110 pounds soaking wet. I've always been amazed at the distance he could hit that little white ball. His rhythmic swing was effortless, but the speed generated by the club head was the real secret to his space accomplishment undoubtedly. It put my hacking, herky-jerky swing to shame. Regina was a plain Jane, prim and proper, true, and honest to the nth degree. She wouldn't win a beauty contest, but she did radiate love.

When I completed my combination office / apartment building in September

1951, my mother signaled her desire to move from our home in Greensburg, PA, to our home in Bay City, MI. My wonderful father had passed on to his creator in August of 1950, premature at age 64 years. His fourth, in a series of strokes, resulted in a massive cerebral hemorrhage, culminating in death. Mother and I struck a bargain. She would sell our homestead, which dad had laboriously erected, and give me the money to build my office building. She would then live gratis in the second story apartment with her dear companion, Catherine Leseman, for their remaining lives. The deal was completed and it benefited both of us magnificently. Mother had the advantage of living near her grandchildren and I reaped the structure for my office practice, which is really paramount in pediatric medicine.

I conjured extensive plans for the office building / apartment in my spare time while I was serving my 27 months duty for Uncle Sam in Alaska, in the Second World War. Mother worked in my office as receptionist and telephone communicator for several years, and did a proficient job. She loved children, as I do, and did her utmost to entertain them and their mothers.

My mother also collected money payments for my services. This was a huge advantage for there was no one more honest. I know several doctors who have been ripped off financially by dishonest employees, and I'm sure that I was one of the goats for large sums at other times. In medical school we were never taught anything about money matters relative to debits and credits. We were greenhorns and sitting ducks for conniving secretaries. Outside of mother, I can wholeheartedly say, I only had two ladies who were strictly honest to the letter, Sue Frantz and Marilyn Vandriesche. My two worst villains were Sandy Gerhauser, and Rose, a policeman's wife who smoked incessantly and didn't know up from down about money. My CPA's (certified public accountants) made excellent salaries but as far as I could surmise, they never contributed to my welfare and let my secretaries get away with murder. At one time, I had over 100 grand outstanding in debts. Literally and figuratively, I must have lost huge sums of money in uncollected insurance claims stuffed in desk drawers uncompleted.

I have no one to blame for my inordinate losses, except myself. Guess I was too involved in saving children's lives and was utterly oblivious to the business nuts and bolts of my practice. It's illogical that I shouldn't realize the importance of monetary values, after surviving the gargantuan '29 stock crash. As a child and youth, I've always been deeply impressed with the biblical dissertations about pecuniary affairs. A special statement is "it is easier for a rich man to go through the eye of a needle than for him to enter the Kingdom of Heaven." Another aphorism is, "think not of worldly possessions, but concentrate on spiritual ideals, which are of everlasting value." Also, "worry not concerning your human needs for God will take care of you." My dear intimate youthful friend, Paul W. Seaton, always reiterated "it's no sin to be poor, but it's damned inconvenient." Anyhow, strange as it seems, I just can't whip up any sweat or passion when it comes down to monetary affairs. Guess I'm just happy with the bare necessities of life, - especially food. Surely, my darling daughter, Melissa, does not inherit her shrewd expert CPA and math talents, by a long shot, from me.

The only person I actually kept in touch with of all my Alaskan army friends, was Carl Olson. Carl was a top notch roentgenologist, and we were closely allied for 2+ years in making difficult diagnosis on brain scratcher patients. When he was extricated from the army in '46, he obtained a job as radiologist at Saginaw General Hospital, only a skip and a jump from Bay City. We renewed our friendship and we got together with our wives for dinners and tete a tete sessions. Carl and I often reminisced about our service in Alaska, - especially concerning the enigmatic back and spinal problem cases. Carl was intrigued to no end about my series of meningococcal meningitis patients. For some inexplicable reason, Carl went off the deep end of reality and ended up in the Veteran's Hospital at Battle Creek, MI, as patient and x-ray staff physician. In Alaska, he was brooding, depressed, and showed cycles of puzzling solitary behavior at times.

In the fifties, we also struck up a liaison with the Medvezkey's and the Connelly's. We reciprocated pot-luck dinners at our residences and shared mutual conviviality. As I previously mentioned, I temporarily established my office practice in Mike Medvezkey's office building when I left Fern Foster in December 1949. Mike was a family M.D. and self made surgeon of no mean ability We entered the army simultaneously and both served in Alaska for a couple years. I lucked out on assignments by being based in Anchorage, while poor Mike served in Cold Harbor, about halfway out on the volcanic Aleutian Island Chain. The weather at his station was totally brutal with a capital B. Mike would say, "It's gotta be the only place on earth where the wind blows in all four directions at the same time." He stated that while heading into a stiff wind with your body jack-knifed forward, a sudden shift of the wind in the opposite direction would propel you forward with a force that would put you on the ground, flat on your face.

Mike was an avid fisherman and hunter, gloriously living with unlimited prey - seal, otter, walrus and fox. There were no trees on these "rat" islands, so one energetic G.I. on Umnak, erected a wooden structure and posted a sign designated, "The National Forest of Umnak".

Mike swore it rained every day at Cold Harbor and after 18 months of duty there, he developed Rheumatic Fever. He was dispatched from his abode of torture to good old U.S.A. I had a steak dinner with him at the Blue Lantern in Anchorage as he was enroute to a Seattle army hospital. He and his buddy, Jim Connelly, (shanty Irish) unfortunately developed a deadly propensity for gin binges. I was a sad pallbearer at Mike's funeral in the late sixties and brother Jim followed in his footsteps circa 15 months later. Jim's first wife died in the early seventies and he remarried a Mercy Hospital pediatric nurse, Mary. He could bake the best apple pie you ever tasted.

One of my most weird and unusual medical relationships was with Bill Reed, who was an erstwhile self educated, pseudo general surgeon. Bill had first class training in surgery under the aegis of the eminent surgeon, Herb Coller, at the University of Michigan. Bill's surgical technique was infallible, but his peers discovered a big flaw in his modus operandi. He was dishonestly operating on <u>normal</u> tissue as revealed by the pathologist and his post operative results were necessarily <u>perfect</u>. Bill married the wealthy, George Reichles' daughter, but divorced her for trumped up reasons. Like the apostle Paul on the road to Damascus, he was suddenly struck by super religious lightening. Bill became an all out super Christian medic, who prayed with his patients in the hospital corridors and operating rooms with every surgical procedure. He became enamored of the Blue Cross/Blue Shield representative in the Saginaw Bay area, Kay Katt, and remarried. They moved to Eugene, Oregon, where Bill applied for medical licensure. There was some investigation by the Oregon Board of Medical Licensure, and they asked me, as long time Bay, Arenac, Iosco Counties' Secretary, for a recommendation for him. I confirmed that Bill was a reputable character who invoked religious principles into his surgery. Apparently, I saved his bacon and he was granted his medical license by reciprocity to practice there.

He and Kay somehow became disenchanted with the "Beaver" state and then moved to Tampa, Florida. Bill obtained his medical license to practice surgery. He had a brainstorm and went off the deep end of religion vis a vis medicine. Along with Kay, he established his dream of a "Christian Medical Foundation". It took roots and he was joined by physicians all over the United States. They would give biblical lectures and talks at medical society meetings in large populated areas state wide. Bill was ultimately successful in recruiting eminent doctors in diverse specialties and formed a solid organization with yearly educational meetings. I have received invitations to each annual meeting and their programs appear very interesting and enlightening. Bill and Kay Reed were able to get a foothold and develop this major project, by deriving monetary profits from a store, selling medical and religious artifacts, in Tampa. They also earned funds from their CME's speeches. I believe their efforts are probably benevolent, sincere, and worthwhile.

One of my dearest and most revered friends of all time was, and is, Harry McGee. Harry is a super conscientious Ophthalmologist, and a fairly decent golfer of no mean repute. He is probably the kindest, most good hearted, truthful person you will ever meet. I'm sure Harry would give anyone in need, the veritable shirt off his back anytime and anywhere. Harry's first wife, Ann, was also very generous and beautiful of thought, word, and deed.

Harry and I were avid golfers and we'd go out to the Bay County golf course every Wednesday afternoon. Usually Harry's father, Clarence, would accompany us. Ann would fix us a culinary delight with sandwiches and fruit. Clarence, in his 80's, was a par and one bogey golfer with a grooved swing. Hiram would hit the ball always down the middle, straight as a dye.

Harry would stop by my house to check on our kitties of which, at one time, we had at least 25 and counting. (We are practically bankrupt with only a baker's dozen now.) We had multiple eye problems with our felines, due to "friend" scuffles. He was always very concerned and would go all out to help restore their normal eye function. Harry had a wry sense of humor and was always somewhat timid, cautious, and leery of offending people. A good golfer, he was usually a one bogey player, but I remember how elated he was one time when he hit 39 for 9 holes.

I attended Harry and Ann's golden anniversary party in '85, at the Michigan House on Westside Saginaw Road. Ann expired in '93, while they were vacationing at their Marco Island, Florida retreat. Apparently, she had fatal cardiovascular atherosclerosis and passed on peacefully in her sleep. Harry was single for three years, and then remarried widow, Eva Hickner. Eva's former spouse was a psychiatrist who committed suicide via carbon monoxide from his car. He also inadvertently killed his daughter, who was sleeping above the garage. Harry and I are staunch friends in the "over the hill" gang of retired medics, who meet at the Holiday Inn in Bay City on the first Tuesday of the month.

Doris and I were also on friendly terms with two Hudson families, totally unrelated. Ralph and Kate Hudson were an eccentric pair, who devoted their time exclusively to running a laundry of repute, on Third Street in downtown Bay City. They had a thriving business and lived on Sixth Street, next door to us. On weekends, they would live it up, in high gear, at the old Country Club. I remember especially one New Years Eve, in about '55, while at a gala club party, about midnight Ralph was really in orbit. He became actively engaged in verbal combat with Joe Hirschfield, who wagered $100.00 that Ralph wouldn't take a dive into the outdoor heated club swimming pool while fully dressed. Ralph was a premier showman and while fully dressed in a tuxedo, fit to kill, actually did this act. Indubitably, he was on a down hill road to self destruction and gave up the ghost during a sudden, lethal coronary attack a couple years later. One of his sons, Jimmie, was stomping in a leaf fire to extinguish it, one afternoon, and sustained a severe extensive 3rd degree burn of his lower right leg. Actually, their two boys had poor supervision, guidance and nurturing. They were odd balls, too, but to a lesser degree.

The other Hudson family is comprised of Nolen C and good wife, Luella. Nolen is a top notch breast surgeon, with no blemishes (lawsuits) yet. He has to pay well over $150 grand yearly for insurance. They call it "malpractice" insurance, but I believe it should be named "mal-lawyer" insurance for greedy, grubber clients. Actually, the counselors get more money than the claimants. One juicy case will net over a million for both miscreants. I suppose I shouldn't be so bitter, but the situation has escalated and grown to gargantuan proportions, way out beyond our Milky Way. It's like dodging a minefield in the dark, going blind.

Nolen's son and his better half are in Montgomery, AL., and they were the proud parents of triplet babies – two femmes and one "stem-winder". In the nineties, the Hudsons invited the Martin Jaffes and us to a dinner celebrating their anniversary. Nolen served a sumptuous beef wellington dinner, made by his culinary artistry. Nolen conducted a weekly meeting, devoted in large part to cancer of the breast, chaired by oncologist David Cook, (one of my patients, way back in the house-call dark ages.) The presentations were scholarly, informative, and creative.

We were also fond of the Tupper family, for many cogent reasons. Tom and Althea Tupper lived in a stately mansion on Center Avenue, a showplace brick building from the lumberman and shipyard era of the late nineteenth century. It was built under the jurisdiction of Virgil Tupper, who was Bay City's number A-1 surgeon. Virgil graduated cum laude from the University of Michigan Medical School, and starred in football for U of M during 1906 – 1909 in his undergraduate days. He showed me a picture of his football team dressed in leather helmets, in bare necessity suits, without pads. The entire squad was only <u>fifteen</u> players. This was when he was on his deathbed in the Tupper home.

Althea has two brothers who are doctors in southwestern Michigan, a dermatologist and an orthopedic surgeon. Tom was a lay minister in the Episcopal Church and was engaged in the hardware business. Althea tells a humorous yarn about a priest who was visiting father Virgil. She was rudely awakened by her two year old daughter; Taffy, age 3 years, who answered the doorbell and screamed, "Mother, there is a man at the door dressed in woman's clothes!" Althea made a fireman's run to the door and offered her abject apologies.

Speaking about Taffy brings to mind a very grave malady involving her shortly thereafter. My bedside phone aroused me from a deep, heavenly sleep at 3 a.m. one night in the early fifties. Tom Tupper was calling and agitatedly reporting that Taffy suddenly was delirious, projectile vomiting, and running a temperature of 105 degrees. I awoke with a startling bang and shouted "I'll meet you at Mercy Hospital, double stat!" I grabbed my red robe and hit the floor running and flew in a whirlwind to Mercy. I met Tom and Taffy at the door and we rushed to pediatrics where I performed a highpoints cursory examination. My original telephone diagnosis was confirmed for Taffy showed neck rigidity, was as hot as a firecracker, and was unconscious and showing early signs of seizure activity. First priority was a stat lumbar puncture with slow release of fluid to relieve increased intracranial pressure which can disastrously jam the medulla (vital centers) into the cervical spinal canal. The spinal fluid was somewhat turbid (cloudy) and under definite increased pressure. A CBC was done immediately, along with a blood culture. The spinal fluid was dispatched urgently to the lab for immediate culture, gram stain smear, glucose and protein determinations. Our gram smear showed biscuit shaped pairs of gram negative organisms and our causative organisms most probably were the meningococci of Weichselbaum.

In young children and infants, bacterial meningitis is caused predominantly by this germ, pneumococcus a gram positive encapsulated diplococcus and by influenza, a gram negative coccobacilus. In 1950, when this illness of Taffy's occurred, Sulfadiazine worked wonders in obliterating the meningococcus at an IV dose of 100 milligrams per kilo per 24 hours. I also had perfect results with sulfa in my meningitis patients in Alaska in the 1940's. But now the honeymoon is over for Sulfa and Penicillin as the crafty meningo and pneumococci have concocted genetic shake ups leading to rank resistance thanks to over usage. Intravenous fluids must be administered meagerly with the utmost care because of causing fatal cerebral edema. If there was allergy to sulfa, we could have used chloramphenicol, but this drug carries the possibility of complete bone marrow suppression and death. If endotoxic shock or papilloldema occurs, Hydrocortisone in high dosage is employed (plus prayer). Frozen plasma helps if there is low blood plasma volume. If there is D.I.C. (disseminated intravascular coagulation), platelet transfusions and heparin IV are employed. Nowadays, 2000era and 21st century, we have the cephalosporin and vancomycin to conquer the meningitic bacteria. The secret in treating bacterial meningitis is early diagnosis and early concentrated treatment to produce a successful outcome. Chronic complications consist of cerebral edema, deafness, cystic formation, blockage of spinal fluid circulation, and reduction of intellectual acuity. For close intimate family exposure, Rifampin fills the bill. For prevention, there is a vaccine for type A, C and Y meningococcus. Many people carry meningococci in their throats but they are usually harmless. Meningitis occurs in groups of persons housed in close contact. Therefore, it is advisable for all college students to be immunized with influenza, pneumonia, meningococcal vaccines before entering college, especially if they are delegated to dormitories, fraternities or sororities. Taffy Tupper was treated with heavy increments of penicillin G IV and made a complete uneventful uncomplicated recovery.

NOTEWORTHY PEER PHYSICIAN ASSOCIATES:

Harris Woodburne, M.D., erstwhile internist and swashbuckling sailor of renown, was Steffie Knobloch's doctor and a good friend of mine. He had a thirty two foot sail boat which served as a posh conveyance for many of our voyages on Saginaw Bay. Harris was a real scholar of the art of medicine, possessing a wry sardonic sense of humor and a great respect for human nature. Besides our sailing escapades, we also had many sessions together of physical fitness, swimming, and exercise at our YMCA. During my high school days, I also spent many pleasant productive hours at our Greensburg Y.

Harris was birthed in Bombay India as his father was a key player in the US Embassy there. His wife Grace was severely handicapped due to arthritis, deafness, and diabetes. They have two sons who are M.D.'s in Traverse City, one an orthopedic surgeon and the other in internal medicine. Harris took his sailing real seriously. One Sunday, I took a radio with me on our sailing excursion to listen to the Lions-Packers football battle. Harris scowled at me and said, "There will be no radio broadcasts on my ship." I got the message loud and clear and readily capitulated to his wishes. I attended his funeral entailing burial from our 1st Presbyterian Church, with a fitting eulogy rendered by a son from Traverse City.

Abraham Kessler was an astute pediatrician practicing his wizard way in northern Michigan's city of Alpena. We became acquainted in the early fifties at pediatric seminars in Detroit and Ann Arbor. Abe was a forceful little guy, an eligible bachelor of 50's passionately wedded to his profession. He married for the first time shortly after we became friends professionally and socially. He became the happy proud father of twins right off the bat. Abe referred several of his puzzling patients to me for consultation and diagnosis.

One little two year old boy in particular referred by Abe is noteworthy of discussion. Billy was moderately mentally deficient due to congenital syphilis and, in addition, he had interstitial keratitis of the cornea. The active syphilis disease had been stamped out by the mother's syphilitic treatment while he was being incubated in utero but, unfortunately, it was too late to obliterate the footsteps of Syphilis entirely. Originally I had done a series of clinical research procedures to try to restore, to some higher degree, a mentally bankrupt child's I.Q. and mental acuity. The methodology consisted of injecting minute doses of typhoid vaccine intravenously daily, over a five day period. The basic reasoning was to create a fever of at least 104 degrees each day to cause an inflammatory reaction to partially living brain cells. This, in turn, hopefully would restore full vitality to their functioning. Kessler referred three patients altogether to me, involving young toddlers who embodied mentally low voltage due to various causations known or unknown. We performed I.Q. tests on these children before and six months after, done by myself, parents, and psychologists. In conclusion, our results on follow up really did not prove any drastic increase in mental functioning of a defining nature. We had to be ultra careful to not cause a speck of harm as incorporated in the Greek Aesculapian Oath doctors take on receiving their degree. The motto is: Treatment must improve but at least not cause any harm or injury.

Dave Bowman, family practitioner and aspiring psychiatrist, was a man of many colors and many wives. He had a magnetism and charm of fatalistic proportions that the female gender just couldn't resist. One of his wives was an X-ray technician at General Hospital who untimely developed Mumps on the first day of their honeymoon. Dave was a physician of average ability, not brilliant. His expertise involved psychosomatic illness and psycho-social matters. One of his live-in members of the opposite gender was a star baseball pitcher who was constructed like a brick chick and lovely too. Bowman moved on to Ohio after a brief practice period in the Allen Building with over 50 fellow colleagues in various specialties and family practice.

Saba and Mana Kessler were inextricably intertwined in my practice with children. Saba was our lone member of the tender gender in general medical practice in Bay City until the advent of Debbie Filek, pediatrician from Canada in the 1980's. Saba consulted with me regarding sick little ones on many occasions, mainly because of a lack of confidence as a family practitioner. Saba invited my wife and me to dinner in her home several times and her cuisine was high caliber and delectable. We all rotated in a carousel fashion at assuming the duties and responsibilities of being president for one year for our Bay County Medical Society. Saba's turn came up during my ten year tenure as Society Secretary and she was reluctant to usurp the mantle of presidency. I assured her that I would exert my utmost to help support her in every way possible to make her year a huge success. Actually, I did perform the lion's share of her obligations and at the end of her year she thanked me profusely and showered me with a one pound box of candy. Her better half, Mana, was an ear, nose, throat, and thoracic surgeon, skilled in the art of bronchoscopy and removal of foreign bodies from the lungs. I worked in concert with him on a few cases of peanut, popcorn, hotdog, and bean aspirations into the bronchi, usually the right main stem bronchus because of its straighter, anatomical relation to the trachea. Mana was rough and somewhat unconsciously brutal with the youngsters.

Hugh Cook, endoscopist, was much gentler and facile in extracting foreign bodies. Speed is of paramount importance in this operation because the child it totally without oxygen while the scope is intratracheal. Hugh is a marvel at speed. My duties were as anesthetist and it was plenty perilous for me.

One of the most unforgettable characters I knew with a cantankerous and irritating modus operandi was Douglas McCrae, family practitioner to the core. Douglas was a strange guy who had weird, unconventional medical ideas and was hard to figure out. The major problem in his life was an uncontrollable love affair with CO2 (carbon dioxide) which he used on all of his patients. Doug had strong aspirations to practice psychiatric treatment on his adults and children. He would employ CO2 gas by mask to a person and it would act like an anesthetic to produce profound somnolence. Regardless of the primary diagnosis, Doug administered CO2 to just about every patient in his office and in the hospital. He hounded me relentlessly to use this modality in treating children in concert with him. The hospital nurses and doctors in his department and the department of medicine were all rebellious, chagrined, and up in arms over this treatment method. It just wasn't acceptable by the hospital administration and it created a combative situation. Hal Shafer, our chief of medicine at General Hospital, was deeply disturbed and worried about possible mortality, especially in elderly handicapped people. Hal practically got into a fist altercation with Douglas. I kept saying "No" to him, making up numerous excuses, but being harassed and haunted day and night. Finally, like a furuncle, the issue came to a head and as Chief of Staff at General Hospital, in combination with the Board of Directors; we kicked him off the staff. We acted after Dr. McCrae failed to pay his hospital dues at a stated time. We called a meeting with him and by due process of our bylaws, we finally, to everyone's considerable relief, rejected him. Douglas had a brother who was a doctor in Caro.

You couldn't meet a nicer guy than Doug. Really, Doug was a brilliant physician, a graduate of the University of Michigan Medical School, but this obsession killed him literally and figuratively. Actually, I tried CO2 inhalations on a six year old patient named Forrest Wiles Jr., in treatment of incorrigible behavior problems. After three inductions with this gas, I discontinued it because of its uselessness, the parent's apprehension, and the child's adverse reaction.

Another very erudite and intellectual acquaintance of mine was George Ascherl, a highly educated neuro-radiologist. George was married for the first time when he was in middle age to a lady doctor who was an emergency room specialist. His wife, Susan, appeared outwardly to be quite amicable, dulcet, and efficient in her professional duties. They consummated the marriage, #2 for Susan, by bearing a baby, George Jr., and seemed to have an ideal, serene marriage. Unfortunately, Susan unpredictable and unreasonably absconded with their young five year old, George Jr., and bolted to Colorado. George Sr. was completely devastated and tried with might and main to come to a legal settlement to retrieve a fatherly relation with his son. The mother consorted with a "filthy rich" lawyer in Colorado, and by some stealthy legerdemain connived with the Judge and a half baked mercenary psychologist to take over George Junior's complete care. I had several long, loquacious sessions with George Sr., regarding this absolutely pitiful situation. I felt deep sadness for poor Doctor Ascherl for being completely robbed of a father-son relationship and for the son who was also robbed. To me, it is unconceivable that any true mother could commit such a dastardly, vile criminal act. George Sr. asked me as an experienced pediatrician to intercede for him by appearing before a Judicial Meeting. I answered affirmatively, but it never happened. I feel strongly that after a divorce, the mother and father should share equal relationship rights with their mutual progeny. After all, their child/children have 50% of their genes and DNA bequeathed by each parent, and a boy especially needs his God given father to fraternize with to establish his identity. In this case, I believe young George could not have possibly been nurtured in all ways by a more capable and deserving father.

My last intimate medical relationship was with Robert Prophater, a jack of all trades as a general family physician. Robert was a proud grad of South Carolina Medical School at Columbia. Robert had practiced for seven years in Greenville, Ohio, before he entered practice in concert with Dave Bowman, a fellow general medical practitioner. Robert was a politician par excellence and had an innate impressive gift of gab to go with a magnetic personality. He had married number two wife just before his migration to Bay City. His partnership with Bowman, like oil and water, was not a congenial mix, and he went solo after two contested, bickering years. These two medical practitioners were definitely grossly incompatible in all ways, you name it.

Prophater was ambitious and promoted himself into the presidency of all organizations he entered into. For some egotistical reason, he strove to always be the head conductor in every coterie he joined. Public relations were his forte' and in 1984 he joined the hospital administrative staff as a problem solver and advisor of all deleterious relations between the physician medical staff and the hospital gurus. He was given a weird title and acted as a go-between the hospital doctors and the hospital governing board, which rankled the doctors. He handled this position admirably until prostate cancer with pulmonary metastasis overtook him in the year 2000. Bob's second wife died from cardiac muscular deteriorization. He then married lovely Nancy Short, a local, well endowed celebrity. In January of 2004, Bob was still a fighting survivor who was on oxygen all day. He succumbed to king cancer in mid 2006, but after a valiant battle.

I would be remiss if I didn't include my very close buddy, Mike Dardas who was a most excellent obstetrician. Mike had the sweetest, mellifluous disposition of anyone I ever knew. He had a heart of gold and was a maximal servant for all of his patients. He was very positive and always smiling, cheerful regardless of the duress and pressure. Mike married a brainy, energetic red headed nurse from St. Louis, MO. They had a beautiful daughter, Karen, who was born with a total loss of hearing (stone deaf). Katie deserves a gold medal for her tenacity and dogged perseverance in successfully teaching Karen to talk, read, and write over a period of 14 years.

Mike's patients loved him like a father for his undying obstetric nurture. He and I worked in tandem and close harmony with the newborns. My wife, Doris, was number one friend of Katie's, and we all had many mutual dinners together. Mike volunteered for service in the medical corps in WWII. He had a rough and tough go in Burma in the Southeast Asian theater of army operations. Mike was converted to general surgery duty there, and walked several hundred miles on the road to Mandalay where the flying fishes play. This arduous physical activity literally ruined his health, and he died shortly after returning home.

My fellow pediatrician brothers and peers were a very happy and congenial group. Of all the medical branches of medicine, I truly believe we are the most congenial, relaxed, and positive in our dealings and transactions with our patients. Children are unique due to the fact they are, or should be, controlled by their guardians. It is advantageous if we have our own children as examples and yardsticks for understanding and judging their actions and reactions. Our prime reason for engaging pediatrics as our life's work is 100% because of our love and championship for all children. Also, we do the work because of our intense desire to help children attain their maximum development mentally, physically and morally. Making money is a necessity for survival, but not an all consuming goal to amass a fortune. My best M.D. friend in pediatric practice was Thomas Benjamin Wright. Our goals and lifestyle coincided to a "T" in just about every way. Tom was saturated with the milk of human kindness for his patients. He was imbued with all out responsibility and was a night and day workhorse with a unique bedside manner. Don Campbell, Dick Bickham, Tom and I, formed the four horsemen of pediatrics for Bay City. We constituted the spine and backbone of service for childhood diseases from fetus and newborn to adults prior to age nineteen or twenty.

Fred Chapin was also an astute pediatrician, who came on the scene to the Allen Clinic during WWII. He sustained a fractured leg celebrating the night before he was scheduled to enter military service. While he served yeoman duty as a pediatrician, his primary consuming interest was in psychiatry. His wife, Margaret, was a renowned Child Psychologist.

Al Ellison joined Chapin and Wright in 1960, and they formed a mighty triumvirate. Al was in his glory in an argument and would always take the opposite side. After he initiated the dialogue and fanned it to its full fury and intensity, he would duck out and let the other parties battle it out tooth and nail. After about seven years, Al moved his practice to East Lansing as he was adamant in being associated with a University. After ten years there, cancer of the thyroid caused his expiration. Al was like the proverbial Harvard Man, "You can always tell a man from Harvard, but you can't tell him much."

Fred Chapin realized his lifelong dream in the '60's when he abruptly bolted Bay City for a course in psychiatry, at the State Mental Hospital in Traverse City. Eventually, he culminated his psych career in Cooksville, TN, at a psychiatric hospital as administrator. He became an erstwhile equestrian and settled on a horse farm. He expired (probably from heart disease) along about August 2006.

Tom Wright rescued Sezai Olgac from the Children's Hospital at Wahjamega and made him a full pediatrician partner in circa 1988. But Sezai had ambitious plans of his own, and dissolved the joint alliance for his own sphere of pediatrics. He employed two Indian pediatricians, Bhaskar Devonagondi and Bilagali Sundara, who were well qualified and real gentlemen doctors just starting out in practice.

After Fred left, Dick Bickham came on the scene in the Allen Clinic and established his Peds dominion. Dick was fresh from his internship at Ford Hospital and cut a Lochinvar swath in our child care practice. As he was winding down toward retirement, Bickham ended up in practice with Olgac, Devonagondi, and Sundara.

We finally broke the spell and did unite for the first time with a stellar tender gender physician from Toronto Canada, viz Debbie Filek. However, it took a Herculean effort for two years by Debbie to manipulate the strings to transfer here. Finally, before I cut the chord of practice, Sue Hendrickson pranced in on the pediatric stage in Bay City, a very welcome addition.

In about 1950, I was instrumental in perpetrating an on call rotation for Dr's. Foster, (on his proverbial last legs), Chapin, and myself. I conceived this idea while overseas as a means of securing precious time off for recreation and family pursuits. It was somewhat patterned after our on call system in the army general hospitals. We each would alternate night and weekend calls from Saturday noon. Fern Foster would answer calls from his vacation residence in Au Gres and Fred and I would cover at the hospital emergency room. This unique plan continued, unabated, for circa thirty years, until our younger, more tender pediatricians decided we should downgrade and take calls from home with the ER physicians shouldering the brunt of the Peds onslaught and calling us for help when needed.

During an assiduous winter weekend, we might service over sixty patients on Saturday and Sunday until way past midnight each evening. This duty certainly was not for the faint of heart. It became especially arduous and perilous if we had real emergencies at both General and Mercy Hospitals synonymously, and our back up pediatrician was not available. This situation did occur for me in the middle of January one time while I was swamped with true emergencies at General Hospital and a ten month old baby boy entered Mercy ER with a totally collapsed right lung due to a foreign body in the right main stem bronchus with hemoglobin of 6 grams. I begged Dr. Grigg to call my backup, Dr. Olgac, but he refused. I was left holding the bag with alligators up to my gluteus maximus. Needless to say, the baby expired after four hours and we all ended up in court. We didn't have a ghost of a china man's chance. Dr. Pelazar, our anesthesiologist, wouldn't operate because of the dastardly low Hg, but in retrospect, surgery, even though hazardous, was really our only slim chance for success. The baby was in extremis with mortal respiratory distress when I first saw her; and transfusion was impossible for several cogent reasons.

Chapter 24

Clouds on the Horizon

Realistically, I had a sliver of doubt on the night of April 1, 1937, that my marriage to Doris the next day might eventually end up on the rocks, but faint of heart ne'er won fair lady. I decided "damn the torpedoes and full speed ahead" to marry her because I was hopelessly in love with the lady of my dreams. I might have had an inkling of possible disaster for the marriage when my mother and father did not show for the wedding ceremony, which was performed in the rectory of St. Boniface Church in Baltimore, because I was a <u>staunc</u>h Protestant. It rankled me <u>severely</u> that I had to sign the birthright of my unborn children over to the Catholic Church as a requirement for our marriage. But I was head over heels, madly in love and I thought somehow things would work out equitably. My heart strings prevailed over my better judgment.

We were both only children and quite immature for the most important decision of our lives. Realistically, Doris was in addition, an only grandchild and <u>most</u> importantly her mother, May, died when she was only nine years old. May picked a pimple on her cheek and it became infected with an extremely virulent bacterium, probably strep or staphococcis with development of cerebral sepsis in 1921, before our miracle antibiotics. Doris' father became a converted pillar of the Catholic Church, and devoted all his energy to Doris as his prime focus in life. An all consuming close father/daughter relationship resulted. She lived with her father's mother, Caroline, for a couple years, but she didn't see eye to eye with the pithy Caroline. She became adopted by Nettie and George Gibson, her father's sister. The Gibson's were childless and superb substitute parents, but Doris was queen and indulged to the maximum. She had everything she desired. In other words, we were both the epitome of "spoiled brats" and fed by a silver spoon with no competition. Our bread was lavishly buttered and literally predigested for us, two immature kids facing a hostile world – sink or swim.

Amazingly, Doris and I were compatible for five years, until I joined the army in July, 1942. In deference to me, Susan was baptized in the Evangelical Church in Marquette, MI. Our four year tenure separation in the army was a huge difficulty in our marriage. But the one prime significant event occurred unbeknownst to both of us, in July 1942, just before I left Bay City for my induction into the US Armed Forces. As you will recall, Dr. Matt Slattery turned his cottage on the Au Sable River over to us for a final farewell get together for a week for us to cement our family relationship. Unfortunately, Doris became pregnant. Doris realized the enormity of the situation about a month after I left but kept it a clandestine secret. However, the truth crushed to earth will rise again and the cat was extricated from the bag when she came to Vancouver, WA to be with me before I was shipped out to an overseas destination. Our first day back together in Vancouver was an inferno of pure "HELL". Doris was burning with unmitigated anger over being pregnant and my pure ecstasy of welcoming her turned to grapes of wrath almost instantly. Apparently, in her mind, I had committed an unforgivable sin. Our mutual relationship during our 3 months together in Vancouver was icy cold until she left at Thanksgiving time for Bay City. We tried to glue the pieces together, knowing it would probably be an eon before we would meet again. It was tough and rugged for both of us to have an unplanned child while being continents apart. However, I believe having the blessed event in absentia was a much harder cross to bear for her all alone. She had to be deeply depressed and it showed in her lukewarm correspondence during the Alaskan era for me.

We did have a most wonderful reunion when I returned from 27 months Alaskan duty. We were blessed with a 2 week recuperation furlough generously donated by the army to the lavish Grosvenor Hotel on Miami Beach. It was an ideal setup to mend two frayed hearts. Notwithstanding, there was one catch. I had come from frigid Alaska to superheated Florida in July. The temperature was over 100 degrees and it felt like we were being boiled in oil except for the cool night offshore ocean breezes. It seemed that during the war schism, while we were living by our own fortitude, that we became hardened, bossy, hard nosed and uncompromising.

My son Tom was 18 months old before I first saw him and I was a total stranger and intruder for years. He was totally attached hook, line, and sinker to his mother's apron strings. Doris and I had bitter disagreements on the proper nurture and behavior problems of our children and the disagreements escalated.

I was working 24 hour call to establish my pediatric practice and earn some money. Doris had exorbitant tastes for clothing and it appeared to me much of our hard earned money was being uselessly squandered. She possessed at least 100 pairs of shoes and dressed to the high heavens, spending money also lavishly on our children's clothes. It was similar to bailing out a boat with a hole in it except instead of water it was money. My pecunia was being incinerated faster than I could make it, figuratively.

I managed by the skin of my teeth to purchase a choice 200 foot frontage lot on the Tittabawassee River ten miles southwest of West Branch, MI in 1960. We dug a 200 foot well and installed a foundation and wooden outside framework for a dream cabin. Doris negated an inside wooden wall and, unfortunately, a heavy winter snowfall caved the roof in and the whole structure collapsed to our chagrin. I ended up by selling it kit and caboodle to pay for my daughter Melissa's final two year business education at the University of Michigan for her graduation sheepskin.

Our financial state deteriorated to the point of no return and I was reluctantly coerced to cancel Doris' credit at the shops and businesses at which she shopped. At about that time, 1962, I was beginning to have increasing anginal left chest pains. I finally made a lifetime decision of necessity to separate from my spouse. I was coming face to face with a possibly fatal heart attack or stroke. It seemed to me like there was absolutely no other choice for survival. Undoubtedly, my love for Doris was still very strong and I realized this agonizing judgment would have very negative repercussions on my four children. However, weighing all positive and negative factors, I decided it was do or die and I was not ready to die so I opted for separation and eventually the odious big D. Nevertheless, I made an all out commitment to our children. I realized that regardless, their welfare must come first, above all other factors. A child is in dire need of both parents to balance the equation and form his/her true image from the composite dyad of genes. My mother contributed a benevolent gift of undying love to our children to moderate the turbulent waves. It was extremely important to our children important that the parting of the parents exist on friendly terms amendable to compromise without strife or blame.

During this period of turmoil and anguish, I did meet my second wife, Mildred Vincent Stephenson, a divorcee with a daughter, Sylvia, who was Greg's age. Steffie was an excellent pediatric R.N. head night honcho in charge of the pediatric department on 2B at General Hospital. We had been associated in the mutual care of pediatric patients for several years beginning at Samaritan Hospital in 1950. We never really became acquainted until the Christmas season in 1961 when I was deep in the doldrums of strife at home. Our romance blossomed precipitously over a three year span and culminated in marriage, April 30, 1964, a year after my divorce became final. After the divorce, which was bitterly opposed by my mother and highly contested by Doris, I would join my former wife, my mother, and the children at dinner on all the holidays.

My divorce had stripped me clear to the bone financially. The vulture lawyers had closed the gates of mercy and collaborated to a settlement of our home and all contents plus $20,000 to Doris and $400 weekly payments for our children until they turned 18 years old. In addition, I had to pay off the mortgage on our home and help support my mother and her consort, Catherine Leseman. Climbing this mountain was a real back breaker and I really cogitated was this life really worth all the blood, sweat, and tears??? Somehow, with God's help and an <u>iron</u> will to survive, I buried myself in my medical practice and "where there's a will there's a way". Fortunately, my relations with my children and my office staff were very cordial and Gregory clung to me like my shadow. I felt guilt to the eyebrows for my separation from our children.

I never had the faintest idea of how severe the consequences of dissolution of our marriage had adversely affected our children, but in fact all of us were involved in this disaster. My mother practically disowned me, my new wife was morose because of the stripped finances, and the children all hated their step mother for her intrusion. Steffie's daughter hated me and my step mother, Marie Vincent, predicted a dire future for Steffie and me. Looking in retrospect, I believe a separation only from Doris would have been the wisest solution of all. "What fools these morals be"! I did consolidate my promise to my mother to support her to the bitter end and to give each one of my children a college education. At least Steffie and I did not add insult to injury by spawning any children as I had a vasectomy by Dr. Orlen Johnson immediately after the birth of Melissa, as advised by Dr. Crissey due to Doris' hypertension during labor.

Greg and Sylvia were identical ages and we took them on frequent trips to Oscar's fireman red cabin on the Tittabawassee River near our ill fated cabin that had foundered. In the winter we often went to Hoyt Park in Saginaw for sledding and ice skating followed by luscious dining. Greg often accompanied me on Sundays to my Presbyterian Church, as well as trips to Mercy and General Hospitals to make rounds on Sundays.

Susan and Tom adapted more readily to the bomb but Melissa remained grossly estranged to the new situation. On one auspicious occasion all my children, Sylvia, Steffie and I packed our bags and headed for Mackinaw Island in the straits of Lakes Heron and Michigan. We drove to Mackinaw City and ferried to the island from St. Ignace after crossing the magnificent Mackinaw Bridge. Cars are prohibited and transportation is by shanks mare, bicycle, or horse and buggy. It was a bright, sunny perfect day in July and our appetites were so razor sharp that the burgers tasted like porter house steaks. Our adorable Pekingese hound, Chet the Jet Hanulok, was with us and he cavorted about on the parade grounds after devouring his burger. We were all in high spirits and took the scenic buggy ride circumventing the island after purchasing some out of this world famous Mackinaw fudge. Everyone appeared quite congenial and our petite excursion ended happily without any hitches.

I've always felt strongly that a child needs a loving attachment with both mother and father. Masculine and feminine humans are vastly different in many ways. Besides the anatomical, the vast differential is between the preponderance of hormones, testosterone in the male and estrogen in the female. Pragmatically, men mesh more readily with men, as females do with females. Reasoning, logistics, decisions, evaluations, and emotions between the genders all are vastly opposing, hence the 50% divorce rate. It's like the simile of the glass of water, one sex visions it half full and the other half empty. A child with a single parent is like a ship without a rudder. Each parent (man and woman) has diverse attributes and this gives the developing child a huge advantage in having them both to nurture him/her. Identity and role modeling for the offspring is established much easier with all the qualities these two parents <u>combined</u> bring to the table. The child's genes are a combination or amalgamation of each parent's genes. This is why he/she reacts one day like his father and the next day like his mother. Diverse personalities nullify boredom and facilitate learning, nurture, and adaptation to life..

The French all say "viva la difference", but in truth this is only one of many major differences demarking the two genders. For another, women's features are much more finely sculptured, and hence generally more pleasing to the eye I believe. Men are more muscular and are basically stronger, can run faster, can jump higher, and can throw further. The fairer sex on the other hand, unbelievably, has more stamina, energy, and endurance. Health wise, females are indubitably much stronger, built tough by nature to mother the human race. Men are more expendable. I definitely remember that when the nursery nurse called me in the middle of the night to report to me that a newborn was having dyspnea and hyperpnea with an O2 tension of 88 I strongly wished "God please let it be a girl" because their chances of survival were much better.

Mentally, I firmly think they each are endowed with <u>equal</u> capacities, the sky being the limit. However, the fairer ones have a definite upper hand mentally early in life, and it takes the ones with "puppy dog tails" many years to reach an equal sagacity. Talents are equally distributed and they are developed to a zenith only by ambition, hard work, hope, and inspiration. The capacity and possibilities are limitless for everyone. Emotionally, I am convinced the tender gender goes a tad deeper with feelings of love probably equally shared. Men are more staid, practical, mathematical, and logical in my estimation. Also, it seems that the ladies have a bit more drive and stick-to-it-ness. Amazingly, they usually control the pocket book and the household duties. It appears to me that men do undoubtedly have the greater sex drive, speak for yourself John. Women prevail on the darker side of life but the men rule as prophets as witness in the Bible. With all these gross diversities in mind, is it any wonder divorce rates are soaring??? It's truly stupefying to realize the immense power and differential hormones can make!! Statistically, the fairer sex generally lives 5 to 10 years longer. The men are much, much deeper into sports events, causing a high degree of dissension, and conflict but the ladies are making rapid strides in developing their sports abilities and tastes. For some reason the girls with hypertrophy of the vocal cords are unquestionably, 10 to 1, more loquacious and articulate. Males usually are succinct with verbiage and express in a few terse words what the opposite gender relates in volumes of words. In other words, men seem to see the forest whereas ladies see the trees. Maybe it's because females are more observant and pick up all the fine details and minutia. Quite often men have eyes that see not and ears that hear not. In conclusion, ladies are vastly more into clothes fashions and cosmetics. They see the forest and men see the trees. There is also a differential in percent of fatty tissues and distribution of upholstery, need I say who is who?!

Chapter 25

Gulliver's Travels

I can firmly acquiesce with the evolutionary theory that all life originated in the oceans over a billion years. Water has always had a deep magnetism and fascination for me. Living in the middle of the ice age glacier carved Great Lakes makes sailing an enticing, automatic option. After deciding to take advantage of the aquatic opportunity dangling before me, I decided to join the Bay City Yacht Club in 1958 and give my family and myself a recreation break from the slavery of medicine. One of my ethereal pipe dreams has been, like Anne Marie Brevig and Martin Vennesland, to circumnavigate the globe in a sailboat. Anne Marie, a Norwegian, was my son Tom's first beloved wife, very muscular, lovely, and loving. However, their temperaments did not jibe. Tom is methodical and thorough, slow motion personified, but exceedingly brilliant in his way. Anne is like a deer, quickness and speed personified. Martin Vennesland, Anne's second husband, is one of the very best sailors in the vintage of the renowned Vikings of yore.

My son Tom and Anne had built the house of their dreams in Vancouver, after going over its infinitely detailed construction for over a year. They were both on the brink of a total nervous collapse. Anne related to me "Dad, I love Tom dearly, but I reached the breaking point because of his utterly slow, stolid movement, and for my salvation I just had to leave him." Actually their separation worked out wisely, for they both are very happily remarried and are the best of friends. To my perspective, Anne is a model of a perfect wife and I harbor fond feelings for her as an adopted daughter.

My love for boating came to fruition when I purchased a sleek, speedy, 18 foot craft at Brennan's Boat Works in 1959. After "wetting" my appetite for two years with this venture, I was a sitting duck for shooting the works and going for a 29 foot Owens Cruiser with twin inboard 400hp Chrysler engines, again at Brennan's. Believe me, this ship would really plane and make fast tracks in the open bay, but there were a few perplexing problems to be reckoned with. The sailing season on Saginaw Bay is dreadfully short. Also, getting from Brennan's to the mouth of the Saginaw River took at least an hour and time was of the essence in an upbeat pressure cooker pediatric practice. Inclement, stormy, windy weather, more often than not, would be a barrier to entering Lake Huron. Monetarily boats don't come cheaply and the upkeep with docking and storage can exact a king's ransom against a poor pediatrician's wages which are low on the totem pole. I've repeatedly thought our take home pay was miniscule and not commensurate with the tremendous responsibility hanging over our heads working with children who are the apple of their parents eyes and the most precious commodity going. Even though getting a ship ship-shape is a labor of love, it is physically a Herculean task, especially a wooden teak craft.

My good friends the Carters, Bill and Mathilde, sailed with me on an overnight trip to Tawas from Bay City, on my "Idyllic Ecstasy" cruiser. Bill was a high school remedial English instructor and his beautiful wife was a kindergarten teacher. We left Bay City at 8 a.m. Saturday in the summer of 1962, and proceeded north by northeast to East Tawas, a distance of approximately 50 miles as the crow flies. We were perplexed that we were the last boat in our safari to dock at Tawas at 4 p.m. that same Saturday. One of my fellow savvy yachtsman discovered my problem was that I carried a handicap of umpteen gallons of water in the hull of my cruiser all the way to my destination.

After a gala fish dinner and dance, we bedded that night on our yacht and set out for the return to Bay City early Sunday. It was a good thing we left at daybreak because we headed into a heavy rainstorm all the way home. The waves were two to three feet high and we dippy-doodled at least ¾ of the <u>long</u> journey to our mooring at good old Brennan's on the Saginaw River. It really was a cliff hanger and nail biter of a return trip, but hats off to the Lord and dear old "Idyllic Ecstasy". We made it!

We often took our yacht out into the Bay for water skiing on Wednesdays and weekends. We also took it out for picnics. On one occasion, on a Sunday with my children aboard, we got marooned a mile off shore. Fortunately, we were kindly rescued by Stuart Milster's yacht which towed us to a safe haven. Another instance had us stuck aground on a mud bar in the Saginaw River offshore. After maneuvering back and forth for seemingly ages, we managed to escape the entrapment. On another juncture, I discovered literally hundreds of huge spiders inhabiting my Owens Craft, after I had taken a weekend vacation to the Bahamas with the Chamber of Commerce as cruise physician.

Doris and I sailed from Detroit to Mackinaw Island on a pleasure cruise in July of 1950. Dr Abe Goldstein, a friend, recruited me to pinch hit as cruise doctor in his place, because of illness. It was a pleasant experience except for an agitated middle aged woman who plagued me morning, noon and night about her cough. She was scared to death of lung cancer from smoking, like her sister had. It was impossible to mollify and reassure her so I gleaned her physicians name and called him from the ship. He informed me that her chest x-ray and sputum were negative for any pathology and that she had an obsession and had bugged him unmercifully also. Finally, to preserve hers and my sanity, I prescribed Benadryl to cut the agitation.

Marshal Alcorn, urologist, took a cadre of six peer M.D.'s on an overnight trip to Caseville on the tip of the thumb of the lower peninsula one perfect August Wednesday in 1952. Marshal was quite the efficient sailor on his 52 foot Chris-Craft. The excursion was very enjoyable and uneventful, except that two of our men became quite inebriated and embarrassed us by unceremoniously spewing their gastric contents in the restaurant after a delicious fish dinner. Needless to say, they were never re-invited for a repeat performance.

On another chamber cruise as ship doctor to Sheboygan, Wisconsin, there occurred a mighty rare fatality. We boarded for the voyage at about 0900 and arrived at the Michigan-Huron Straits around 2100 on a perfect starry moonlit night. All was serene on the horizon while everyone participated in sane merriment. I retired at about the witching hour and all was well and copesetic. Along about 0300, my phone interrupted a deep slumber. An agitated, tremulous voice blurted out, "Doctor, we believe we have a dead passenger in our suite." This message electrified me and I was off at the crack of the bat. Sure enough, when I arrived at the designated room, my most horrific fears were translated to brazen reality. The corpse was a middle aged dentist from Midland, who had had a previous coronary assault. My informant was absolutely correct; he was deader than the proverbial doornail. The narrative evolved that he had imbibed the major portion of at least a pint of alcoholic beverages. This situation presented a dilemma of gigantic proportions. We were six hours from Sheboygan and we were urgently in need of a mortician and the nearest relatives (whomever they were) had to be notified at once. I woke the ship captain at once and we decided to wrap the body in blankets and inter it in the freezer. We dropped the bomb on his wife, who didn't seem to be overwhelmed with grief or surprise. The body was properly prepared by an undertaker in Sheboygan when we made port, as authorized by his spouse. Then he was planed to MBS Airport where the Midland mortician and his wife took charge. Aside from this episode, we all had a rollicking good time with no further untoward happenings.

Chapter 26

More Meanderings and Travels

My son, Gregory Haines, was a habitual companion for me in my travels during my estrangement and remarriage period from 1962 to 1972. We planed to Vancouver, British Columbia, twice to visit my son J.H. Thomas and wife, Anne E. Brevig. While there we explored the famous Stanley Park, played a couple rounds of golf, and took a couple long hikes in the beautiful British Columbia Mountains.

Melissa Mary, my younger daughter, also accompanied me on three memorable excursions. One was to a CME at Duke University in Durham, NC. While we were there we attended an Easter conference at the Tarheel University Planetarium in Chapel Hill, N.C (University of North Carolina).

A second trip was made to Aspen, CO, where I rekindled my friendship with Sidney S. Gellis, my ageless mentor whom I had last seen in Anchorage, AL, while in the army. Funny thing, there was a span of 15 years between these two meetings but he recognized me immediately as though just one day had passed. Indubitably, Sidney was number one Pediatrician nationwide for several decades. As I previously mentioned, Sidney published "Pediatric Notes" weekly for at least 30 years (and I never missed one) until his untimely demise in 2001. I still enjoy it immensely as published by his erudite student, pediatrician Richard Goldbloom, M.D.

Getting back to our escapade, Melissa and I flew to Denver, rented a car, and drove to Aspen via Leadville, the antique capital of Colorado. We had a sumptuous steak dinner (Melissa's favorite) in Leadville and visited the ancient Opera House and Museum there. On the way to Aspen, we passed Mt. Elbert which was 14,433 foot elevation, the highest point in Colorado. We navigated the dangerous Independence Pass and the roadway narrowed to barely a two car passage. It was raining, there was no outside guardrail, and there were numerous rockslides but, by Gods' help and the skin of our teeth, we made it! Surprisingly, I was gritting my teeth and had a stronghold on the steering wheel. Melissa was undaunted and sightseeing the whole route which included a sheer 2000+ foot drop.

At Aspen the teenage Philharmonic Orchestra was in prime session. It is a haven for the beginning musical artists, similar to Interlochen in Michigan. Regardless of their youth and immaturity, they played the classics of Mozart, Rachmaninoff, Brahms, Beethoven and Tchaikovsky to perfection. Blindfolded you would have sworn it was the New York Philharmonic playing.

The third trip Melissa made with me was in 1986 to Baltimore to my venerable fiftieth Maryland Medical School class reunion. Melissa is really and truly a beautiful young lady and all my classmates thought I was exceedingly fortunate to have such a comely escort. Actually, Melissa is a chip off the Knobloch resembling her stately, statuesque mother but favoring the Knobloch kin in her facial physiognomy and constructed with a classic chassis. Be that as it may, there were thirty two of my dear young hearties of our '36 class in attendance. We enjoyed a good old fashioned supreme Chesapeake Bay oyster and crab cake dinner the night before our formal reunion. Lucky me, I was the only one in full active practice. We toured the new inner harbor business development and inspected the majestic elderly ship, the Constitution of John Paul Jones fame. Each night before retiring, we would have a tete a tete conference, sharing reminiscences of yore, over a Southern Comfort cocktail.

My first born daughter, Susan Caroline, was my partner at my 55th Medical School reunion in Baltimore. One of the noteworthy features of our abode at the Sheraton Hotel was free champagne at the happy hour. This time there were only twenty two (out of a 100 member graduating class) of my gallant happy comrades enjoying our get together. Brother Morris Nicholson was instrumental in organizing our societal appointments. Susan and I toured the historic sites of Lord Baltimore, had dinner at the Maryland Museum, and went to the Pimlico Racetrack. We had dinner there and some idiot ordered a filet mignon dinner instead of the revered Maryland crab cake feast for which we persons out of Maryland were salivating. Susan bet on the horses. She picked out a couple of winners relying on her magical woman's intuition. She really had a ball at the annual crab fest conducted for all the alumni. That night we toured the Davidge Hall morgue and cadavers. When I bid her fond adieu at 0600 a.m. at the hotel entrance, it dawned on me, dressed only in my robe, that I was locked out of my room. No problem, I secured a key at the desk.

Tom and I had a rendezvous at my 60th Medical School Class Reunion, May 23rd 1996, and we resided at the Marriott Hotel. The evening of arrival, Tom must have had a ravenous appetite for he totally devoured the biggest porterhouse steak you ever saw. When he was an orderly at old General

Hospital in Bay City, the nurses observed that he would inhale all the residual food left on patient's trays. I was dead tired, but after our evening repast, my son was quite adamant that we go to see the Baltimore Orioles home baseball game at their new Camden Field, which was within walking distance. Finally, I decided not to be a party pooper and acquiesced, against my better judgment. Our seats were in the upper deck and it was cold and windy. After the third inning of shivering, I decided to depart Tom's company and go inside and I watched the game on television until Morpheus overtook me.

On Friday night our '36 class held a private dinner party at a palatial residence within a stone's throw of the famous Washington Monument. There were eleven venerable classmates answering the call to celebrate the year of their dreams. Son Tom, a photographer first class, took a photo of our majestic group and a copy hangs in my bedroom. Also hanging there in the same frame, compliments of Tom, is a picture taken on Friday afternoon of myself standing on Edgar Allen Poe's tombstone. Poe's burial site is located in the courtyard of the First Presbyterian Church on Greene St, two blocks north of Davidge Hall. In the early 30's, his grave was situated in a field of unkempt weeds just south of the church. We walked past it every morning on our way to Medical School. At present, he is the most famous amongst over a hundred other gravestones on the church grounds. Poe had an insurmountable fondness for cognac and on his birthday at 3 a.m. every year, an unknown admirer comes and places a 4/5 bottle of cognac on his grave and disappears pronto.

Tom did himself proud at our annual crab fest on Saturday night, following our second Orioles baseball game. On Sunday morning we decided to put the icing on the cake and drove 50 miles northwest to Gettysburg. We toured the hallowed battle field in the p.m. and then obtained lodging in a hotel on the square, originally erected in 1798. On Monday we walked across the street to the lawyers home where Abraham Lincoln slept the night before his immortal Gettysburg address. Actually, we sat at his four poster bedside and meditated. The miracle was how dear aged Abe fit his carcass in that diminutive bed.

The piece de resistance was a visit to the "Jennie" Wade house on Baltimore Street. On July 3, 1863, "Jennie" Wade was the only female civilian killed outright on the second day during this monumental battle. She was kneading dough for biscuits for the Union Troops at her sister's home when she was killed instantly as a bullet passed through two wooden doors and penetrated her heart from the back. Her body was not cleansed, embalmed, or clothes changed, and she was placed in a wooden casket made by Confederate infantry men for a Mississippi rebel general killed in the wheat field battle at Gettysburg on day two. She was interred the same day in the back yard of sister, Georgia Wade McClellan's home. A year later "Jennie" was moved to the courtyard of the German Lutheran Church and finally planted in Evergreen Cemetery at the top of Cemetery Hill about 100 paces from the grave of her sweetheart, Johnston Hastings Skelly Jr. (Johnston was a soldier in the union army, mortally wounded at Carters Woods, Virginia, on June 15, 1863. He met his creator shortly thereafter.) A statue of Jennie was erected at her gravesite. People who visualized her corpse at her final interment swear that her body had literally turned to stone, mummified. She carried a letter and picture of her betrothed in her bosom. President Lincoln sat beside Georgia Wade at Gettysburg on November 19th, on the day he spoke his immortal Gettysburg address. It was the dedication to the fallen heroes in the combined Union / Confederate Cemetery.

There were two trips to Oba, Canada, that I made with my gnarled and doughty second father-in-law, Oscar Willis Vincent. The Algoma Central Railroad travels 100 miles due north from the Canadian Sault St. Marie to Oba, Ontario. Oscar was an avid big game moose hunter as evidenced by a huge prize moose trophy which hung in his garage office. He was a car dealer and repairman who could change a tire in the blink of an eye and was an incessant cigar smoker, at least 6 or more a day. One really needed a gas mask to weather the smoke storm he created. He had the constitution of a Gorilla. Oba was prime moose hunting territory but Oscar's hunting in the wilds of Canada was terminated. Our first sojourn to Oba via the Algoma Central Railroad included Oscar's son and grandson in the middle of July in 1965. We had rented a cabin and a boat on Lake Nipinnissing, ten miles southwest of Oba, at the headwaters of the Oba River. We had a pleasurable vacation together as all parties were compatible. The fishing was par excellante and Oscar was a tolerable culinary chef. Our fare consisted of walleye, crappies, sunfish, and perch. I taught "Tar" and Brad, Oscar's son and grandson, to play solitaire and we had a solitaire festival for one solid week at nights and on the train. On our return train trip I was anxiously summoned to attend a young man who had "passed out" about midway to the Soo. He was a newly wed bridegroom who had previously had occasional febrile epileptic seizures in childhood. While we were talking, he spontaneously regained consciousness, T.P.R. and breathing normalized and my diagnosis was a mild harmless grand mal seizure caused by the stress of taking on the responsibilities of a wife and the drastic changes in his life.

Oscar and I made a second fishing excursion to Oba. It came about in the last week in May of 1972. About fifty miles before we made Oba, it began to snow, becoming heavier until it reached a veritable whiteout as we attained our destination at the Oba hotel. We became literally buried in snow as a total of 30 inches fell in circa 18 hours. Fortuitously, thanks to my father-in-law, I had packed a pair of high top rubber galoshes. The following day we painfully realized that our piscatorial activities were stymied. We decided to take the train northward to Hurst, which was at the end of the Algoma Central line about 100 miles north. Oba also was a whistle stop for the Canadian National Railway which spans the continent. We had a hearty beef tenderloin dinner and attended a rock and roll session at a Hurst bar. The steel string guitars were painfully deafening, requiring using our fingertips as earplugs to restore sanity. Our return trip to Oba was uneventful. We journeyed to a fairly large waterfall near Oba, but my golf clubs were useless as the local course was invisible due to snowfall. The highlight of our trip was the purchase of a huge Russian wolf skin from the hotel manager for a reasonable $75.00 in cash. He had shot the mammoth, beleaguered wolf with his rifle as it was crossing the railroad tracks a couple miles out of town. After our return to Bay City, I took the wolf skin to a taxidermist to cure for a rug for posterity.

I almost forgot the idyllic vacation escape Doris and I made to Williamsburg preceding our bond cutting. As mentioned, Dr. Crissey (the great dictator) admonished me in no uncertain terms to cease and desist from any further procreation activities due to Doris' hypertension following the birth of our fourth child, Melissa, who he delivered in 1951. After deep cogitation over time, I decided to make sure the inevitable hypertensive diathesis did not happen and I had my Vas Deferenses severed by my buddy, surgeon Orlen Johnson. After a proper waiting period for the prostate to expel all the HTK sperm, we embarked on a repeat honeymoon to a haven of which we had always dreamed. Indeed we surely did have a true ecstatic week of unmitigated pleasure. I even took along my new golf club which could be formulated into putter, chipper, iron, and driver by adjusting the toe. After envisioning all the colonial treasures we would have a luxurious dinner and have heart to heart dialogue. At that period, I never had even the foggiest idea that we would ever cut the cord.

There was a sortie in Detroit my first beloved and I went to with Frank and Regina Bearsch to commemorate the fiftieth birthday of the American Academy of Pediatrics. For some inexplicable reason, I became separated from my party. We searched anxiously for each other for nearly 18 hours before we connected. I still have a souvenir Frisbee disc I got there.

Our headline speaker at the meeting was none other than the renowned comic Bill Cosby. There had to be at least 1000 in attendance at this banquet and outside there was a deluging downpour rainstorm of gigantic proportions. We all had raincoats and they all looked alike. I couldn't locate mine and took what resembled it. When we retrieved the solace of our hotel room, to my consternation, I had purloined a woman's raincoat, but it did the trick!

In relation to the academy's birth rite celebration, Tom Wright and yours truly were present at a dedication ceremony for the American Academy of Pediatrics at Harper Hospital in Detroit, in 1980, where the academy was first formulated by several venerable local Pediatricians headed by Eddie Wishropp. The gathering pediatricians designated me, as the eldest living member of the academy present, to hold up the flag of recognition. After the assemblage completed the ritual, we adjourned to the hospital physician's dining room for sustenance. Many of the past presidents of the American Academy of Pediatrics have come from Detroit, Ann Arbor, and even Saginaw, including Harry Towsley (A.A.) and Bob Heavenrich (Saginaw).

There eventuated a most indelibly memorable journey to the New Year's Rose Bowl I made with staunch undying Wolverine fan Pat Brilinski. This event occurred in 1990, just two years following my castigation surgery by Nephrologist, Peter Fujewara, for prostate cancer. Pat was a nursery nurse who discovered that I was a dyed in the wool supporter for UM pigskin sports, having been inducted in the fall of 1938 during my first resident year at UM Hospital. It had always been my fervent desire to travel to Pasadena CA, to enjoy a Rose Bowl extravaganza. It was a bonanza for me while recuperating from the shock of a diagnosis of cancer, which is always a potential death sentence, and my surgery.

Anyhow, we kicked up our proverbial heels and lived it up for three festive days. We toured Hollywood (tinsel town) and environs. We arose at an ungodly hour to catch a bus to Pasadena for the famous Rose Bowl Parade. Our seats at the bowl were in the end zone where we were taunted and upbraided unmercifully by the enthusiastic rooters for the Trojans of the University of Southern California. We carried on a counter friendly, good natured bantering with our hosts. Pat warned me about the Trojan Band hurling slanderous epithets about our University at her previous Rose Bowl encounter with them. To our deep consternation, our team was defeated by a close margin. Bo Schembechler, our football coach, always had Herculean difficulty in defeating the West Coast teams in our post season skirmishes. I firmly believe that weather played a major role, along with all the frills and thrills our players experienced. We were fattened immeasurably for the kill. Bo was one of the best ever coaches, but he couldn't overcome the West Coast media and festive holidays and the long layover from the end of the regular season. He had a coronary attack while preparing his team for combat in the 1980's. Bo was a total task master who put tremendous pressure on himself, as well as his players.

One of the most unforgettable characters I have ever met was Edward James Kaake, Chief of Police in Essexville. My introduction was a wee bit ominous. It happened one rainy, foggy night on Borton Avenue in 1958, near Main Street when my daughter Susan was driving. We were blind sided by meteorological conditions and struck a parked car on the south side of the street. Lo and behold, my good friend to be, Chief Kaake himself, came out of nowhere to check out our fender bender accident. Bill Hewitt, who's car she hit, was quite understanding and courteous. Fortunately, Susan had an active driver's license and all our credentials were in order. Shortly thereafter, as the roll of the dice would have it, on a fateful evening I introduced myself to Kaake's lovely wife, Betty, while collecting yearly pledges for my First Presbyterian Church. Betty presented in a bathrobe at the door when I rang the bell. We both blushed and I wanted to crawl under a rug, but Betty was very gracious and we had a good laugh. When a person unexpectedly gets into a squirmy situation, he or she can always be extricated by a shot of good humor. Edward and I had a bond of common ground, for we both soldiered in WWII. He was a doughty marine and was involved in heavy fighting in the Italian invasion.

Ed had fairly severe asthma with lobular emphysema. He elected to go with my advice and medications to ameliorate his asthmatic attacks. He also frequently called me to prescribe therapy for his daughters, Linda and Nancy when they were ill. I rendered all these services gratis for the Kaakes were the salt of the earth. They invited me to frequent dinners, for my second wife was adverse to cooking with a passion. Betty was a superb chef and her carrot cake and key lime pies were inferior to none. Ed was a master at preparing turkey for the holidays, to which I had a perennial invitation. I often dropped by their home on Main Street to exchange tete a tete dialogue about global issues, especially on weekends. I never did forgive Linda for rejecting me as a pediatrician in preference to my protagonist peer for the care of her children. However, the bright side was that her sister, Nancy, had the sagacity to call me for pediatric issues for her two infants. The Kaakes and I had many card games on rainy dreary days. Betty developed a malignant brain tumor along about 1972. It regrettably was a medulloblastoma, tantamount to galloping consumption, rapidly aggressive, and 100% fatal.

Ed, Irv Hacker, Ed's two brothers, and I made an annual pilgrimage to Beaverton to engage in deer hunting during the Nov 15 to 30 time span. Ed's father owned a 50 acre tract of land which was well endowed with antlered, ruminant wild animals. I was and am a <u>very</u> lukewarm hunter and prefer to spell these beasts by the appellation, "DEAR." However, I do relish venison in a pinch and the camaraderie, fellowship, exercise, fresh air, card games and relaxation were always quite enticing and enjoyable. I remember on one occasion while hunting with my buddy Ed, I flushed a fallow deer approximately 10 yards away from us and I veritably froze. Ed yelled, "Shoot, Doc" in a stentorian voice whereupon I responded, "I can't pull the trigger, my hand is paralyzed."

In another incident, we were rabidly listening to the Michigan State vs. Notre Dame football game of the year and I excitedly, during the heat of the game, bellowed, "Go State" and thrust my arm upwards. To everyone's dismay, my fist penetrated the wall, leaving a large gaping hole. Ed spoke up and said, "Cool it, Doc." Embarrassment set in, in big chunks, and I did succumb to reality. Ed survived his good wife's untimely demise, but he was a lost soul until his final reckoning. He went through the motions of life with a ruptured spirit even though basically, he was a rugged human.

There was one instance of discord between us. I had entrusted my prized, new 16 gauge shotgun in his care, but when I endeavored to reclaim it, inexplicably my rifle had mysteriously disappeared?! Ed offered no excuse. However, he did refer me to a gunsmith who made me a gorgeous .06 gauge rifle for $75.00 which Ed coveted. It eventually ended up in son Greg's permanent possession, for his hunting prowess. During Ed's habitation at a condominium in Frankenmuth, I visited him a couple times and we had dinner and some pool games together. My final encounter with my buddy was as a pallbearer at the turn of the century.

Another liaison brings into focus Stanley Cousins. In 1950, Stan was our last intern at Mercy Hospital. Aloysius Zaremba was the first Mercy House Officer at the turn of the 20th Century and S. Franklin Horowitz preceded Cousins just before the outbreak of WWII. I was an advisor to Dr. Cousins during his internship at Mercy. Stanley was an erudite, honest, dependable, and hard working general practice physician. In his extracurricular activities, he was vitally interested in golf, which was right up my alley. So, I was nominated to purchase a gift for him as a going away present from Mercy Hospital which was a set of brand, spanking, new golf clubs. Stan wasted no time in breaking them in and joining the Bay City Country Club of which I had a membership. Needless to say, we enjoyed many, many good golf outings. One of our prime cavorts was the annual Follis Open Tournament at Lewiston, which he won twice and I won once.

Chapter 27

My Most Intriguing Pediatric Cases

One of my utmost thrilling and rewarding pediatric cases was a dangerous intussusception in a 1 ½ year old asthenic female baby around 1954. Carmen was admitted with a diagnosis of probable iliocolic intestinal disorder, characterized by acute intermittent sever spastic abdominal pain occurring every 2-4 hours with vomiting. X-rays, barium enema, flat plate, palpable sausage like tumor, rectal bleeding, and bowel obstruction were all absent and she presented a perplexing enigma. Intussception usually involves telescoping of the ileum into the ascending colon with incarceration of blood supply causing bleeding. Coincidentally, after three days of intractable symptoms, the chief radiologist at the University of Michigan Hospital appeared on the scene to deliver an address to our medical staff on "Intestinal Obstruction", of all subjects.

We summoned him to examine our writhing little girl and her x-rays. He was stumped for a clean cut solution to her problem and commiserated with us. My consulting surgeon on this patient was Arthur D. Allen, our foremost surgeon. A.D. was a general practitioner basically and a self developed surgeon through years of the vicissitudes of medical practice. There is a joke concerning A.D., as related by raconteur Hal Shafer. Arthur was making a house call for an old farmer in Auburn who had a large abscess on his leg. The farmer had been applying manure poultices to the sore for two days and asked Dr. Allen if this was an appropriate therapy. Whereupon A.D. said, "Yes, but you must sterilize it first."

To get down to the nitty gritty of my little lady patient, I confronted A.D., also known as "Bill" to his cohorts, on a Sunday morning while making my rounds. I said, "Bill, enough dalliance. We've got to take the bull by the horns and open up her belly and see first hand what the problem really is, and hopefully correct it. She'll die if we don't do something positive, right now." Bill cogitated for a minute and said, "Yes, you are absolutely right, we've been dragging our feet too long. I'll call surgery to set it up immediately and we'll hop to it." I gave the anesthetic, good old, dear, smelly, and inflammable ether. Upon cracking the abdomen, we found, to our amazement, an ileal-ileal intussusception with gangrenous ileum from almost stem to stern, about 4/5 involvement. There were only two small viable segments of ileum remaining, circa 4 inches at the origin and 3 inches terminal. We looked at one another in awe for a minute, our minds deeply querulous. A. D. said to me, "Can you handle this awful mess?" and I said, "With God's miraculous help I will give it my best shot." We created a 'short bowel syndrome' in an infant who requires maximum food calories for growth and development, let alone sustenance to stay alive. Carmen did live and she did grow and develop. However, it was a gargantuan struggle with umpteen glucose IV's and two transfusions. The nurses and dieticians deserve the lion's share of credit for their laborious, unswerving, and loving care. Heartfelt prayers from all of us contributed vastly to be sure. I last saw Carmen two years later for a respiratory infection and she appeared to be growing and functioning at least fairly normally. With the short bowel, food transits the intestines at a rapid pace, permitting incomplete digestion. It produces intractable diarrhea with multiple stools daily and electrolyte loss. We were precariously on the edge for months, but we sweated that one out, without lawyer intervention. In time there was always the possibility of growth of new ileum.

Another lulu of a presenting congenital defect was a case of "prune belly" syndrome. It occurred in a term male newborn one dark night. The designation of the term "prune belly" is descriptive of a flat to scaphoid external abdomen with multiple rolls of wrinkled abdominal skin. But the real crux of the problem lay with the kidneys and ureters. It is a form of idiopathic (unknown cause), hydronephrosis indicating an enlarged pelvicalyceal system in the kidneys and hydroureter, due to obstruction of urinary outflow. The ureters are deformed, shortened and not connected to the bladder due to absent cystro-ureteral valves bilaterally. As a result, the urine flow is zero and there is increasing back up pressure on the glomeruli and kidney medulla if not relieved by diversion implantation of the ureters externally in the back to enable voiding. If this situation is not apprehended at birth, total renal destruction will ensue within two weeks. Nowadays, as of 1986, there are two tests to determine kidney function and assess urinary obstruction. They are the pressure perfusion study and the diuretic augmented renal scan; having an accuracy of 90%. The urinary system normally transports urine at a rate of 10cc/minute without concomitant elevation of the intra pelvic calyceal framework. When I saw this patient at delivery, he presented with anuria, (no micturetion), a dearth of amniotic fluid, and intrauterine starvation. The main visible diagnostic feature was the characteristic prune belly configuration of the abdomen, which really hit me between the eyes and said in a loud voice, "Here I am." We had immediate consult with the eminent urology surgeon, Dr Livinius Stroia. The ureters were exteriorized immediately creating a big relief and saving the life of the kidneys. Stroia also performed a life saving operation on Harry Jarkey by relieving a kinked right ureter at the ureteropelvic junction to salvage his kidney.

On another occasion, I tended to a case of Potter's Disease. This baby also showed anuria (unable to urinate) at birth. I consulted with surgeon, F. Pitkin Husted, on this newborn male. It was a real brain scratcher and we decided after 24 hours, to open his abdomen and take a look. To our rank consternation, he had no kidneys whatsoever. Knowing full well that living without kidneys was impossible; we closed the belly and let nature take its course. There were no renal vessels either or we might have considered renal transplants.

I cared for two interesting cases of tuberculosis meningitis in the 70's. One was for Dr. Floyd (Bud) Stevens, and the other child was for Dr. Ray R. (Railroad) Cook. Success smiled on me with Cookies 2 year old diminutive boy, at Mercy Hospital. I did a lumbar spinal tap when I discovered cervical rigidity in combination with fever, marked irritability, lassitude, and septic manners. The spinal fluid was noticeably cloudy, turbid, and under increased pressure. With a family history of TBC, positive X-ray, recent weight loss, elevated spinal fluid WBC's and proteins, and positive smear for tubercle bacilli, a diagnosis of acid fast meningitis was a cinch. A new treatment of the intraspinal injection of Streptomycin was curative for him. Tuberculous meningitis is invariably fatal. Ray and I were on cloud nine when he recovered and felt that we really salvaged a life, a real feather in our caps. My only beefs with Ray Cook were fraudulent evasion of army service in WWII and his blatant, continuous bragging about his accomplishments with his patients. Apparently, Ray had a formidable inferiority complex but otherwise he was deeply sincere, honest, and conscientious to an admirable degree. He did nip me in golf too.

My other patient with TBC meningitis in private practice, was diagnosed, unfortunately for me, at University of Michigan Hospital in Ann Arbor. Dr "Bud" Stevens called me in consultation for a five year old little girl at Bay City General Hospital, early in 1980. There was a history of an acute episode of high fever, headache, anorexia, depression, and lethargy for 48 hours. In my examination, after studying her for a few moments while she was resting in bed, I put my left hand under her occiput and lifted her head slowly and forcibly against resistance, and surprisingly her entire body rose in one stiff as a board unit to a sitting position. I exclaimed immediately in amazement, "She's got meningitis" in the presence of Dr. Stevens, the nurse, and her parents. The spinal fluid did indeed bear out our snap diagnosis. However, the stained smear and the culture were negative, there was no family history of contagious disease, and hers was not a chronic illness by a long shot. I thought I must be losing all diagnostic acumen when the lab findings didn't signify an explicit, acute bacterial meningitis picture of the meningococcal, pneumococcic or influenzal variety. Tuberculosis, the great imitator of disease in all body systems, should have hit me as a beacon light, but it never entered my mind. We were stumped, literally up a creek without a paddle. I should have tumbled to the correct diagnosis here, for her eyes did not exhibit signs of an acute illness. The eyes are the only visible extension of the brain and they are always tell tale signs of the nature and depth of sickness. By scrutinizing the orbs of an ill person, we can detect innumerable diagnostic clues.

True Diabetes Type I occurs customarily in mid childhood, 6-10 years. However, it surely can occur at any age from birth as witnessed by my little patient, Emily, who developed full fledged Diabetes Type I at birth. She was a profound challenge because her blood glucose levels fluctuated in extremes like a yo-yo. She required constant care and supervision by nurses, diabetologists, physicians, dieticians, and parents. Her mother, of necessity, needed an intensive, crash course in all of the ramifications and nuances in diabetic diagnosis, therapy, laboratory techniques, diet, and insulin injections. Somehow, the Lord smiled on us dumb and blind humans and with a Herculean effort we managed to get Emily's blood chemistry regulated. Along with a breast milk diet and insulin fine tuning, she did survive and actually thrived with proper growth and development. With blood, sweat, and tears, I assumed her total care through the medical vicissitudes of childhood and adolescence. At present, she is a mother of two gorgeous children who, to my knowledge, have not developed diabetes yet. Infants and children are inherently resilient and tough to the nth degree and Mother Nature is the greatest doctor of all. I have conducted treatment of innumerable children with diabetic acidosis. It is a precarious situation and demands the utmost expertise and proper decisions. Providence has been my buddy in guiding me through all these hazardous patients without a fatality. The innovation of intravenous insulin has been a huge help.

I saw three cases of tetanus in my early days of practice, before the tetanus vaccine. Vaccines for almost all the acute contagious diseases of childhood have been the greatest discoveries for the preservation of human life in pediatrics. We have practically, completely nullified polio and small pox. Influenza B, mumps measles, chicken pox, and rubella have been dealt mortal blows. Pneumonia, meningitis, diphtheria, typhoid, pertussis, rabies and influenza have all been mainly neutralized by our most wonderful vaccines. I believe they vastly save more lives than the vaunted miracle antibiotics which can be wiped out by resistant mutating organisms. Truly, they are our foremost contribution to earthly civilization.

A serious problem with children (as well as adults) is overfeeding, inertia, and obesity. Television, with all its positives, is the number one etiological cause to be sure. It leads to laziness and critical lack of exercise to burn up the calories consumed. Besides this, the enticing culinary advertisements on TV are conducive to high calorie food ingestion. Also, instead of being a boon, TV contributes to distractions at mealtime and bedtime and can actually be a curse of the first order. Those attractive video games our offspring play on the 'tube' to while away the hours contribute unmercifully to lassitude and inertia.

Automobiles, a most wonderful transport invention, are another potent contributor to a dearth of activity. The 'wheels' negate shoe leather propulsion to school and the art of good old fashioned walking has become long lost. School lunches also may be a factor, as they contain a diet of magna caloric foods to quench the huge appetites. A further distraction to the ideal diet is the easy access and availability to the countless 'fast food' restaurants which are heavy on calories, light on true value, and dripping with saturated fats, sugars, and salt. Alas, cooking has become a lost, antiquated art in a majority of homes. The 'soda' drinks extravaganza is sweeping roughshod on all children now. Except for providing fluids, they are valueless.

We had practically an epidemic of nephroblastomas or Wilms tumors of the kidneys in the late fifties and early sixties. There are a dozen or so cases that cross my memory. Apparently we had a fabulous success rate, for only one patient died two years after chemo treatment, with vincristine and actinomycin D followed by export surgery. Survival is linked to tumor histology (type of cells), cachexia, and degree of stage of the Wilms disease. Diagnosis is dependent upon abdominal mass, hypertension, and hematuria. My beloved surgeons were the Alcorn brothers, (Kent and Marshal), Hugh Shields, and Charley Rogers. As of 2004, only Shields is living but with terminal Parkinson's disease.

Inflammatory bowel disease (IBD), especially Crohns disorder, is a curse of the first order and occurs during adolescence, the most crucial time of life. Two of my fellow physicians had sons with this hated Crohns affliction. Apparently there are inheritable factors with a specific 'intestinal constitution' at risk for developing IBD abetted by untoward environmental influences. The worst possible outcome of Crohns disease happened with Stan Cousin's son. His lot was a severe, unremitting series of relapses of excruciating abdominal pain, massive rectal bleedings, and nutritional failure due to failure of medical management. He had several colectomy surgeries along with total parenteral nutrition until he ran out of bowels. There were temporary, periodic ameliorations of the disease process, but his course was persistently downhill eventuating in death over a period of about three years. The other instance of this dreaded lifetime disorder occurred in Tom Wright's son, W. Kenneth. His involvement was minimal and he has survived to live a fairly normal life with mild recurrences of symptoms at lengthy intervals. Tom himself has had a few bouts of massive rectal hemorrhage.

One of my most notable patients with this intestinal problem was Barney Balcer's daughter. We almost lost her at birth due to intestinal hemorrhage corrected by multiple transfusions. Her diagnosis was confirmed at Ford Hospital in Detroit by colonoscopy and imaging intestinal studies. She had many moderate recurrences and relapses, but managed to survive with her parent's deep loving care and help from Jehovah.

Another special instance of IBD appeared in a sixteen year old young lady with whom I was called into consultation. Inez Lopez was in extremis when I first saw her. Her family doctor, Gary Bomphray, referred her to me with provisional diagnosis of acute infectious mononucleosis. She had lost about 20 pounds, hemoglobin was 6.5 grams, 15 plus bloody stools daily, and unbearable cramping. I ordered two units of 500cc blood stat and I'm humbly sure it was veritably life saving. She responded remarkably positively almost immediately, but her intestinal bleeding, excruciating belly ache, diarrhea, and psychological problems persisted for a couple weeks unremittingly. I called Varin Kule, an expert gastroenterologist in consultation the first day of my take over. He performed a colonoscopy but he leaned toward a diagnosis of entomoeba histolytica. This is an acute parasitic amoebic infection which mimics Crohns disease almost to a T. It is a tropical disease, usually obtained person to person or by contaminated food or water. However, Inez gave negative history of contact with Asians or ever having been in any country outside of her native America. Also smears and cultures were negative for entomoeba. I was undoubtedly convinced our diagnosis was dyed in the wool Crohns disease. After two weeks of indecisive non-positive progress in her disease status, I decided to consult further with the gastroenterologist at University of Michigan Hospital. I had strongly wanted to order cortisone for her primary treatment, but my consultant advised against its usage for questionable reason. Anyhow, she went to Ann Arbor pronto. The medics there took over her management completely and never sent me a report, nor did they send me follow up instructions regarding her continued treatment. The Ann Arbor GE doctor did send a letter to our chief ER doctor, criticizing and berating the 'slovenly' treatment she received at Bay City Medical Center. Thus, they seriously undermined our treatment of Inez, reducing to zero confidence our case handling in the eyes of her parents and setting us up for litigation if any untoward event occurred. They treated Inez with high doses of cortisone for a couple months without tapering the dosage properly. I did not see Inez until she crashed suddenly one night, and blew out her entire colon.

She was taken to the ER where she was seen by Drs. Kule, Jaffe, and Tom Burk. After three plus hours of ER confusion, I was called in consultation. I could see that she was in an extremely ill state and immediately called her Ann Arbor physician and ordered a helicopter, magna fluids, and blood IV. She made it to Ann Arbor but died shortly after arriving there.

My next contact with Inez, after a visit to the funeral home in Bay City, was a lawsuit as a defendant involved in her demise. It was not understandable to me, why the mother didn't sue the Ann Arbor doctors who were really responsible for her death, because they were in total command of Inez's illness the entire period after she was discharged from Bay Medical Center. My deposition for Inez proved my 100% innocence in her management to the U of M Hospital gastroenterologist physician and J. Kule and I both were completely exonerated.

We humans are not perfect and we all have at least about ten glitches in our chromosomes and genes which do not show as nature surreptitiously conceals them. Visible malformations and congenital faux pas occur in approximately 7% of newborns. Congenital heart defects and brain aberrations causing seizures rank highly as major contributors to natures foul ups in human inheritance. The constitution states that all men are created equal, but pragmatically and genetically it ain't so. Humankind, through billions of years of natural evolution and time, has developed from the one celled paramecium to the first human over about eighty thousand years. Man has progressed in rapid stages from the crude cave man to the present, highly intelligent version today (homo sapiens) mainly through the intricate development of the brain. He has metamorphosed from predominant physical prowess to a sophisticated, scientific state. However, his life can be terminated by his innate genetic killer, warlike instincts, the atom bomb, or natural cataclysmic events. There is a precarious existence due to meteorological imbalances, possible ice age destruction of the ozone, and being struck by meteorites (like the one that cold cocked the dinosaurs), tsunamis, hurricanes, rain storms, tornadoes, mudslides, snow avalanches, and you name it!

Seizures are caused by paroxysmal electric waves, probably due to defects in synapses and neurone conductions in the cerebral cortex, especially the temporal lobes. I have witnessed innumerable grand mal, petite mal, febrile, and partial seizures, but one special patient is preeminent in my memory. Megan Wilinski, granddaughter of Mel Smith my Lincoln car dealer, was a freshman in high school with intractable grand mal seizures of temporal lobe origin. They occurred with hop, skip, and jump irregularity, at any time of day or night with several days of escape between episodes. I gave her plight my best shot, but it was fruitless and maddening. So, I sent her to

Ford Hospital in Detroit, for possible resolution of her vexing problem. After numerous electronic studies there to localize the source of the disturbance, they decided to surgically do a temporal lobotomy (total removal). Following this extirpation at Fords, she did have lessened intensity seizures at less frequency for several months, and thereafter they gradually petered out to practically zero. At present, Megan is thriving. Her mother apparently had implicit faith in my ability and needed iron clad reassurance from me before she would give her consent for the brain surgery. I am brimming with jubilation to ascertain that Megan had such a happy "all is well that ends well" outcome.

Brain tumor management has come a long way since I graduated from medical school in the antiquated year of 1936. Now we are able to diagnose the type of tumor (histology) by E.E.G. (electro encephalogram), ultrasound or CT guided stereotactic biopsy, and magnetic resonance imaging of brain tissue. Stereotactic radio surgery of these tumors is replacing the crude, cave man removal by knives done previously. I've seen many patients with malignant and benign neoplasms of the central nervous system. Every time a child entered my office with a chief complaint of "headache", the titillating etiology of brain tumor reared its ugly head. The children's mothers had lurid visions of brain tumor firmly entrenched in their cerebrums and I had to strive arduously to dispel these anxious thoughts. Much less than 1% of "headaches" are caused by increased intracranial pressure.

Two special premature newborns come to mind as interesting cases. They were the daughters of Harry and Jenny Jarkey, named Julie and Linda, and were born at Mercy Hospital. Harry was a comedienne of extraordinary caliber and he often commented, "How can Jenny and I bequeath such puny undeveloped babies?" The girls survived like gangbusters without a hitch in spite of their puzzled parents. Jenny was taken by the grim reaper suddenly one night in the early 60's, probably due to myocardial infarction. Harry profoundly mourned Jenny's tragic demise and never remarried. He nurtured his two girls proficiently like a mother hen.

A most unusual disease, Reyes' Syndrome, haunted us the late 50's. It mysteriously appeared out of the blue and seemed to be associated with influenza A, varicella, hepatitis, and aspirin. It was a stealthy and treacherous killer causing morbid increase in intracranial pressure and metabolic derangements resulting in coma. Diagnosis was by serum electrolytes, osmobility, blood sugar, B.U.N., amylase, and toxic screen. The patient showed peculiar excitability alternating with lethargy and rapidly deteriorating to a comatose state. My only morbid case occurred about two hours after I first saw him, a 7 year old. The undertaker and I diagnosed the disease with a postmortem liver biopsy, with parental permission. After a few agonizing years with combating Reyes, the culprit was discovered and the cause was our fever reducer, common acetylacitic acid or aspirin. The syndrome almost immediately disappeared when all aspirin treatment for fever was replaced by tylenol.

Attention deficit hyperactive disturbance, ADHD, is a common childhood affliction occurring predominantly in boys. School based academic problems, social discord, and behavioral difficulties are prominent characteristics of this disorder. The school teacher usually is the one who makes the diagnosis because of the overt disruption imposed on class conduct and discipline. Pediatricians are well aware of the vast differences between the two genders. By basic instinct and hormone differences like testosterone levels, boys are definitely more impulsive, aggressive, active, practical, and warlike in contraindication to their counterparts. Girls are naturally more patient, passive, emotional, intelligent, and governed by estrogen as their basic hormone. In life, the males are the hunters and pitchers, whereas the softer females are the homemakers, catchers, and bearers of the human race. Therefore, nature makes girls tougher physically and more disease resistant. I recall the striking differences in the sick newborns. If there was a postnatal problem with the heart, lungs, or kidneys, the girls were definitely tougher and stronger. They had a much better chance of survival; therefore, I would pray for any problem newborns to be a girl.

Realistically, the girls use their brain and the boys use their muscles to settle arguments or disputes. Parents are cognizant of the combative nature of boys and often fail to differentiate the fine line of distinction between normal hyperactive behavior and ADHD. Probably the tendency to over diagnose this disease is in the ascendancy. Assessment medically should embrace thorough physical, neurological, and psychiatric examinations. It seems like almost every child with cerebral palsy, brain damage, or severe head injury develops this syndrome. Treatment consists of pharmacological, behavioral, and psychological therapy. Social service investigation of the family functions and organization is also quite important. If the illness is uncontrollable, pharmacologic approach with methylphenidate, amphetamine, and trcyclic antidepressants can be employed. Apparently, these drugs act on the central nervous system dopamine, serotonin and norepinephrine systems. Dose levels have to be calibrated individually and are usually given at breakfast and noon. Mild side effects are moodiness, irritability, and appetite suppression but are controllable. Most parents are worried that the meds given to help dampen the over-activity and overdrive will have an opposite stimulating effect and will contribute to insomnia and anorexia. Actually, their fears are logical and well founded, for this behavior is true for a normal child.

Sometimes I wonder if parents and teachers aren't confusing hyperactivity with normal activity limits, especially with the male gender. Since colonial days, our lives have become greatly more complicated with magnification of pressure and stress. It's possible that this present lifestyle has an increased sensitivity effect on the child supervisors' reactions to the child's hopped up activities. Also, the stabilizing effects of child rearing have been somewhat ruptured because of single or working mothers, divorces, and strained marital relations. Realistically, it's conceivable that nearly all children have a little ADHD. A gargantuan number of these children require remedial reading, writing and arithmetic assistance. In my childhood days, no one ever heard of hyperactive disease. Girls have an attenuated version of ADHD, quite often controlled without medication. Also, ADHD usually abates in adulthood to almost zero.

Asthmatic children are multiplying by leaps and bounds, most notably, in the latter quarter of the 20th century. Asthma is a chronic disease of the lungs, characterized by increased spasticity of the airways and manifested by recurrent episodes of airway obstruction and asphyxia with chronic, persistent night cough and expiratory wheezing. Pollution and contamination of air, soil, and water by chemicals and noxious gases are major contributors with industry and automobiles the main culprits. The allergic triggers of asthma are extremely multifactorical consisting of pollens, molds, tobacco, foods, cold weather, bacteria, dust, rubber, exercise, insects, animals, and genes. In other words, all environment and inheritance factors play a vital role. Overpopulation also can contribute to the duke's mixture of causation factors. We've advanced exponentially in our armamentarium of modes of therapy. The most notable advances in treatment are the adrenal corticosteroids and inhalation masks to combat bronchial and tracheal inflammation. There are all degrees of severity embodied and expressed in asthma. Morbidity and mortality caused by this scourge is unfortunately on the upside. Probably, I have tended thousands of asthmatic children, have seen many seriously ill hospitalized asthmatics, sometimes on the edge hovering between life and the grim reaper, but thank Jehovah, none have given up the ghost as far as I am aware.

Dental cavities in children are an entirely preventable problem, controllable by proper hygiene (brushing), non carcinogenic diet, fluoride, and complete avoidance of sugar in nighttime bottles. The discovery of fluoride has prevented at least 60 to 75% of dental cavities since 1945. Coincidentally, it was a dental doctor in Detroit, who discovered the life saver for teeth from his experimentation in the early 40's. For a long time, he was not exactly a prophet in his own country and his revelation of the salient benefits of fluoride were pooh-poohed and condemned because of its injurious effects when taken in over dosages. Finally, the dental and medical professions saw the light at the end of the tunnel and accepted fluoride for its true worth as a life saver for nature's choppers and chewers.

My anesthetic prowess was put to the test on many occasions during surgery for week old infants with pyloric stenosis. The newborns with this ailment were in precarious straits because of starvation and vomiting, which violated their electrolytes balance. At their young age, growth and development are paramount, absolutely necessary aspects. Actually, it is a battle of life and death for survival. Medical management over a protracted period of time can be successful, but sometimes exacts a price of maximum suffering, starvation, and cachexia. I always felt that where terrible suffering was involved, we shouldn't mess around and should take the proven short cut to success even including surgery. However, I was basically diametrically opposed to surgical solutions under any circumstance unless it was the mother of necessity.

Another feature of time honored post operative feeding regimen, which got my goat, was the piddling, time consuming restoration of full diet. It occurred to me to try full preoperative diet after 12 hours of slowly increasing quotas of 5% glucose water. This regimen was quite successful because the babies were quite hungry and didn't vomit any more than they did using the time honored, antiquated, and complicated method of restoring diet. It also shortened the hospital stay of the babies as they regained weight and good health more rapidly. Of course, the mothers were also happier and that is the proof of the pudding.

One most notable pyloric stenosis happened in a 4 lb. premature male infant at 4 days of age. Ed Miller performed the operation under my light ether anesthetic and it came off without a problem or hitch.

A new disease appeared on the medical horizon along about 1950, called Kawasaki syndrome because it was first discovered in Japan. It started cropping up in America shortly thereafter with increasing appearance.

Mucocutaneous lymph node disease (Kawasaki) awaits discovery of an identity and pathogenesis. After an acute febrile period of about 12 days, a second stage of arthritis, skin rash, carditis, and large artery aneurisms (especially coronary) pervades for approximately 20 days, along with high risk of sudden death. Stage III lasts from clinical recovery to normal sedimentation rate of 10 weeks or so from onset. Repeat EKG's throughout the illness detect the most deleterious complications of coronary thrombosis and aneurysms and are a prime necessity. Treatment consisted of aspirin, IV gamma globulin daily for a couple days and supportive care. Even though there is a predominant vasculitis throughout with a proclivity to platelet aggregation and clotting, corticosteroids are blatantly contraindicated. A special incidence of this weird syndrome occurred in a corpulent 6 year old female. Her diagnosis was a nightmarish enigma for she presented a few vague, positive symptoms but nothing definite. I called Dr. Don Campbell in consultation and he said it was a brain scratcher, but ruled against Kawasaki syndrome. After a few days of agonizing and worrying about possible coronary heart disease development, I decided to take the bull by the horns and initiate aspirin and gamma globulin therapy for a definitive diagnosis of Kawasaki. She responded at once to this treatment and made an uneventful, albeit protracted recovery because we dilly dallied in our diagnosis.

Non-accidental violence, injury, and neglect of young children by parents or guardians, is a major health and social problem. Starvation and exploitation contribute to damaged minds and bodies of infants and children. There is a greater awareness of these issues but it still happens to an astounding number of youngsters. Health professionals have become more alarmed and attentive to battering of helpless children with state laws mandating a report of child abuse and neglect to designated public child protective agencies. It is unofficially estimated that several million children per year undergo this barbaric attack. Five percent of all children give histories of sexual abuse by depraved relatives or supposed "friends". The most severely maltreated children are the infants below age two years. Quite often sexual assault by the father is ignored or tolerated by the mother.

Henry Kempe, professor of pediatrics at Colorado University, became the champion and father to the rescue of all abused children. He was the kingpin who carried the torch constantly to alert the health professionals of the extreme, serious, and noxious repercussions of child abuse. Apparently there are certain characteristics of parents or guardians who abuse the defenseless kiddies. Single, overburdened, immature, poverty stricken young mothers are understandably out of control due to the vicissitudes and pressures of life. In my limited experience, the "<u>boyfriends</u>" of these lassies are quite often the prime offenders. Men are much more intolerant by nature and the constant crying can be a key factor. The abuser many times has been abused in childhood, instilling a large chunk of anger and aggressiveness which negates compassion and the milk of human kindness. Another way of detecting the person who abuses is by making detailed inquiries into the circumstances surrounding the explicit evidence of bodily injuries. Quite often the abuser paints a bizarre, flawed, impossible, or incomprehensible picture of etiology of the body injury. "He fell off the couch and fractured his skull on a rug." Or, a circular depression ½ inch deep on the hand was "caused by a stove contact (more probably a cigarette or cigar)" or "I just left her for a second to answer the telephone and she broke her arm." I'll believe some of these falsehoods when elephants fly.

Little two or three year old brothers can be a mighty hazard to a newborn sibling also. Several instances of fractured skulls have occurred in my practice, probably due to sibling jealousy, rivalry, and necessary over attentiveness of the mother towards her golden newborn. These two year old males must be watched and scrutinized like a hawk constantly, until adaptation and natural brotherly love set in.

One occurrence of severe head injury in a six month old female infant vividly comes to mind. The poor little one was brought in to my office in extreme coma, practically on her death bed, by a guilty, agitated father. I immediately grasped her in my arms and said to her dad, "Follow me to Bay Medical Center, now". Time was of the essence and on the way out I instructed my nurse to call ER to set up for an emergency spinal tap and normal saline IV When I did the spinal, the fluid was grossly bloody and shot out of the needle like a volcano splattering against the wall due to tremendous, increased intracranial pressure. This maneuver had to be life saving for she almost instantaneously regained consciousness and began "music to my ears" crying. The daddy claimed her injury was due to a fall from the diaper station, which is fairly common. But I was positive there was a more obvious solution and made a stat maltreatment report to the child protection agency. The child was admitted to the hospital as all possible child abuse incidents should be, to escape a lethal situation at home. The abusing father was arraigned in court and I testified for the baby as I have done on numerous occasions.

I saw one seven year old female child involved in a sexual abuse relation with her father, which came to litigation before an arbitration tribunal. The mother brought the 6 year old Fisher child to my office with a chief complaint of "itchy privates". On examination, there were small pearly blisters on the labia, which I considered as herpes simplex and prescribed specific antiherpes ointment, which was curative. However, I made two mistakes in not ordering a culture and in not reporting this predicament as a possible instance of sexual abuse. My logic here was that the herpes lesions were self inoculated to the labia from fingers picking herpes mouth sores. The child was in good health, well adjusted, acting very nonchalant and the mother was completely unperturbed. On inquiring about the father, I was answered that all family relations were on the up and up and copesetic. I saw Amy once thereafter, about six months later and there was no recurrence of the herpes. To all intents and purposes, she was thriving. After several years, the mother finally came to her senses and discovered the father's overt role in the rank sexual abuse of her daughter and she consulted with a lawyer. The rest is history and I learned a costly, but valuable, lesson of a $125,000.00 settlement. Later we cultured the external genitalia and it was negative.

Chapter 28

Pediatrician Lawsuits

My only four lawsuits occurred after 1978, when the lawyers, insurance companies, and litigants went crazy for the almighty dollar and grandiose expectations of perfect outcomes in all treated cases of illness. The medical profession is at a decided disadvantage in this battle, because the lawyers make the laws to their advantage, the insurance companies set the exorbitant malpractice protection fees, and the medical regulating systems set the fees and skim the cream of profits off the top.

My first dazzling shocker was a most impossible situation. I felt like a mouse caught in a trap. Around 1970, on a Sunday evening at 18:30 while eating dinner at home, I was interrupted by a phone call from Dr. Grigg demanding an emergency consultation on a nine month old baby girl named Delaney. She was having gasping, rapid respirations (dyspnea and hyperpnea) due to a foreign body (bean) lodged in the carina of the main stem right bronchus causing complete right lung collapse. Her hemoglobin was a very low 6 grams. I just happened to be on call that entire weekend for all pediatrics at both Mercy and General Hospital emergency rooms (ER's), which entailed seeing, on the average, 60 plus patients per day split about equally between the two ER's. I explained my strenuous duties to John and recommended that he enlist Dr. Olgac's services as he was my back up on call. Dr. Olgac, unfortunately, was unavailable, so yours truly was the gored goat and I acquiesced under extreme pressure.

On examination at Mercy Pediatrics, I found a beautiful little girl breathing deeply and constantly at probably around 100 respirations per minute (violent hyperpnea) for oxygen, apparently in the throes of death. History was that she had aspirated beans from the dinner at approximately 13:30 that fateful day, while her mother left the table to attend to a sick father in the basement. The mother called the child's family physician, Dr. Charlie Schisler, who upon examination referred the infant to Mercy ER at about 15:30. After dragging their feet for a vital, interminable three hours, I was their last resort, but I should have been their important first consideration. The ER physicians ordered lab and X-ray studies and then consulted with Dr. Grigg for bronchoscopy removal of the right main stem bronchus obstructing baked bean foreign body. John called in the anesthesiologist, Dr. Walt Pelzar and they kicked the ball around for a couple hours and unwisely decided against going after the foreign body because of the 6 gram hemoglobin which was exactly the reason they should have operated at once. Her only chance of salvation, certainly, was extraction of the bronchial plug which was completely blocking O2 from entering the collapsed right lung in consortium with the very low O2 carrying capacity of the RBC's. It was comparable to air entering or escaping from a cork in a bottle. As a horrible result, she suffocated to death at 10 p.m., 3 1/2 hours after I saw her. I called John and begged him on bent knee to go after the villainous plug. I immediately ordered blood for transfusion after my rapid exam. However, although blood was available through a Saginaw blood repository, there was snow and ice a foot deep on the roads. One thing I deeply regret was that when I took her in the treatment room, I decided not to do a cut down IV reasoning that it might cause cerebral edema and possible heart failure, so my brain reasoned wait until the blood comes over from Saginaw. Hindsight is truly better than foresight and reviewing post mortem thoughts I'm fully convinced that the one and only solution to her rescue was to have gotten that swollen bean out, pronto (her only chance) even though she may have died on the operating table, the crucial compulsive issue in every surgeon's mind. As you might anticipate, the lawyers had a ball with this case and the hospital and I were plundered for $60,000.00 each. Grigg settled for $50,000.00, unbeknownst to us, three months earlier.

I firmly believe the mother must have contributed to the baby's demise because of her squalid state of health before the aspiration incident. She was remiss for not giving this little one any of the life saving, readily available immunologic vaccines and apparently the infant was on a fairly strict milk diet which is very feeble in iron content. It is so easy to give in to the infant's intense desire for milk to constitute a complete meal. It's much easier to drink a meal. Milk has been the mainstay food in the child's diet for the entire first six months of life. I have administered many transfusions to the 8-9 month old "milk babies" in my early practice days. Proper baby diet foods (vegetables, fruits, and meats) have now been initiated at proper ages; thank the Lord, thanks to proper dissemination of sensible, dietary information.

My fourth and most dramatic instance of liability involvement was the untimely death of barely 13 year old Stacy Yanna due to pulmonary embolism in 1998, I believe. Stacy was a corpulent, 208 pound heavyweight adolescent, who sustained a simple undisplaced right tibial plateau fracture in school gym class caused by a fall while engaged in a game of "kick ball" with her classmates. Following the accident, she was directly transported to my office around noon. My staff, Terry Collier and Jane Parr, realizing the gravity of the situation, referred her immediately to General Hospital ER. There she was seen by the very efficient Dr. Terry Cherwin, orthopedic surgeon. A cast was applied and she was given pain medication and observed for several hours for possible complications. Stacy was then dispatched to home care by her grandmother (since her mother was working), with explicit warning and instructions to avoid immobilization and keep her very active and in frequent body movement to obviate vascular or fatty stasis, deep vein thrombosis, and finally dreaded embolic thrombi formation in vital organs. Pulmonary embolism in a thirteen year old is rare as hen's teeth. This case is unique in the entire history of hospitalized teenagers in Bay City. Indeed I could find no such case in the <u>entire</u> medical literature of pulmonary embolism occurring in a child 18years or under. Ordinarily, children are constantly in motion, which is the diathesis of blood stasis developing. Many times heparin is administered to complex fracture patients to prevent clotting and embolism, but she was prescribed none by the orthopedist.

I had been Stacy's pediatrician her entire life and had seen her on at least 25 occasions for laryngo tracheo bronchitis (LTB). After over a month's stay at home, she was rushed in to my office as an emergency by a disturbed, worried mother. She showed signs and symptoms of LTB, as she had done at least 2 dozen times previously. An antibiotic (penicillin) was prescribed and she was encouraged to be up and around and to do honest to God physical exercise at numerous times daily for substantial periods. It was evident that she was of the indolent habitus and her grandmother, behaving like a grandmother, could not force her to get out of bed. A week later she came back to my office in a state of full blown pulmonary failure at about 17:00. She was panting, breathing very deeply at about a rate of 70 per minute, and gasping for oxygen. Her respiratory efforts were relieved by mask O2 and she was dispatched stat to Bay City Medical Center as an urgent emergency for intensive care, CBC, x-ray, blood gases, and stat pulmonary consult by our capable Dr. Vincent Haroon. The x-ray was visualized in detail by roentgenologist Tyre Jones and myself and a diagnosis of pneumonia pervaded. Tyre reiterated positively that it could not possibly be pulmonary embolism and the blood gases came back as "normal". Tyre also reassured me, "It would be crazy to do a lung scan tonight or even consider lung arteriography". Vince Haroon was contacted by the pediatric nurse by telephone directly after receiving the emergency report, and he stated that he was busy and would see her later. I rechecked her condition late that night and decided with normal labs to observe her overnight. I was rudely awakened by my "friend" the telephone at 05:20 a.m. by her agitated nurse stating "Dr. K, come quickly, Stacy Yanna has ceased respirations and the respiratory therapy team is in here trying to restore breathing." I hightailed it to her bedside and found Stacy to be dead as a door nail. Vince had never seen her and I was the prime scapegoat left holding the bag.

I called the parents and reported the catastrophic state of affairs. How can you explain the sudden death of a presumably healthy, vibrant, young adolescent, to her parents? I was well acquainted with her mother but this was the first time I had ever seen the estranged father. I gave it my best shot but I could plainly envision the "doubting Thomas" look in their eyes that they, in their heartfelt grief, were unconvinced and unsatisfied that we had done all possible to save her life. In this present world of unmitigated frenzy of litigation and greed, it seems that all logic and reasoning has veritably gone out the window. She had been in the hospital as a patient perhaps for around 10 hours. Looking back retrospectively, I could have insisted firmly that Haroon see her at once or else she would be referred to a pulmonologist at Saginaw or Flint. But, I was somewhat lulled to sleep by Jones positive x-ray assurance and the "normal" blood gases. Actually, after a couple hours in the hospital, Stacy rallied and her breathing became fairly normal. Anyhow, the inevitable lawsuit was dropped in my lap, as well as the hospital's lap.

As a defendant, my lawyer was Bill Martin, whom I had collaborated with in defense of my suit against the herpes case described previously. We thought we had a reasonable chance for success on this one, and we were supported by a brilliant pulmonologist at Beaumont Hospital, Royal Oak, MI. However, the claimant's lawyer was a very astute young Hebrew lady from the Bronx and she really grilled me in my deposition. Her consultant pediatrician was a renowned doctor authority at Jewish Hospital in New York named Schaffner, specializing in pediatric pulmonary diseases and litigious cases. Martin, she, and I went to New York to interview and depose our adversary, Schaffner. He was known as a "suer's whore" as he had testified for the claimant in hundreds of lawsuits and virtually made it his prime source of income. Naturally, Schaffner painted a black, demonic picture of me and with all his might and main really thrust the dagger in deeply to the hilt - the more incriminating his testimony, the more moola for his "shaft". Our opposing lady lawyer was shrewd and put in hours of arduous labor to prove beyond a doubt that Stacy's life could have been saved hands down, just like shooting fish in a barrel. This nightmare eventually came to trial and the mother cried constantly in her bereavement. My lawyer, I, and the hospital attorney could obviously see that the members of the jury were being swayed increasingly, emotionally toward the mother. Several of them were truly weeping. We held a conclave and quickly decided that we should try desperately for a settlement. Even though we thought that we honestly had a fairly fool proof case, we could plainly perceive that our case was going down the tubes in a basket. We pleaded with Mrs.Yanna and persuaded her, after a sweat, to settle for 125 grand. We twisted Judge Bielawski's arm and finally were in clover. I was ecstatic and embraced Mrs. Yanna (I knew her well) and her lawyer (sealed it with a kiss). The hospital lawyer had words of adulation for me as a solid human and physician and volunteered to take all the defendants to dinner at the Bay City Country Club in celebration afterwards.

I recall the catastrophic Wenonah Hotel fire in the late sixties. All physicians congregated at Bay Medical Center ER and were stationed at their relative medical departments in the hospital. There were an abundance of burn patients and fractures from jumps and falls. There was bedlam, panic, and hysteria to the nth degree. The hotel was a famous landmark and meeting place for Bay City. It was a devastating tragedy for all Bay City residents. The hospital charity ball was staged annually in early December at this grand location. It really was our heritage. We held many rousing Bay County medical meetings there. The hotel was dedicated to the Princess Wenonah of antiquity.

One of my most thrilling experiences was a helicopter ride with Tom Wright in about 1980. The professor of pediatric cardiology at University of Michigan had come to Bay Medical Center to see and retrieve a cyanotic, congenital heart afflicted newborn for a work up at Ann Arbor. Pediatric physicians at Bay Medical Center had a closely knit liaison with the pediatric cardiology department at University Hospital, Ann Arbor. They would send one of their cardiologists to Bay Medical Center monthly to consult, examine, and make recommendations on all of our heart patients. This service was in vogue for a span of years in the fifties, sixties, and seventies; and it was predominantly due to the strenuous efforts of my buddy Dr. Thomas Benjamin Wright. It was sort of a pediatric cardiac clinic.

One of our main sources of post graduate education was the formation of the Northeastern Michigan Pediatric Society in 1949. I distinctly remember our first meeting at the Washington complex at the foot of our main business drag on Washington Ave. Our first speaker was Wolfe Zeulzer, professor of pediatrics at Detroit Children's Hospital speaking on the Rh factor, isoimmunization in newborns. As an added incentive, yours truly was elected president of this organization. It was ably supported by Ross Company who is earnestly and vitally interested in pediatric formulae and education. Bomfray and Linda Leach were their representatives and they remunerated the speaker, furnished the libations, and did the social amenities. Pediatricians from Flint, Midland, Saginaw, and Bay City convened at alternating city restaurants twice a year.

The presiding officer called the shots on the speaker, usually a renowned professor from medical schools or hospitals. In the afternoon preceding the evening meeting, Dick and Dottie Bickham and Linda Leach and I would meet at a nearby country club for a rousing game of golf for "duffers", all except Dick Bickham who was almost eligible for the P.G.A. championships.

In 1971, it was my explicit pleasure to attend the International Congress of Pediatrics meeting in Vienna. Prior to embarkation, I bought a $900 Leica camera, to enhance my photographic library. My younger son, Gregory, accompanied me. Tom Wright and his wife, Florrie, also made the trip from Windsor, Canada. Greg and I debarked from the plane in Paris and flew from there to Wiesbaden, Germany, to visit my daughter Susan, and her better half Ekkehard Paul Prengel, and their son Jon Paul.

After a glorious couple days partying in Wiesbaden, we entrained for Vienna, Austria, a distance of 350 miles and nine hours travel time. We stayed at a hotel on the outskirts of Vienna in Baden, the site of the Kaiser Wilhelm's former playground. Our classes and lectures were held in the palace; and we made several bus trips to Haydn's grave and Luxemburg. I was especially impressed with the stork nests on the roofs of houses in the towns we passed through. On our last day, due to a plumbing fallacy, our hotel room was flooded as were several other rooms. One of the doctor's wives had a miscarriage. We passed by Amadeus Mozart's statue, everyday on our way to the palace where the grounds were resplendent with the most beautiful flower gardens. We managed to go to the Vienna Opera one evening and attended "The Bartered Bride" musical by Santana.

Dr. William Oliver, Professor of Pediatrics at the University of Michigan accompanied us on the plane to this congress. On the second day in Vienna, out of a clear blue sky, he was paged by none other than the head ruler of Morocco to come at once to be the neonatal delivery room physician for his daughter's first newborn, an expected male. We Michiganders all were brimming with pride that our chief should be summoned for such a prestigious duty. In fact, he sold me his return plane ticket at a bargain for my son, Greg, and asked me to be lookout for his precious wife on the return voyage to Detroit. I purchased several books depicting the various organ system diseases and they are a perspicacious addition to my library.

I made another happy visit to Wiesbaden in 1986 to see Susan and my wonderful grandchildren, Jon, Lisa, and Sara. We traveled to Hamburg to see the Tutankhamen memorabilia. Susan had a young girl, May Yelverton from Limerick, Ireland, assisting her with the household duties. One memorable occasion during my stay was when better half Ekki returned from an educational meeting in Columbia, South Carolina, unexpectedly in the dark side of the night and roughly railroaded a visitor resident, Terry, kit and caboodle out to the street. I remember while there, taking a very pleasant and eventful train trip to Florence, Italy, to see all the famous paintings, carvings, and sculptures. The rail trip back to Wiesbaden over the Alps on a perfect day was breathtaking and really out of this world. I anticipate making one more flight to Germany to see my beloved great-grandchild, Lisa's first little one, the Lord willing.

My mother was a veritable rock of Gibraltar, while fulfilling the duties of receptionist in my office. She was exceedingly amorous with children and was in her glory when children entered my office. She served in this capacity for at least 15 years and was as honest and trustworthy as the day is 24 hours long. She developed severe osteoporosis, (she hated milk) and in 1971 became a basket case, unable to stand erect. She became a patient at the county nursing home. I visited her daily and took Greg to visit her every Sunday after church. Harry Vail, one of the nicest ever family doctors, took superb care of her. She succumbed to heart and kidney failure, May 27, 1971. My mother had rheumatic fever as a child and indubitably it insidiously contributed to heart damage and life shortening. She was the most wonderful mother a son could ever have. She was the stabilizing and motivating factor in my life and I bequeath any meager success I've had to her angelic influence. We had our disagreements and she blatantly disapproved of my two marriage partners (she voiced her decision notably by being in absentia at both my weddings). She was always very positive, determined, resilient, astute, and had a great sense of humor. My first born, Susan, is almost an exact carbon copy of her grandmother in physiognomy, conduct, behavior, articulation and so full of the love of human kindness. Incredibly, when I look at my daughter, I envision my mother. She lives as long as Susan lives and I'm tempted to believe in reincarnation. Mother's live in lifelong lady friend, Catherine Leseman, stayed on in my apartment above the office for an additional four years, under my tutelage. Her only daughter lived in Washington, D.C., and would have no relationship with her. Catherine was a very kind, understanding, and lovely person and seemed almost like a second mother to me. She capitulated to diabetes after amputations of both lower extremities in 1975.

My office building apartment was nearly like a designated hospice. My second wife's parents moved in and stayed there until the Grim Reaper cut their life cords. Oscar Vincent, my father-in-law, was really quite a character. As I previously mentioned, he smoked around a half dozen plus cigars daily and embodied the airs of a languid southern gentleman. Steffie's mother, Marie Liebrich, was a generous, hardworking person who was the breadwinner of the family. Later, Sylvia, my wife's daughter, and her family, moved into the apartment but stayed for only about a year. Her husband Bill had been discharged from the Navy following the termination of the Vietnam War and they needed a temporary home. Sylvia gradually became estranged from her mother for some unknown, weird reason. She suddenly became understandably enamored of her divorced father, who remarried but never formed any kind of kinship with her after she was born. Now Sylvia lives in Illinois but, for several years, has not had any communication or contact with her devoted mother. Apparently, Sylvia is confused as to her identity and has mixed priorities as to her maternal allegiance. To my knowledge, Steffie always was all a mother could ever be to Sylvia, while nurturing her as a single parent. Sylvia had a sour taste for moi.

Chapter 29

Nurses and Staff Personnel

I never met a nurse I didn't like. I take my hat off to the many countless numbers of nurses who have so nobly, honorably, and arduously devoted their services in my behalf. I'm impelled to state that throughout my entire practice, I have always worked with benevolent, caring, cognizant, and cheerful nurses. In my estimation, they deserve a seat next to St. Peter in the next world. They knock themselves out working long hours with tremendous responsibilities for barely a living wage. Pediatric nurses warrant special acclaim for their intense and motherly fidelity to the infants and youngsters.

Evelyn Lewicki comes to mind as the zenith of virtuous nursing attributes. She was head pediatric nurse at Mercy Hospital. Evie always smiled in the face of adversity and ran a tight ship impeccably. "Tessa" Marlene Tasiemski was chief pediatric nurse at General Hospital and was equally qualified to manage the little ones. She always baked me a chocolate cake on my birthday and her staff would have a little celebration ceremony with me. Margie Goik deserves very special attention for her "beyond the call of duty" services to the children. Margie was an LPN and was shanghaied to orthopedics from pediatrics at Bay Medical Center, by a wicked chief nurse because only R.N.'s were qualified to work in Peds. This really fractured poor Margie's heart as she was undyingly in love with kids and she only had six of her own at home. Other faithful hospital nurses who crowd my memory are Linda Jezak, Lynn Bergevin, Rebecca Vermeesch, Jan Mont, Ann Kovaleski, Marlene Cole (Kevin's sister-in-law), and Mary Kay Freel, (Dr. John Freel's daughter). All the nurses working in my office were very high caliber, honest, and trustworthy. Mary Kay was distinctively Dr. John's 13th baby as his other 12 kids were all male (stem-winders).

The nurses who worked directly for me also were all dear angels of mercy for my little patients. My first elegant nurse hired after returning from my tour of duty in WWII, was "Fee Fee" Burdick. Fee Fee was quite a naïve, what you see is what you get, type of person. One particular instance tweaks my memory. She related a tale concerning her first lesson while playing golf. Her partner was the golf pro at the Bay Valley course. Fee Fee stroked her ball into a virtually unplayable lie. After cogitating the options for a seeming eternity, she decided to employ the pro's expertise. She gently approached him and pleadingly said, "Will you please knock me up on the green?" Enough said.

When I moved into my new building on 1102 Columbus, my new nurse was Genevieve Malecki, who was available after clinician Clyde Tarter retired. Jenny was a plump, good natured, no nonsense, industrious, and all business worker – a practical nurse. One particular happening stands out in bold relief. She was authorized to give penicillin shots on occasion. This time it was a five year old boy who had a high fever, (diagnosed by the best way of determination - my five fingers on his forehead). In spite of the discomfort, rectal temps are most reliable, unless the thermometer is rinsed in hot water. Not withstanding, almost instantaneously following her injection into the right femoral triangle, his leg turned an alarming deep blue purple color and he was unable to move the leg. We called for an ambulance stat and transported him to General Hospital and had emergency consultation with renowned general surgeon, Peter McGee. Apparently, the needle had struck the femoral artery and nerve accidentally. We employed heat, massage, passive exercise, elevation, and sedation. Thanks to God, he made a complete recovery of function after a week of blood, sweat and tears. It's a wonder that my hair did not turn entirely white. Thereafter, all shots were administered deep in the mid lateral leg muscle mass. Actually, I gave almost all the shots. Steffie and I gave Genevieve a Bedlington terrier, Molly, who didn't see eye to eye with our beloved Pekingese dogs.

Ester Bergman was my right hand helper for a few years. She embodied all the favorable qualities of a nurse and was imbued with the milk of human kindness. My last benevolent nurse was Jane Parr. Jane had a fantastic memory for names, places, and epithets. Her recall of my patients was unbelievably accurate and this was really a boon to me. I am on target with figures and diseases, but severely lacking in remembering people's appellations. When I would introduce friends, I often drew a blank for names. Sheepishly I would ask the parties to introduce themselves. Jane was very virtuous and strictly adherent to the "rules of the road" regarding ethics and morals. She was a damsel of few succinct words, a real stickler for details in all dealings, and a tower of strength at work.

Generally speaking, nurses are well deserving of all the kudos possible for their unswerving devotion to duty. However, in my experience and observation over an epoch of medicine, it is my deduction that they generally shun household duties and the culinary art. To be perfectly reasonable, we must consider their multiplicity of jobs. Working with doctors is a gargantuan job in itself, let alone working oddball shifts, taking care of husbands, and efficiently mothering children. A nurse is kind of caught between the "Devil and the Deep Blue Sea" and is expected to be pleasant and smiling at all times. They are absolutely indispensable – and a real joy to boot.

I am well aware of exceptions to my downgrading critique of their cooking ability. One very special, lovely nurse, Joan Cummings, a graduate of the University of Maryland School of Nursing, comes to mind. Joan is the wife of Douglas Cummings, an urologist extraordinaire. She has superbly mastered to a science, the art of making crab cakes, oyster patties, and shrimp cocktails. In Michigan, anyone rendering sea food edible is as rare as hen's teeth. In the first place, procuring fresh seafood here is a Herculean task. Nevertheless, Joan was born and bred in the good old Chesapeake Bay country of Maryland's eastern shore and knows the magic secrets of fixing crab cakes supreme. Also, being a Terrapin, she bears an unbroken bond of mercy. We are church pals too.

Another premier exception in the gourmet cooking department is a very dear friend, Nurse Patricia Brilinski, whom I previously mentioned. I have had many sumptuous holiday dinners at Pat's home. I talk about our close friendship in more detail later in the book.

Fortunately, I employed two crackerjack bookkeepers and they were Marilyn Van Diesche and Terri Collier. Marilyn was formerly Bob Prophater's ace secretary and she was, next to my mother, the most trustworthy accountant in my office practice. My cash flow was never so great; and I was able to liquidate my office and house mortgages. Unfortunately, I lost Marilyn to fellow practitioner, Terry Cherwin, a top notch orthopedic surgeon who wooed her with a massive salary incentive. In retrospect, it would have behooved me to appoint her as my office manager.

Terri Collier was my Girl Friday, chief cook and bottle washer, acting like a manager, accountant, receptionist, and cleaning lady - a veritable jack of all trades. Her versatility was cum magna appreciated, especially after the hatchet job Sandy Gerhauser did, leaving my office books and papers in a veritable shambles and disarray. Terri was a faithful and intense worker who paid no attention to overtime. She was a veritable diamond in the rough. I was confident Terri would go through a mine infested field to discharge her duties for my patients and to maintain my reputation. In fact, Terri may have had hearty feelings for me - not reciprocated.

In the 60's, I constructed a room in the basement of my building and rented it to a group of anesthesiologists, headed by Walt Pelczar. Walt had been a family clinician at Unionville for over 10 years and decided to become an anesthetist by a three year study course at Ann Arbor. Up until the time he appeared upon the scene in 1962, anesthesia had been delivered by me, Chapin, Wright, Otto Jens and other family practitioners. Ether was antiquated and the gas anesthesia corps was augmented by experts John Geneczko, McSherry, Wan, and Garry Bundy. Each one had distinctive personalities and all were intensive care specialists. After about seven years, they decided to move out and as secretary of the Bay Arenac Iosco Medical Society, I designated this room for our monthly meetings for several years. Finally, following a violent rainstorm, the room was practically knee deep in flood water and thus ended our rendezvous and a hoard of patient charts.

Chapter 30

Awards, Honors, and Tributes

It was via Dr. Thomas Benjamin Wright's doughty effort that in 1975, I was named a delegate at large from Bay City to the Michigan chapter of the American Academy of Pediatrics (AAP). I cover this activity in more depth later in the book.

It has been my good fortune to receive recognition and acknowledgements in my later years, for my pediatric and community services. On my fortieth year in practice, 1980, tricky Dick Bickham chaired a dinner celebration in my honor at the Lantern Restaurant across the street from St. Laurent's "Nuthouse" and on the east side of Saginaw River. There must have been a gathering of at least 80 to 90 nurses and doctors present, including Senator Barcia and Hans Jeppesen, Jr., our hospital administrator.

Hans succeeded his father, Hans Sr., as CEO and COO at General Hospital. I was Barcias' pediatrician when he was a child, as well as doctor to many physicians who are now practicing in Bay City. Remarkably, among the present practicing M.D.'s, that I served in their childhood, are the Dardas twins, Gary and Terry, Mike Gruber, and Charlie Schisler but to name a few.

After the big affair honoring my fiftieth year in practice in 1990, I had a total front page write-up in the Bay City Times by Gay McGee, Peter's wife who toiled as news editor after Pete's untimely death. I also had a citation from Michigan's governor, Blanchard, and was given the keys to Bay City by our mayor at City Hall in a special ceremony. This party was to proclaim my retirement but I didn't retire in 1990. I always stated I would persevere in helping my kids until I crashed physically (Ides of March was in 1999).

My most prestigious honor came in July, 1996, from the Michigan chapter of the American Academy of Pediatrics when I was named Pediatrician of the Year for Michigan. I was unable to accept this most worthy honor at the annual meeting of the Michigan chapter at the Grand Traverse Resort because my second son, Gregory, was married on that same fateful day in Atlanta, Georgia. Greg's nuptials were a gala affair, enjoyed by all his siblings. There was only one faux pas during the ceremony. The benevolent minister, who was facing retirement, mistakenly pronounced Gregory's appellation as "Herbert" when he pronounced the wedded couple as man and wife. Diane, Greg's wife, is a gorgeous belle from Oak Ridge, site of the famous barber shop quartettes. Diane works at Georgia Institute of Technology as an expert in the nutrition department. For some inexplicable, psychological reason, she has become estranged from the Knobloch family after two years of affability to the nth degree.

In 2003, I was accorded a superb honor as Education Doctor Supreme (EDS). I have always been intensely interested in learning and have taught nurses, interns, residents, and fellow practitioners ever since my graduation in 1936. This EDS honor is in my name and will be awarded annually to the outstanding medical teacher of the year by Bay Medical Center. This plaque I bequeathed to my faithful daughter, Melissa, who also is deserving as a prime student of art and accounting. Melissa has accomplished Herculean feats in accounting as a partner with Deloitte, Haskins and Sells (predecessor to Deloitte and Touche), and as Vice President with BET plc of England and National Service Industries. She retired at the tender age of forty-five years and now enjoys art and facilitates creativity workshops. Her husband, Martin, a nuclear physicist and Professor at Georgia State University, is also retired. To her absolute credit, she engineered her first husband, Douglas McAlpine, monetarily through Emory University Law School. Unfortunately, the marriage went asunder and they divorced ten years later.

One other most coveted award was my name being attached to "DDD Day", (Doctors, Dentists, Druggists Day). This day is one of the happiest, most fun loving days of the year. Camaraderie is at its zenith and anything bearing a hint of worry is taboo. As before mentioned, I had a brainstorm idea about combining the three professions in a day sports outing. I consulted with Robert H. Criswell about the practicality of this venture. He too thought it was a pregnant idea worth activating. So, I notified the local dental and pharmaceutical societies and we were off to the races with our inaugural meeting after Labor Day, 1948. We had a renowned cardiologist from the Cleveland Clinic lecturing on "The Cardiac Constellation" that day. Luckily, my good health has enabled me to attend each and every annual meeting (54) since its inception. During the 2003 get together, it was my good fortune to receive a handsome plaque designating my name officially as the founder and originator of this blessed event.

The protocol for the meeting is as follows: 1. We meet on Wednesday at 11a.m. at Bay Valley Resort for a one hour learning exercise, usually presented by the hospital pharmacy. 2. We gather on the golf course at 1p.m. and pick up heterogeneously designated partners for an 18 hole round of "best ball" golf in teams of four containing at least one long ball hitter, good chipper, and capable putter. 3. On the course, we have bratwursts and varied beverages for quenching thirsts and soothing jangled nerves. 4. We return to the resort center, wash up, and engage in an hour of fellowship while partaking of hors d'oeuvres and imbibing drinks to wet the whistle and enliven the conversations. 5. We have a sumptuous salad, steak, and baked potato dinner topped off with delicious apple pie. 6. Then we have prizes - awards for skill holes and probably 20 drawings for gifts of golf balls, golf clubs, golf bags, and golf clothes. 7. Now pleasantly exhausted and happy, we depart for home hoping our good partners are in a personable frame of mind. Indubitably this is one of my cum laude, happiest days of the year, barring none. Turnout is usually around 80 to 100 personages.

One other truly unforgettable person that it has been my good fortune to know is John Edmands. John is truly a unique person, a brilliant graduate engineer of the University of Michigan with multiple skills and talents to compliment his work ethic. I recall with sardonic bliss, the time I received a phone call from his mother, Margery, 10 minutes before Doris and I were to plane to New York for a CME and booked musical plays. She said, "Doctor K, my 3 year old son John is just post ictal from a grand mal seizure and has a fever of 103.5 degrees. My agile cerebrum quickly rehearsed all options and I told her, "Give his body an ice cold sponge bath, have him take ½ an aspirin tablet when he regains consciousness, and when he is stable transport John to the General Hospital ER. I will notify the on call doctor of your plight." On we went on our merry flight to the Big Apple and all's well that ends well. John never had another febrile convulsion.

John is a superb engineer. His father, Jack, also was a first class engineer and had his own company which John later joined.

My son Tom and John were classmates and playmates. Father Jack Edmands put in a personal appearance at my office one day when the boys were in their early teens and reported that they had been caught throwing paper airplanes from the tower of the First Presbyterian Church on a Sunday. Jack and I coolly plotted our strategy to combat this mischievous behavior, each of us addressing our own son. This episode was relegated to limbo and never recurred.

My son, Tom had a fatal fascination for cars. One time he blew out the engine of my prized six month old Chevy Impala while drag racing on Euclid Avenue. He tried to shift without the clutch. Needless to say, he never got to drive my car for another such performance. Tom also built a hybrid Oldsmobile by amalgamating different car engine and body parts. He gave up when it was fully assembled and refused to move it off the blocks. Tom and John were roommates all four years at the University of Michigan. Tom majored in history and then took a position in the insurance business as an adjustor.

John has resurrected an antiquated home and converted it into a mansion filled with unique antique furnishings. He is the proud owner of several rental homes, including his mother's home, and has a gorgeous home on Lake Superior just west of the Soo. John is a true builder and is constantly at work erecting buildings around this 'cabin' up north, including guest houses and a sauna warm up for the frigid waters of Lake Superior. John is single, having lost his lovely wife to a tragic, accidental gunshot wound. He does have a distinct preference for male relationships. I have celebrated several birthday's with parties at John's beautiful residence on Fifth Avenue and McClellan. John does a great job caring for his infirm, lovely mother.

Chapter 31

Family Matters

My number one wife, Doris Mathilde Meyer, succumbed in October 1984, from probable coronary and myocardial infarction. She was afflicted with hypertension for umpteen years, had a fatal proclivity for nicotine, and had become overweight in later years.

Following our divorce, Doris developed a happy circle of tender, gender friends, including auditory champion Katie Dardas, Jean Medvezky and Roz Blumenau. She was living it up in Bay City in a cozy apartment and we maintained a luke warm friendship. I would get together with her, my mother, and the children on practically every holiday despite considerable resistance from second wife Steffie. I made a determined, heart rending decision to attend her funeral with all my children in Atlanta, in spite of strong spouse opposition. My dear friend, Alice Ward, rendered staunch support, favoring my resolute decision. In spite of the sad circumstances, the Knobloch family had a glorious reunion with all of my children and grandchildren present.

The circumstances surrounding her demise were rather mystic and weird. Melissa had dinner with her on a Saturday night and then they attended a symphony. Doris appeared completely normal throughout the evening and Melissa dropped her off at her residence. The following Monday, Melissa and Doris had a shopping trip planned. When Melissa came by to retrieve her, she found the Sunday paper lying on the doorstep. She climbed in a window and found Doris peacefully dead in bed. There was no post mortem but the cause of death was evident – heart disease, the number one killer.

One unique and ethereal happening was related by my son, J. H. Thomas. On the night of her passing, at about 3 a.m., Tom swears he was awakened by a dazzling bright light and an apparition (his mother) appeared and beckoned him to follow her. Tom froze and resisted by saying, "No". The figure disappeared and nothing further transpired. Tom always was the apple of her eye in life and apparently she wanted to bid him goodbye.

Since the loss of our benevolent maternal figure, we have had several scintillating family reunions in summer seasons. My dear children and I have grown much closer each succeeding year from 1984 to the present. Even though my kids are spread all over the globe, we manage to communicate rather intimately as much as the phone, pen, plane auto, and computers will permit. Nowadays, Atlanta; Vancouver, Canada; and Wurzburg, Germany where they live are just a hop, skip, and a jump removed. I have finally realized with my maturation, that my direct genetic descendants are the absolute, most wonderful possessions and heirlooms that the Lord has ever bequeathed to me. Our intense love for each other has grown by leaps and bounds as precious moments we are together melt away. Evidently, I am trying desperately to make up for lost time in my retirement for all those good times together I sacrificed while I was "saving" the Bay City environs brood of babies and juveniles.

My reminiscences recall one special occasion (although they all were) in the fall when we were all together in Sterling, MI, and had a delicious chicken dinner at Iva's. Speaking of chicken, it seems that we have a big hankering for Zehnders in Frankenmuth (little Bavaria) and their special chicken dinners – capital of the universe.

Since the turn of the century, in July each year we have celebrated my birthday with a huge extravaganza reunion and birthday party with all the trimmings and fanfare at this restaurant. John Edmunds and Pat and Marvin Brilinski have been extremely gracious in furnishing lodging and kitchen for many of our get togethers.

Greg made a collateral series of pictures of my 90th year of life in one framed photo. Susan and Melissa were with me in the 90's, in separate years, on St. Patrick's Day and we viewed the big Bay City St. Patrick's Day parade together. This parade is probably the largest parade around on March 17th. One time Susan and I visited the people who own our former home at 1911 Center Avenue. They were in deliriums of enthusiasm about restoration of the house to its old realm of glory. It seems as though Bay City has a magnetic attraction for all my kinder. They seem to relish returning to their roots and scenes of their childhood, which doesn't make me feel bad. They all grew up there, went to Washington Elementary School, and graduated from Bay City Central High School with honors.

Chapter 32

Further Highlights on Sundry Diseases

Rabies vaccine a la 1936 embodied 21 injections in a combination of all components of the rabies virus, grown on guinea pig embryos and antibodies from horse serum. Naturally, this method of immunization conjured up all possible forms of serious reactions and repercussions imaginable, including anaphylaxis severe central nervous system injury, serum sickness, stunting of growth, paralysis, and mental retardation. Now we administer one shot of human rabies passive immune globulin (RG) immediately and then administer human diploid cell strain active rabies vaccine stat. We repeat this on days 3, 7, 14, and 28 after the first dose. We do not mix the vaccine and human serum together in the same syringe and do not inject these two entities at the same site. This mode of immunization produces a minimum of mild local reactions and seldom ever causes any harmful adverse effects. Bites and human contact with wild dogs and cats are the main reasons for rabies immunization in youngsters. The disease is most hazardous for humans from bats, foxes, skunks, and raccoons. Bats can be especially hazardous because they get into attics via chimneys and even the slightest contact (even their breath) can cause transmission of rabies. I have ordered rabies prophylaxis for many youngsters, usually because of wild animal bites but fortunately have never seen the real entity. The RIG and human hiploid serum have caused no adverse repercussions in my limited experience. Rabies is diagnosed by exam of the animal's brain.

Vaccine reactions and anaphylaxis are rather rare but there really is no greater emergency in pediatrics. They demand a cool head and a plethora of action. With every injection of vaccine or drug, epinephrine 1: 10,000 dilution must be available by syringe at a seconds notice. This is especially true when injecting penicillin medication IV, Vaccine 1M, or local anesthesia anywhere. Seconds are equivalent to minutes and hours and time is of the essence. These untoward occurrences are totally unanticipated but the person responsible must always be prepared for this cataclysmic event and respond like lightening automatically. It is productive, as in golf to rehearse in your mind your swing, the exact course of action to counteract a serious reaction. I've only had one profound reaction to a vaccine injection, in a five year old boy who was in perfect health. He became heliotropic almost immediately, convulsive, apneic, and severe shock prevailed. I gave him 2.0 ml of 1:10,000 epinephrine sub q, l ml in the deltoid stat and 0.2 ml by bag and mask in the supine position. I also put him on an IV of normal saline for 100cc wide open. Finally, the nurse prepared a syringe of antihistamine for IV injection. By the grace of God, he regained consciousness after an interminable period of about 5 minutes. There is nothing to make you feel more helpless with a total sickening feeling of stark anxiety than one of these torturous crushing events, believe me.

Another similar emergency that can deduct several years from your life is a severe, immediate I.M penicillin reaction which fortuitously is relegated to the past tense. This horrendous event must have occurred at least a half dozen times to yours truly. As with the above vaccine encounter, I would similarly prepare medicinally to counteract and reverse the anaphylactic state while inwardly suffering the agonies of pure HELL until the morbidity dissipated. We did have a pseudo test to uncover penicillin allergy but it was not trustworthy.

Continuing with the transmission of zoonotic infections, Lyme disease comes in focus. For a while there was a Lyme disease 'craze' (everyone had it) conjured up by fertile imaginations. There was a practitioner in Saginaw in the 60's era who was obsessed with Lyme disease and treated almost every patient he saw for ioxodes damini spirochete infection. The deer tick in Michigan is rare as dinosaur teeth. It is mainly confined to the New England states. To my knowledge, I have not seen an actual case of Lyme disease malady, but have been suspicious of the illness in children in whom ticks were found on their body or head by the mothers while bathing them. The prime diagnostic sign occurs in the second stage of sickness which presents with erythema chronicum migarans (ECM) 3 to 32 days following the tick bite. Actually, there are no written, in stone, infallible diagnostic tests and the whole thing is a jigsaw puzzle. In 1/3 of patients, ECM is a large red bull's eye, 4 to 10 cm in diameter and is absolutely specific for Lyme infection. It lasts for weeks to months and is accompanied by systemic acute symptoms. It arises from a papule and spreads centrifugally. If not treated by penicillin, tetracycline, or erythro there are three major morbid manifestations, notably myocarditis, meningoencelphalitis, and recurrent arthritis.

"Cat Scratch" disease is transmitted usually by kittens from razor blade nail scratches of the epidermis through the lymphatic system to lymph nodes mainly in the axilla. It is usually a benign self-limited acute/chronic infection in young children with spontaneous resolution over a two to four month period. A note of caution is warranted for any trauma to the enlarged nodes can result in dreaded abscess formation. There really is no specific treatment via antibiotics for this cat scratch affliction and culture of lymph nodes for organisms is negative. Sterile, hot, normal saline packs and pain medication are the essence of the treatment. If the nodes become supperative, aspiration is required. Surgical excision is by all means to be avoided, if possible. I have treated many cases of cat scratch disease and in the majority their outcomes were benign – all's well that ends well. Patience is a virtue and the keynote of success here. The use of antipyretics for fever is debatable. Certainly they are needed desperately for discomfort, throbbing headache, and where convulsions are a possible hazard. But suppression of fever has its drawbacks. Fever is nature's warning and alarm signal of the presence of active infection. I believe the febrile response also stimulates the immune system and helps mobilize the body defenses including phagocytosis. There is one thing for sure and that is infants and toddlers should not be unprotected for a second with kittens and small dogs. Larger breeds of canines, especially the labs and golden retrievers are more phlegmatic, much safer as guardians for kiddies.

Streptococcus aureus bacterial pneumonia, usually of the lobar type, occurs in children between one month and five years of age. In the sixties, I had several cases recognized by lobar presentation, underage six months with pneumatoceles and purulent empyema. IV oxacillin and or vancomycin worked well in all these infants. This initial therapy is followed by oral cloxacillin or oxacillin for a period of weeks during convalescence. If the organism is a methicillin resistant staph, vancomycin plus rifampin can be antibiotics of choice. These children are often deathly ill and they do require oodles of supportive, constant care. The onset of this disease is strikingly abrupt and virulent. Early diagnosis is imperative.

Tracheotomies early in my practice were not uncommon. There were many indications for (in the vast majority) this truly lifesaving surgical procedure. Any cause of tracheal blockage or obstruction compromising the airway to a large degree must be relieved immediately to avoid brain injury. Diphtheria, the most dramatic etiology of tracheal restriction, was at one time the most common cause until the vaccine for it was available. At first diphtheria vaccine (active immune response) and diphth antitoxin were derived from horse serum which sensitized the donee to allergic reactions. As I previously mentioned, I received this diphth vaccine shot when in the first grade after Edna Mae Cousins died of this brutal disease. As a result, I was eternally subjected to horse serum anaphylaxis. I always carried a sterile, curved beveled trochar in my bag in the forties for the purpose of emergency tracheal intubation below the cricoid cartilage. Other indications for this operation are aspiration of unremovable coins or other solid foreign bodies, epiglottises, retropharyngeal or bilateral tonsillar obstruction due to abscess, acute infectious mononucleosis, and severe laryngotracheitis. IV or /.M. decadron was a godsend in acute Epstein-Barr, (kissing disease) viral infections and spasmodic croup.

In my experience, viral meningoencephalitis comprised about 25% of the cases in infants and children over one month of age. My pediatric care also encompassed cases of about 60% H. influenza and 15% strep pneumococcal bacterial meningitides. Of these three bacterial ogres, the S. pneumococcal is probably the most virulent and results in the most serious post recovery sequelae, mainly deafness. I'll never forget one of my patients who had severe life threatening meningococcic (weichselbam bacillus) meningitis with adrenal hemorrhage. His mother carried her lifeless three year old son into my office out of a clear blue sky one morning in 1951. He was comatose and in deep shock with a stiff neck, raging fever, and an hemorrhagic rash over his face, chest, and trunk. I sensed that the grim reaper was hot on his trail so, without the loss of a second, I grabbed him from his mother's arms and headed stat for old General Hospital with mom in my car. While on the way, I had my nurse alert the Peds nurses at the hospital that we were in a mad rush heading in their direction with the sickest child this side of heaven. The Peds nurses instinctively set up a normal saline IV with penicillin G 300000 u/kg in 6 divided doses, ice bags, and readied for a spinal tap. On admission, he received immediate gigantic doses of IV gamma globulin, penicillin epinephrine, and a transfusion of compatible RBC's. After checking his CBC, platelets, blood factors II, V, VIII, and fibrinogen and fundoscopic eye exam, I performed a lumbar puncture to obtain turbid spinal fluid. This fluid showed over 4000 WBC with 82% polys, low glucose, high protein content, and gram negative biscuit shaped diplococci on smear. Spinal fluid and blood cultures on blood agar were indubitably positive for meningococci susceptible to good old penicillin. The diagnosis was as plain as the nose on your face - acute meningococcic meningitis, fulminanent with friedbuchsen syndrome, disseminated intravascular coagulation, and purpura fulminans. By the grace of God, he did recover in a couple weeks of intensive care by the prodigious efforts of the nurses in attendance. However, the price he paid was the loss of a few fingers and toes due to gangrene from coagulation of small arteries in the terminal phalanges. Dieter Roloff, Chief Resident M.D. at University Hospital, was mesmerized by this story and was intensely interested in our protocol and mode of armamentarium for saving his life. He said, "Salvation of life in a case like this is rare!"

Parents of autistic children use an empty gaze and a failure to use gaze to regulate behavior and to engage in the social games of infancy. Autistic children when presented with two spatially adjacent stimuli, show few back and forth movements. By implication, deficits in early developing processes of visual attention can underlie the restricted temperamental styles, atypical social communication, and aberrant behavior of autism. Kanner first described this disorder in 1943 and at first it was classified as an emotional problem. Autism is defined by Webster's Dictionary as absorption in fantasy to the exclusion of interest in reality. Diagnosis of the autistic child is dependent on cognitive delays and bizarre behavior, and is generally not a subtle discovery. Work up is best done by a multidisciplinary approach. This disorder is generally noticed in the first year of life and its hallmark characteristic is the lack of interest in other persons. Etiology is elusive but evidence points to an organic cause. It can be associated with perinatal complications, congenital rubella or tuberculosis, structural brain abnormalities, genetic disorders (Fragile X), and metabolic derangements. Asperger syndrome is a developmental disorder on a continuum with autism and is characterized by paucity of empathy, naïve and inappropriate interaction, speech egocentrism, poor nonverbal communication, and ill coordinated movements. It is similar to autism but is less likely to have delayed speech or stereotypical behavior. With Asperger syndrome, the child tends to have normal intelligence and onset is usually after 24 months. The focus of treatment should embody communication skills, cognitive strategies, adaptive functioning, social skills, and physical and occupational therapies. Autism therefore is purely a problem for neurodevelopment pediatricians. I have purposely mentioned no drugs with respect to its treatment as there are none worth their salt.

Dyslexia also is another one of those ephemeral unknown entities with intangible resolution. It is characterized by jumbled, misplaced, smorgasbord words and body movements. They are spatially disorganized in helter skelter fashion, probably caused by cerebral cellular synaptic electrical conduction and chemical derangements in formation and development. I'm sure I've seen numerous instances of children who have exhibited this pattern.

With respect to lead poisoning (PB), in 1985 the CDC promulgated a blood lead level of minus 25 as fairly safe to prevent lead encephalopathy anemia and brain injury. In the 1990's, this value was remarkably reduced to 10 minus for brain safety and integrity. In fact, perhaps any concentration of blood lead is unhealthy and possibly harmful. The main priority in elevated blood lead levels is the identification of the source of the lead. This is most commonly from wall paint, plaster chips, lead pipes, lead coated cooking utensils, automobile exhausts, pulverized fragments in household dust, outside ground dust, and the paint of buildings built before 1950. Demolition and renovation of old homes can be a potent source of poisoning if specific precautions are not observed. Dry sweeping inside homes must be avoided, especially when there are children. Deficient ingestion of calcium, magnesium, iron, copper, or zinc and excessive dietary fat, increases absorption, toxicity and retention of lead in the body. Lead soldered seams in cans may be the origin of lead leaching especially in those containing acidic foods such as fruits, fruit juices, tomatoes, and soda drinks. Chelating agents like EDTA are not metabolized in the body but are excreted, unchanged, by glomerular filtration in the kidneys and are very efficacious means in the deleading process. EDTA must be withheld if these are anuria or dysuria for obvious reasons. Also, any kidney disease elevated Bun or creatinine or hepatocellular injury, are indications for holding EDTA in treatment. BAL Rx can be employed in cases of anuria, high PB blood levels (<100) and PB encephalopathy. I have had many cases of lead poisoning >25 PB that have had EDTA therapy with excellent success and no really serious consequences. Blood lead levels should be monitored periodically from birth, especially if there are any environmental factors which might cause a rise in blood lead levels.

Attention deficit disorder (ADHD) is a mixture of behavior related difficulties including academic and social relationship difficulties. It may involve rank, aggressive behavior and mood lability resulting in discipline issues and poor peer relations. Psychological testing will help to determine academic problems and point to remedial measures. Structured classrooms are generally preferred to open classes. Ideally, specialized personnel such as psychologists, nurses, tutors, speech therapists, and social workers can contribute immensely in the assessment and management of these children. Medical assessment should embody thorough physical, neurological, and psychiatric examinations. Family environment and nurture should also be appraised. Problems with family discord, substance abuse, and dysfunctional interpersonal relationships with all family members must be investigated. Basic behavioral and psychological therapy should be thoroughly explored. ADHD is deeply rooted in the male gender, primarily because of their innate aggressive behavior. But the female children are not exempt from this malady. The school teacher is a prime diagnostician because of their intimate contact with these afflicted children. Mothers are at a disadvantage here, because of their inexperience and multitude of household duties. Mother is also with the child all day and too much familiarity breeds a bit of contempt for discipline in the home. By her inborn passionate and sympathetic nature, mothers can be "pushovers" for a stubborn, dominate, and aggressive male child. Actually, mothers understand and can deal better with daughters, and vice versa for fathers with the male ruffians.

Pharmacological therapy can be a God send in the treatment of ADHD or a curse if not properly administered. Each case is unique and the drug (amphetamine or methylphenidate) must be dose titrated for each child. Methyl phenidate is the drug of choice because of its lesser effect on prolactin and growth hormone. But both drugs are pretty much equally effective if used for the appropriate diagnosis. Twenty percent of these children can show lack of motor coordination, enuresis, encopresis or EEG abnormalities. Medication is best given in the morning and at noon because methylphenidate can cause sleep deprivation, anorexia, and loss of height growth temporarily. However, I've never felt that addiction was the slightest problem. Boys naturally show more aggressive behavior and diagnosis depends on its degree and intensity. Many are classified falsely as ADHD kids, especially when their mothers are intolerant and not understanding.

Gastro esophageal reflux (GERD) and hiatal hernia are extremely common in the pediatric population. In fact, to a certain degree, it is accepted as a normal phenomenon in newborns and young infants. However, pyloric stenosis can be a pitfall and must always, in every case, be seriously considered as a possibility, especially if vomiting is forceful or projectile with weight inhibition. A palpable pyloric tumor is summa qua non for diagnosis of an organic problem. The upright position for feeding is definitely pragmatic and hypo-allergenic foods are preferable viz soy formulas. Frequent, smaller portioned feedings are advisable to meet caloric requirements and typically solids or thickened gruel-like feedings with added cereal are much less apt to be regurgitated. Infants on breast feedings have an advantage because their food is always ready, 24 hours a day, on demand. Elevation of the bed head is recommended to negate Isaac Newton's law of gravity. When not feeding, the supine position is in order. Overfeeding is to be strictly avoided and the prime signal to decease feeding is when the baby pushes the nipple away with the tongue. Due to hiatal hernia and difficulties with obesity, weight reduction in older children may be a central issue. Antacids, by their buffering effects, coat and alkalinize the esophagus to counteract the acid regurge flow. Sucralfate, an aluminum salt of sucrose, is a non absorbed chemical with several unique properties and is a strong buffer. It presents a protective barrier effect. One gram is best given 1 hour before meals and hour before sleep. Motility stimulating drugs have been tried, but due to serious side effects like respiratory problems or esophagitis, they are employed almost exclusively for infants and children with significant failure to thrive. Surgical treatment is not considered unless there is definite failure of medical measures.

Mother Nature, I'm sure, intended 100% for babies to be fed by breast alone or mainly at least. It is the species' sustenance and the advantages are incomparable to the bottle. But there are exceptions to all rules and a small percentage of babies are unable to do well on the breast. Also, mothers with HIV or hepatitis should not breast feed.

Celiac disease falls under the heading of chronic diarrhea and malabsorption syndromes. It is a small intestinal disorder, with a gluten sensitive enteropathy similar to non-tropical sprue. The presentation of celiac malabsorption syndrome is usually in the 6-12 month age period with irritability, growth failure, and diarrhea. The basis of this disease is believed to be hypersensitivity to alcohol soluble gliadin fraction of dietary gluten, a component of grain flours. It usually holds sway after cereal is admitted to the diet when primary incisors erupt and solids are added into the dietary regime. Gluten containing foods, such as teething biscuits, bread, or cookies, may cause gluten sensitivity when absorption of intact micro molecules occurs. A familial disposition towards this disease has long been recognized. It appears to be more common in those children of Scotch or Irish descent. There also is a strong association with histo-compatibility Type III.A.-B8. The diagnosis is confirmed by finding the characteristic histologic pattern of small intestinal villies atrophy and chronic inflammation of the mucosa on suction biopsy. Treatment consists of stringent, dietary gluten restriction and generally accomplishes symptomatic improvement, normal growth, and correction of histologic abnormalities. A similar celiac disease picture presents in cow's milk or soy intolerance, immunodeficiency, tropical sprue, iosinophilic gastroenteritis, and giardasis. In any case, foods containing wheat, rye, barley, and oats are to be strictly avoided like the plague.

Sudden infant death syndrome (SIDS) is defined as sudden or unanticipated death. Even after exhaustive post mortem examinations and intensive studies, we come up empty for a diagnosis. This phenomenon peaks between the second and third months of life. The unexpected nature of this event as it strikes apparently healthy infants in their sleep, produces deep repercussions of psychopathology in the entire family. Intense counseling is required and a thorough autopsy is imperative. Reassurance of the grieving parents, grandparents, and siblings immediately following this tragedy is an absolute must to negate any guilt feelings.

We believe SIDS is basically a problem of immaturity. Polygraphic techniques for sleep disturbance are now available in Bay City at Bay Regional Medical Center (its new moniker after amalgamation with McClaren Hospitals). Hurley Hospital was formerly our selection for use with suspicious or near miss SIDS problems, especially with prolonged apneic episodes. Home monitors for apnea have been in vogue since the 60's. Infants at risk for SIDS fall into two main categories, obstructive apnea due to oral and throat abnormalities and CNS medullary breathing center lack of development. Infants at increased risk for SIDS are premature babies, twins, males, history of sibling death due to SIDS, sleeping in prone position, and strangulation. Sometimes I wonder if apnea monitors in home don't cause more anxiety for parents than reduce anxiety. Diagnostic pneumocardiograms can be helpful in detecting possible SIDS. As a rule, SIDS rarely occurs after six months of age, and the suspect baby is home free.

I have had several infants with profound, frequent apneic attacks and have been unable to determine any rhyme or reason for them. But usually, Dr.Time causes dramatic improvement. I am cognizant of a breathtaking incident which occurred with my first born child, Susan, when she was about eight months old. We were living in a garage apartment at 2018 Center Ave. I awoke at about 2 a.m. one night and heard a choking, gasping noise in her bedroom and rushed there in a split second. I found her struggling vigorously and gasping for air with a covering laced tightly around her neck. She was salivating. At once I ripped the covering off her and threw it out the window. My heart was beating at maximum speed and I'm convinced it was a life saving experience.

I was very sorry when aspirin was sounded the death knell as a drug due to its connection to Reyes disease. I must have seen at least a half dozen cases of Reyes disease. It was fatal nearly 25% of the time. Intensive care is mandatory in treating it. Serum transaminase ammonia, prothrombin time, Bun, and glucose values are mandatory. Treatment is pentobarbital, IV infusion 10-15T dextrose, IV albumin, and intracranial pressure monitoring. I am reminded of one special twelve year old young man who died suddenly before I could get him hospitalized. Clinically, I was quite suspicious of Reyes disease. However, the parents refused an autopsy. So I went to the funeral home and convinced the funeral director to do a liver biopsy and draw blood for serum determinations of the appropriate studies to diagnose Reyes disease. Sure enough, all studies were positive for Reyes disease and I informed the parents who happily exonerated my actions in his care.

Renal stone disease (nephrolithiasis), afflicts over a ½ million Americans per year. Men are predominately affected with this curse by a 3:1 ratio as compared to females, until after age 70. Incidence predominates in the 4-5th decade. I was 55 years old in the summer of 1966, when my first attack of renal colic ensued. High humidity and high temperature seem to be definite contributing factors, and in 1966 the summer was a true scorcher. Diet and fluid intake are important factors in the development of urinary stones. Sodium and protein foods must be restricted because their intake will increase calcium excretion and monosodium urate saturation. The vast majority of stones are formed of calcium oxalate and calcium phosphate. Genetic factors may be contributory, especially cystinuria and sedentary occupations. My first experience with these odious critters came in the middle of my car drive from Midland to Bay City one afternoon in July of '66. Onset was with instantaneous, unbearable, jackknifing, piercing pain in my right flank, just below the ribs. On a scale of 1to 10, intensity was at least a 10. I put a death grip on the steering wheel and prayed to the Supreme Being to please send down the endorphins stat. Wisdom ordered me to pull off the road and stop instantly. After about 10 minutes, which seemed like an hour, the pain subsided and I decided to head directly to Mercy Emergency ASAP, hoping fervently the renal colic wouldn't recur on the way. I had had plenty of prior run-ins with renal calculi, and recognized it immediately. At the hospital, my renal studies were not conclusive and I didn't pass any stones. I did have gross microscopic hematuria, some urgency, and frequency of urinary function. However, at this time in medical history, CT Scans, MRI's and the stone crushing technique (extra corporeal shock wave lithotripsy) were unfortunately unavailable for me. So, after 3 more renal attacks, Dr. Pete Fujiwara, urologist, decided to send me to University Hospital in Ann Arbor for definitive diagnosis and therapy. At the fountain of learning, I was given the royal treatment by the beloved interns. They did several cystoscopies up to the right kidney in the pelvis and discovered a large 'rock' obliterating ¾ of this area. An astute decision was made by the chief urologist to make an incision in my right flank and directly dissect to the renal pelvis and extract the stone. This operation was carried out successfully and finally my kidney woes were over. My gracious neighbor, Floyd Natzmer, kindly made several trips to Ann Arbor with me during this ordeal, but not without remuneration. Diuresis in medical treatment of urinary calculi is counterproductive and causes an exacerbation of renal colic. Metabolic analysis of my stone was evaluated and it turned out to be calcium phosphate.

Chapter 33

Meltdown Years

As my medical career wound down due to physical limitations, my patients gradually retired me. A host of speed bumps descended upon the medical profession in the guise of HMO's, lawyers, insurance companies, and big businesses. Our professional control was voided almost completely - thrown out the window. Medicaid and Medicare reared their ugly, gorgonistic heads and our pediatric economics were raped disastrously. We always were the low guys on the totem pole. It became almost impossible, literally and figuratively, to make ends meet. For about the last ten years of my practice, it seemed like Medicaid patients multiplied with leaps and bounds, until practically ¾ of my work was engulfed in cases having substandard monetary remuneration. However, I never, ever refused to take care of any patient who wanted my services. And I rendered my pediatric expertise to the best of my ability regardless of their social status. Actually, I strongly felt that my real joy and recompense was in helping the little ones regain their complete recovery, low pay was not their fault. My finances got so low in the last several years, that I was forced to borrow pecunia (money) in large amounts from the bank and dip deeply into my savings to pay my quarterly income taxes. In pediatric practice there are no surgical procedures involved, and office patients are the backbone, bread and butter of the practice. Remuneration is grossly over weighed on the surgical side of medicine. In the past twenty years, hospital practice has dwindled to a trickle and bare minimum in pediatrics.

In September 1997, I made an ironclad agreement with Bay Medical Services to transfer my entire pediatric practice to the Doctors of Osteopathy Family Clinic in the medical mall and teach the osteopathic resident doctors, interns and medical students. My supervisors were Carmella D'Addazio (Chief) and Floyd Stevens, second in command of the clinic operations. I relished my duties at the family medical clinic, because I really love teaching and educating the medical students and young physicians.

I have been a teacher to nurses and doctors all of my life. I taught pediatrics to the University of Michigan Saginaw Hospital (General and St. Luke's) interns and residents for about fifteen years. I was elected Associate Clinical Professor of Pediatrics at Michigan State University College of Human Medicine in 1982. I was also honored by Bay Medical Center in 2002, with a plaque designating me as Education Medic Guru of the Year, to be awarded in my memory to a physician each succeeding year. My greatest honor of recognition, hands down, was being named by the state of Michigan as the "Michigan Pediatrician of the Year" in 1996. However, it just so happened that my #2 son, Gregory (or Gregoravitch as our dear Mrs. Boelte used to call him), planned to have his nuptials with Diane Smith on the precise date I was to be bestowed with this honor. Naturally, my family was numero uno, so it was off to Atlanta on that red letter date.

I carried all of my patient's charts to the Doctors of Osteopathy Family Clinic and this maneuver afforded me a blessed avenue to escape storing them in my cellar or attic after retiring. Likewise, I transferred my entire library, examining tables, and Dr. T.B. Wright's infant weighing table to the new location, lock, stock and barrel. The blessed residents would always kindly pick me up and escort me to their journal club meetings every second Tuesday night throughout the year. Notably, Pat O'Malley with whom I formed a close family relationship, Rachel Monroe, a brilliant doctor, and Genevieve Stuber, an astute competent D.O., were my benefactors in this exercise. At journal club meetings, we were wined and dined at the elite, culinary eateries in our area. At each meeting we would have dissertations by pharmacy representatives and interesting medical renditions by rotating physicians.

I had perennially hoped and prayed that at least one of my descendents would follow my footsteps and dive deeply into the field of medicine, emulating my career. However, I was not a shining knight of armor example to my children. My 24 hour on-call profession, with all its arduous work, emergency calls day and night, and frustrations which negated family get togethers, made medicine unappealing as an avocation to all my children. Actually, they were all straight A students, had pleasant personalities, and were physically able to tackle any medical career of their choice. But why swim upstream? My son, J.H. Thomas, gave it a brief whirl as a hospital orderly for a year or so. But the only fulfilling passion he developed was an overpowering love affair with food. Hospital food never really swept me off my feet. However, Tom cleaned up numerous patient food trays with a voracious appetite second to none.

My last hope for a descendant in the medical profession turned out to be my granddaughter, Susan's third child, Sara. I attended her graduation from Pacific Lutheran College in Tacoma, WA, where she was an honor student in Women's Studies, Anthropology, and Art. Sara worked as a waitress through her college years to earn some shekels for her post graduate education. Fortuitously for me, she unexpectedly chose to go for a medical career. My fervent hope that one of my descendants would take up the baton and follow in my footsteps was a pipe dream realized! I was in 7th heaven and was really dumbfounded when Sara revealed her final decision to go all out to become a physician. Sara has a striking natural beauty and can strike up meaningful dialogue with any person she meets. She possesses a keen, perceptive intelligence and possesses great empathy and the milk of human kindness. (My mentor "Coop" in Marquette used to emphasize the need for the milk of human kindness.) I am positive of few things; but in this instance, my basic intellect tells me in loud intonations that Sara has all the necessary qualities and ingredients to become a stellar medical doctor. She is living in the lap of luxury, because in going to medical school at Mainz University in Germany, she gets a six year "free ride" economically except for food and lodging. As I now am composing my memoirs, she is at the end of her third year of all out dedication and passing all courses with laudable grades. I couldn't be happier with her success. I thank the Lord for her toughness and compassionate blood, sweat, and tears in accomplishing her goals.

Chapter 34

Notable R.N. Acquaintances

Through the passing years, I have made binding friendships with four very special nurses with whom I have worked. Actually, I have been incorporated or adopted as a foster member of the families of all these wonderful medical partners. My association with Rindy began at Bay Medical Center in the 60's through the 70's, in the outpatient department where I medically managed and cared for pediatric patients weekends and nights on call. Rindy was one of our stellar R.N.'s. We seemed to mesh gears with coinciding outlooks on life in general, as well as patient care. She was extremely capable, intelligent, forceful, and possessed a striking pulchritude and charisma. Religiously, Rindy was a dyed in the wool 7th Day Adventist, which emanated from her grandparents. Having married a Catholic girl and had a high school / college love alliance with a dear Christian Science femme, I had learned the value of tolerance and the negative effects of prejudice in religions even though my nurturing was of the old fashioned, adamant stance of Martin Luther.

Rindy transferred to the ER in the 80's and, while there, unfortunately had a losing disagreement with a doctor anesthetist which resulted in her release of duties at Bay Medical Center. Her battle was regarding her mother, following surgery. Her first husband was a rank lothario. I attended her 2nd marriage to a Pinconning EMT which also failed because he was homosexual. She ended up in Chattanooga, TN, and was hired in diverse capacities at various hospitals. She remarried number three husband of similar evangelical faith there. She now lives in an elegant new home, located on the peak of famous Lookout Mountain, TN. (This is the same location of the Civil War battle engineered deftly by our unflappable General Ulysses S. Grant.) Rindy now resides in the home of her dreams, constructed from scratch, with surrounding flower rock gardens, and a pool with a fountain. She is a strict vegetarian and grows her own organic, natural vegetables. As a full fledged R.N., Rindy has worked in surgery, surgical recovery, heart research, obstetrics, intensive care, and ER.

She has now found her niche in night shift obstetrics, which she really enjoys to the hilt. We have been corresponding and touching base for several years. I did pay her and present better half, a visit around about 1990. I have also seen her briefly a couple times in Bay City when she visits her sister. Maybe on some propitious occasion, I can see her castle in Chattanooga first hand.

My second nurse alliance was with Pat Brilinski. Pat invaded my life in the mid 80's when she transferred to Bay Medical Center nursery from Saginaw General Hospital nursery. Patricia is a most excellent nurse in all attributes, but our staunch friendship is bound by our fervid feelings for the University of Michigan, notably their football program, as I previously mentioned. Her husband, Marvin, is a U of M graduate, and a certified CPA of renown. Marvin had been a stellar grid iron performer in high school at Alpena. Unknowingly, I had seen him as a player in the Alpena – Bay City Central football game here around 1960. Pat has only one outstanding failing and that is a torrid love affair for food. Perhaps her mother helped to create this by admonishing her to "eat all you want, but be sure to clean your plate of every crumb", as all good mommies were want to repeatedly proclaim. Along with Pat and Marvin, I would attend all the University of Michigan football games for at least 15 years. As I related previously, in 1996, Pat and I attended the Rose Bowl, one of my life long dreams. Pat invited me to join their Pinochle club in the 80's and we convene on a Saturday night once each month. Off and on I've been an avid Pinochler since college days – taught me by my dear Terrapin classmate, Charles Gassaway Spicknall, at College Park, Maryland.

Marvin and Pat were great for camping on weekends and I made several sorties with them to various lakes in the environs. Camping has never been my strong suit, but I do love nature. However, you can't really escape our toys and wonderful modern inventions of living for longer than an eye blink. As I said before, Pat is a genuine sumptuous culinary artist. I am always an invited guest at Christmas, Thanksgiving, and for various holiday dinners. I can really attest with veracity to her excellent cooking abilities. She and Marvin have one adopted son, Matt Their son, Matt is a superb athlete and physically built like a high bred stallion. Matt had a host of academic problems but his physical prowess is beyond reproach.. Now the apple of their eye is Brady, their two year old New Year's 1st grandson. Pat has a heart as large as a whale's. She graciously opens her home to all of my far distant children and grandchildren during their visits to their roots in Bay City. Actually, I have a close knit kinship with the Brilinski's.

I would be remiss if I didn't mention my brief platonic relationship to nurse Karen Taylor who was in charge of the nursery in the 2000's. Coincidentally, our birthdays meshed and we are both "gems" (Gemini signs). We were tuned in intellectually by our hospital relations. We did have a couple birthday celebrations together, but never got romantically involved. Karen is divorced, has two children, and doted on her son, the apple of her eye. She was a beautiful lady and was endowed with charisma and high moral bearing. During her tenure at Bay City Med, she attained a degree as ARNP (Advanced Registered Nurse Practitioner) from Grand Valley State, in Grand Rapids, by commuting. Shortly thereafter, in 1998, duty called her to Ocala, FL to work with three family practitioners. Karen is a sure shot to attain success.

My last enduring nurse alliance is with Joan Cummings. Her husband Doug's medical alma mater is the University of Arkansas, preceded by West Point graduation and 20 years Army service as Colonel. I was medically allied in pediatric urology with Doug when he first came to Bay City from the University of Maryland Hospital in Baltimore and Chestertown, MD., in 1992. I first met his wife, Joan, in 1994 when I escorted them by car from a Midland Medical Society meeting back to Bay City one night. Then along about five years later, Doug invited me to dinner to his old home on Center Avenue, two blocks east of my old lumber home on Center Ave. It was there that Joan and I discovered we were both dyed in the wool, fellow Terrapin graduates from the University of Maryland; she in nursing in 1970, and me with 1933 BS and 1936 M.D. degrees. That night, Joan displayed her culinary prowess (as previously mentioned) as a master crab cake queen purveyor and our relationship was sealed.

About a couple years later, I had a gnawing, irresistible hankering for oysters. I mentioned my desire to Doug, who passed it along to Joan, and she transmitted it to her folks in Chestertown, MD. Presto, I had a quart of delicious oysters in no time. Then lo and behold, I was an invitee to a dinner with her visiting son and daughter (by a former marriage) and their families. I have been a member of First Presbyterian Church for well nigh on to 64 years and our paths often cross there. One Sunday a couple or so years ago, I sat with Doug and Joan during a church service. Then Joan and I became spiritual buddies at church. During the golf season, Doug is an inveterate golfer and Joan, a church elder, still regularly attends. We both have been engaged in giving communion to the handicapped and sick shut-ins of our congregation.

When Susan and Val were here on vacation in Bay City in the summer of 2004, Joan invited all of us out for a crab cake dinner at her home on the Bay City Country Club (BCCC) grounds. When the menu calls for crab cakes, she has no superior to titillate the taste buds. Needless to say, she earned her expertise having spent her childhood at Chestertown on Maryland's eastern shore alongside the Chesapeake Bay, crab central. Her well deserved epithet is heralded as "The Crab Cake Queen". In Bay City our chefs lack experience in preparing seafood and it is well nigh impossible to obtain really fresh sea creatures.

In October of '05, Doug and Joan Cummings sponsored me on the trip of my life to the football homecoming game between the University of Maryland and North Carolina State at College Park, Maryland. It was my 68th anniversary of graduating with the Terrapin class back in '33, in the dinosaur age. Joan, is called "Nana" by her exquisite grandchildren, Nick and Jordan, who live with her daughter Jill and husband Scott Bramble in a home on Chesapeake Bay. Joan's parents, Ed and Loraine Fry, met us at the Baltimore airport on Friday and escorted us 70+ miles by car to Chestertown in a continuous driving rain. My accommodations at the Chestertown Comfort Inn were most excellent. After a recuperative nap, Joan picked me up for a rendezvous with her family at a unique, honest to goodness seafood restaurant in Rockport, a stones throw from my abode. Following a hearty wine toast, we were served heavenly rock fish, crab cakes, and oysters. Upon devouring one half dozen brawny raw oysters on the shell, I ordered another ½ dozen of the oysters, they were so good. The rock fish was also literally out of this world. Of course, "them 'sutherin' folks" know how to extract the fortissimo flavor from the Chesapeake Bay catch.

On Saturday morning, Joan's brother Ed Fry and wife Maureen transported us to College Park for the festivities there. We were taken on a tour of a gargantuan alumni building of 60,000 square feet which was in the midst of construction. We wore our "hard hats". Then we were treated to a sumptuous pregame feast in Cole Field House, the hallowed basketball court prior to the brand new Comcast Sports Center.

Brother Ed Fry, a 1971 University of MD graduate, belongs to the Colonnade Society comprised of 500 Maryland Alumni members who each contribute 1000 greenbacks yearly to the university. Ed was instrumental in placing me on the speakers' agenda preceding the game to address the Colonnaders on the subject of how the University of Maryland became known by the soubriquet of Terrapins. I did deliver an impromptu oration on the evolution of the nomen "Terrapin" to timely replace the luke warm designation of "Old Liners" for Maryland sports teams. After my extemporaneous discourse, I was showered with plaudits and handshakes. Notably, our esteemed head basketball coach Gary E Williams was one of my prime hand shakers and every Colonnade member was somewhat taken aback. There were numerous exclaims, "He never shakes hands with anyone". Maryland had a national college championship in basketball two years previously under his expert tutelage.

After my dissertation, we adjourned to the Press Box of the stadium to witness the pigskin festivities. As each member of the Maryland football team emerged on to the field, he patted "Testudo" lovingly on its shell. Howsoever, the charisma of the terrapin deserted us and N.C. State eked out a 17-13 victory. In the glass enclosed, cozy Press Box, we were happily protected from a couple of rain showers. We also were treated to a luxurious banquet of hors d'oeuvres fit for royalty. On Sunday morning we attended impressive church services in Chestertown with a brilliant lady minister presiding. We then met up with Ed Fry and were observers of a fox hunt on horseback with the hounds howling. Apparently there were many foxes in this terrain of beautiful rolling hills by the Chesapeake Bay. These lovely roller coaster hills are reminiscent of similar ones in southern Maryland around La Plata and Hughesville, my haunts with Phi Sigma Kappa fraternity brother, George Matthews, during those luscious pre-med days in College Park.

We spent Sunday afternoon and evening with Jill, Scott and the grandchildren in their gorgeous, brand spanking new home by the Bay. Scott is the Lacrosse coach at Washington College nearby. They all gave us red carpet treatment. Nick was especially entertaining with his energetic athleticism, love of football, and card games. Poor Jordan was ill with a fever and signs of viral pneumonitis. We also took a Sunday midnight tour of downtown Chestertown. I was utterly amazed to see historic buildings erected way back in the 1790's. At this time my ardent wish was for daylight to really see these antique structures.

On Monday morning, Jill and Jordan drove us to the Baltimore Washington Friendship Airport for our uneventful homeward journey back to Michigan. Airline security was good, but not overwhelming and being ensconced in a wheel chair has its advantages. All in all, it was quite a blast of friendship all the way. Joan was my caretaker both ways on the plane from Tri-City (MBS) and performed a noble job with the wheelchair at all stations.

Chapter 35

Association with the D.O. Residents

As I previously mentioned, while working at the Doctors of Osteopathy Family Clinic, I was in association with doctors Bud Stevenson and Carmella D'Addazio who were in charge of the D.O. students, interns and residents. My swan song final years, 1997-1999, in pediatric practice were devoted to my own patients plus teaching the basics and rudiments of pediatric practice which encompasses <u>all</u> diseases of children. Bud Stevenson had relinquished his thriving family medical practice in Auburn, after about a quarter century, and taken on instruction of the doctors in the practice of osteopathy in the hospital.

Osteopathy was first promulgated by Civil War Dr. Still. Actually and realistically the D.O.'s now get virtually identical medical teaching and training courses in their four years in medical school as that given to the M.D.'s, except they are immersed in the Still chiropractic tradition. Prior to WWII, osteopaths went their way and M.D.'s went our way. Now these two medical spheres have amalgamated and are practically inseparable in all phases. Each one is exceedingly proud of its specific identity, wrought within the cauldron of time. These two giant bastions in medicine duly remind me of the differential between Michigan and Michigan State in sports. One is a staid, supercilious, sophisticated and "cool" as a cucumber, while the other is like a joyous, energetic puppy full of fire and brim stone and just firmly planting its feet on the hallowed ground. Personality and empathy wise, the D.O.'s win thumbs up. One thing is for sure, there were no D.O.'s serving in WWII and they made hay while the sun shone in civilian practice. My relations with the doctors of osteopathy have <u>always</u> and forever been most amiable, brotherly, and respectful.

Carmella D'Adazio was nominally head of education at Bay Medical Center and hence was in charge of the D.O. resident program. Carmella is quite erudite in medical knowledge but, unfortunately, she has a pithy, abrasive, demanding, and demeaning manner and personality. This was not acceptable by her protégés. Eventually, she faded out of the picture and Bud, who was more pragmatic and congenial, assumed the drivers seat. Bud has a keen sense of humor and is very adept in the kid glove handling of the multiple woes and problems of his young medical trainees. His theme song was "keep them happy, carry a big stick, but yield and compromise wherever possible with their demands". Albeit immature, each trainee was a prudent, rugged individual with his own distinct personality and character. Harmony, friendly camaraderie, and respect bilaterally were the prime keynotes for consensual relations betwixt master and pupils.

My patients reluctantly accepted the change of venue to the clinic setting where they did not receive quite the warm coddling, personal love, and red carpet treatment they had received in my office. It was more of a business by the numbers at the clinic. I luxuriated in my instructional duties and figuratively had a ball in teaching the pristine basics of clinical pediatric practice to these eager, intense, enthusiastic, serious, and affable young people - literally a "piece of cake" for me. We actually fit like a glove, and developed an ironclad, mutual, lasting friendship. For me it was a reincarnation and reliving of my own beloved freshman internship at Union Memorial Hospital in Baltimore, only this time my role was reversed and the shoe was on the other foot. Unfortunately, my tenure as trainer with these "eager beaver" trainees possessing an insatiable appetite for medical knowledge came to an abrupt halt literally on the Ides of March of 1999. I suffered a dandy congestive heart failure and was hospitalized at Bay Medical Center. My career at Doctors of Osteopathy Family Clinic was immediately, reluctantly, and justifiably terminated in toto. This ended sixty three years of arduous, enjoyable, and faithful service as champion for my kids.

Chapter 36

Special D.O. Residents I Have Known

My most amiable, academic, and platonic relations with the D.O. chief residents via their commendable journal club meetings began when I joined their ranks in 1997 and persists now and, hopefully, ad infinitum. My first close alliance is with my good friend Patrick O'Malley. Pat is a brilliant student with an undying thirst and hunger for medical knowledge. Pat is a dyed in the wool "Badger" from the great state of Wisconsin. He and I are somewhat bitter sports antagonists, as Wisconsin and Michigan have an innate Big Ten rivalry, preeminently in football and basketball. Patrick married a very beautiful, lovely, and talented South Korean lady, A. Young. Proudly, I was their pediatrician at the births of their son Sean in 1998, and daughter Amanda in 2000, both at Bay Medical Center. (In fact, I rendered my medical services to several of the D.O. residents children for a majority of them were happily married.) After wrestling with several opportunities for group and private family practice, Pat decided, with a little nudge from me, to establish a solo general family oriented practice in Oconomowoc, Wisconsin, near his parent's home. Pat and I were <u>very</u> good friends. We often had dinner together and went to journal club every two weeks. He invited me along on his visits to his parent's home on numerous occasions.

My second friendly relationship is with Rachel Nixon Monroe. She is one of two well known past osteopathic resident presidents. Rachel and I have a blessed, symbiotic, trainer-trainee relationship. She has a fervent desire to learn, and a positive, take command, happy, and bright attitude. She doesn't lack one bit of pulchritudinous personality, to be sure. Her marriage partner, Bruce is a civil engineer and erstwhile airplane pilot. She was chief resident '02-'03 and was a wise, compromising, whip negotiator. Unfortunately, during her adolescence Rachel had to undergo extirpation of her most important uterus because of uncontrollable metrorrhagia. After her graduation, she opted to join forces with a medical group in Fondulac, WI, as a family practitioner, and a darned <u>good</u> one.

My third resident union is with two third year D.O. married residents - Nanette Myers and James Cobeen. We entertain a very affable, friendly, and somewhat familial relationship. Both are in their late thirties and are quite knowledgeable and mature. Nan was chief resident but her whip is comparable to a wet noodle. James is of equal intelligence and is brilliantly hyper-loquacious. Nan has a penchant for the Wolverine football team, to the consternation of her peers, and veritably bleeds blue, whereas a high majority of the D.O.'s bleed Spartan green. Nan and James have invited me several times to their modest abode for dinner and a few of the "Big Ones" with the Wolverines. They make a yearly pilgrimage to Guatemala for a couple weeks of medical missionary work with the natives. Wisely, they decided upon graduation to go into joint practice in Bay City at Dr. Kohler's office building on Mulholland, near the hospital. They bought this building and also put a down payment on an elegant home on McKinley Street. They have adopted two hounds. Undoubtedly they have the acumen and personalities to succeed.

My favorite fourth pleasant chief resident alliance is with Genevieve Struder. She has a great sense of humor but actually is <u>all</u> business and seems able to furnish answers to all questions posed by her fellow students. Her recent conjugal partner, Walter, is a Presbyterian Minister, a graduate of Princeton Seminary College. He has an excellent ecclesiastical personage and personality to burn. They make a great couple. One or the other will chauffeur me to the journal meetings. Genevieve is quite medically passionate and bubbly verbose on all subjects pertaining to medicine. Walter executed his ministerial duties at Presbyterian churches in the thumb at Yale and Saginaw, Michigan. Upon graduation, Genevieve hooked up with a medical clinic in Rochester, NY, as a general family practitioner and Walter landed a job as assistant pastor in Rochester. Inevitably, they are bound to be a resounding story of unlimited success.

My ongoing, fifth connection to the 3rd year residents, is with chief resident Tessa Schisler and Tim Volm as I am writing now, Sept 13, 2005. Perhaps my undying happy relation with these residents is one of ironclad, brotherly love, and my recapitulation of my own intense and hectic intern days. Truly, at my tender young age of almost nine and one half decades, I am amazed that my D.O. resident friends accept me with so much ardor and respect as one of their own group. They come and go, but always our bond and union remain staunch as steel. At the moment, I am awaiting New Year's resident Justin Klaassen, a medical student.

I must also acknowledge my affinity with my good friend pediatrician Susan Hendrickson, M.D., during my retirement phase. Sue has been a bastion of support in escorting me to CME's sponsored by Reps from sundry drug companies at various educational clambakes in the environs. Susan has a severe, life threatening allergic sensitivity to all rubber products and multiple food restrictions. She has had innumerable, mortally threatening anaphylactic attacks when exposed accidentally to unknown sources of rubber in balloons, gloves, hospital instruments, clothing, and toys. In fact, she has abrogated her hospital practice completely because of fear of unknown exposure to microscopic rubber containing materials. She is single and leads a lonely, protective existence en garde by carrying emergency packets of I.M.epinephrine at all times. She has an extremely close relationship with her father. He is a CPA, residing with her mother in Detroit, but comes to her office on Euclid in Bay City several times a week to balance her books and render any other needed assistance. Sue lives and breaths asthma in her pediatric practice, and many of our seminars are devoted exclusively to this subject. At one of the meetings we attended a humorous incident occurred. While we were seated at a table of eight for dinner in very subdued light viewing the slide show, our waiter approached me and said, “Sir, would your wife take the lobster or the filet mignon?” I corrected his faux pas convincingly while everyone at the table stared and chuckled in disbelief. We both got a big kick out of it, for Susan probably is in her early thirties.

Her partnership with Van Gelderen was incompatible her first couple years in Bay City and she moved to Midland for a few years, before returning to Bay City in solo practice. She has an arrangement with her fellow pediatricians to take care of her hospital patients until they recover. Sue is quite passionate about her pediatric patients and constantly bubbles over in describing her encounters with them. Sue had her pediatric training at Buffalo Children’s Hospital under the tutelage of Mitchell Rubin, who was my venerable instructor when I interned in Children’s Hospital of Philadelphia way back in ‘37/’38, eons ago, just a drop in the bucket of time.

Chapter 37

Potpourri and All Skate

"Potpourri and all skate" is Bill O'Reilly's (FOX News) favorite squib to describe that everyone participates actively in the show activities. This seems an appropriate segue into the subject of music.

Music has always been a formidable part of my repertoire. It has been my prime solace in stormy times, my inspiration when solving problems, my torrid pleasure at concerts, and my venue for soothing relaxation and romantic dreams. My ultimate enjoyment is derived from the classics, and especially the piano and violin concertos. At the top of the list for favorite composers are genius Mozart, the 3B's (Brahms, Beethoven, and Bach), Rachmaninov, Tchaikovsky, Schubert, Grieg, and Sebelius. Actually, I never heard a classical composer I didn't love, but the romantic ones take the cake. Next for unadulterated sheer pleasure come the "Big Bands" of the 30's, 40's, and 50's. Glenn Miller is tops, followed closely by Benny Goodman, Tommy Dorsey, Duke Ellington, Ted Weems, Wayne (the Waltz King), Artie Shaw, Mantovani, and Lawrence Welk. My all time favorite melodies are Star Dust, Rhapsody in Blue, and at least a hundred other yum-yums. My number 1-A pianist of all time is Rudolf Serkin; and my favorite orchestras are the Ormandy Philadelphia Symphony and the New York Philharmonic. After fifty plus years, I have grown to appreciate the operas. For voices, the sopranos take the cake. The tenors are breathing down their necks. I'm also very fond of opera music, but wish the words were anglicized. I like good jazz, Dixie, country, and polka in that order. But, rock and roll gets almost a big fat zero from me.

Melissa loves the symphonies and thereby is my complementing partner. On her visits to Bay City for my 93rd and 94th birthday celebrations, she booked high caliber Detroit Symphony Orchestra concerts for us. Her superb birthday present was a weekend stay at the Twin Towers hotel in the Motor

City. Along with her better half, Martin, we attended a memorable Beethoven symphony during my visit to Atlanta in May, 2005.

Also a highlight of that visit, was an excursion to the Center for Disease Control and Prevention (CDC) orchestrated by my eminent son, Gregory, who works there as a full time professional photographer. The CDC has over 2,000 employees and over twenty massive buildings at present. A new administration building is under construction and Greg will finally have his very own office there. Greg is passionately in love with his job and apparently the powers that be share a mutual feeling for him.

Every time Melissa and I get together we usually parry umpteen sessions of our favorite card game of cribbage. Melissa is a chip off the old "Knoblock" and is a most worthy competitor and paddy for me. We enjoy the intense games and virtually split the wins evenly. They are pro-friendly and when the smoke clears, we kiss and make up.

I have had innumerable happy, rollicking, frolicking summer birthday reunions with my irreplaceable, inimitable children over the past 10 years, usually in July. Our headquarters often are John Edmands home and Marvin and Pat Brilinski's home on Cedar off Old Midland Rd. Usually, Susan and Val (second groom merry-go-round) cross the Atlantic from Deutschland or La Madelena (an island in the Mediterranean off the coast of Italy) and all my other progeny with their spouses (except one estranged wife) come and throw a big birthday bash for me. The Edmand's or the Brilinski families, my pediatrician peers, and sometimes the Cummings also often enter into the gala festivities. Susan is a renowned culinary artist and she, John, and Marvin (two also proficient chefs) prepare a feast fit for royalty. My cake is usually adorned with numbers because if realistic, yearly candles are employed it will necessitate the firemen to douse the flames. Marvin is a grilling whiz and John is adept in preparing fish and desserts. There is much frivolity, good humor, and rehashing of golden moments from previous get togethers.

On two memorable occasions in the late 80's and early 90's, we all convened in San Antonio at Susan's domicile and veritably "hung one on" sans alcohol. My memory resurrects a killer pumpkin pie Susan manufactured with her cooking wizardry. At all our gatherings our activities and personalities are photographed by my professional camera wielding son Greg in his unique style. He is most impressive with his monkeyish athleticism and gymnastic ability to catch everyone in realistic and truly relaxed positions. He is an astute, prudent, flashy (camera) actor, deep thinker, and philosopher with quite the Irish wit. Son Tom is a <u>deep</u> thinker and analyzer taking his time to decipher all the details of a given problem or situation. Daughter Susan is a true facsimile and dyed in the wool version of my mother in will power, physiognomy, character, mood, personality and behavior - the works. Daughter Melissa is the epitome of grace, sensitivity, and passion, a true artist in every way. Apparently the parental DNA contributes an optimal mixture and combination of genes and characteristics to create maximally endowed human beings and my cup runneth over. The grand parents, ad infinitum, deserve their hallowed congratulations as well.

Chapter 38

Delegate to Michigan Chapter of the American Academy of Pediatrics

For several years from 1980 to 1994, I was the elected delegate from Bay City to the Michigan Chapter of the American Academy of Pediatrics (MAAP) and would attend annual meetings predominately held in July of each year, to conduct all business matters relative to the academy and for Educational, fellowship and family vacation purposes. We would meet for four days (Thurs thru Sun) at a plush summer resort in Michigan, - quite often at Grand Traverse Resort, at Acme, Shanty Creek at Bellaire, and Bay Valley near Bay City. We had a healthy heart breakfast, conducted our business session and had a CME until noon. After the noon repast, we had three hours of educational topics promulgated by pediatric professionals from Detroit Children's Hospital, Wayne State University, the University of Michigan, and Michigan State University. On Saturday we engaged in golf, hiking, horseback riding, shopping, and trips to wineries and various points of interest. At the Grand Traverse Resort, master golfer Jack Nickless has formulated an intricate, challenging gold course; and at Shanty Creek, Arnie Palmer had put his stamp on a grueling and frustrating links course. Tom Wright and I usually traveled together to these meetings for he was a member of the executive committee. We would delve into the chapter's problems and play our favorite classic music cassettes of the masters en route. Tom was a concert pianist and was head over heels into the classics. His daughter, sweet Sue, also is a highly talented pianist and has conducted the symphony in Honolulu.

A hilarious incident involving Tom's son Benjamin comes to my memory in bold relief. Benjamin and yours truly attended the famous '83 Ohio State game in Ann Arbor, won by the maize and blue Wolverines (U of M). After the game you never witnessed a bigger traffic jam of 105,000 plus people sparring to extricate their cars from the parking lots.

I left Benjie in charge of my Mercedes while I tried to establish telephone contact with my friend, Ken Barker. Benjie was besieged by umpteen agitated drivers to move our car but he unwaveringly and adamantly stood his ground, refusing to move until I returned. Ben was complimented by me for being a tiger, in spite of hell and high water.

On another memorable occasion, in '86, my great architect grandson, Jon, while on vacation from college in Germany, drove Tom and I north to our academy meeting in Shanty Creek. In several instances, Tom and I would visit with our good acquaintance and fellow pediatrician Sezai Olgac and his lovely wife at their posh summer home on the peninsula in the eastern arm of Traverse Bay. I assumed the duties of delegate to the MAAP for 24 years, and reluctantly resigned when my health crashed in 1999. It was a duty of love and good times.

Chapter 39

Seniors, Seniors, and More Seniors

Rheumatologist supreme Walter Howland, in charge of the retired physicians in the Saginaw Bay area, extended several invitations to me to join their hallowed group. I finally took the bait and hooked on to this prestigious club in 1999, when I finally gave up the ghost and unequivocally retired. In fact, I was bereft of options to retirement for my heart sent me a loud and clear message of complete congestive cardiac failure. My blood pressure shot sky high at 260/140 that first day in Bay Regional Hospital and I developed an acute multivariate bacterial urinary infection. On entering my office, my good friend and mentor Carmella addressed me excitedly, "Oh my God! Howard, you look awful and I'm calling 911 now." Anyhow, with Jehovah's help and my tenacious genes, I did recover and came home, to stay home, 3 days later. While I was encased in the hospital, I received a supportive call from my Bickham and Cummings buddies who were then in Fort Meyers, FL.

Dr. Howland's rover boys meet on the first Tuesday of each month at 12 noon at the Holiday Inn for lunch and a good old fashioned memory trip. We are a group of a duke's mixture of retired family practitioners and virtually all the medical specialties. There is Joe Loree, a surgeon of lofty virtue, Tom Wright, erstwhile pediatrician, Vanasupa, neurosurgeon par excellente, John Langin and Tom Cajegas, erudite pathologists, Sam Midas (touch), a roentgenologist, Lou Berta, of general practice fame, Harry McGee, our esteemed ophthalmologist, Johnny Grigg, our double indemnity combo lawyer and ENT doctor of renown, Nick Tsonka, our somnambulistic anesthetist expert, Tyre Jones, X-ray and aviator supreme. Until recently John Campbell, our stately and accomplished orthopedist and Don Campbell, our pediatric, Evangelist also joined us. We discourse and toss over old times, present news events and juicy stories, brag about the virtues and noble endeavors of our blessed children; and review past adventures and unusual medical cases. Joe Loree is especially prominent in our tete a tetes for he was a Canadian Air force bomber with 12 sorties in WWII and was shot down in mid air to be imprisoned in a prisoners camp for a year.

The second senior's organization I attend regularly for evening dinners is the "Happy Hearts Hampton Hall retirees". It is a closely knit group that shares conversations of their illnesses, politics, religion, progeny, old times, ill members, and dietary fares. It has been my good fortune to become inextricably acquainted with several partners at my dinner table.

One dinner companion, John Scantleberry appears to my consciousness in bold relief. John, age 91 years, is a retired Episcopal minister, who was in this capacity at our renowned Center Avenue Episcopal Church for several years until our surgeon, Peter McGee, blew the whistle on him in 1980. John is overboard, narcissistic with an undying fervor for his birthplace, glamorous New York City. Unbelievably John and I are fraternity brothers in Phi Sigma Kappa, he at City College of New York and I at ETA Chapter in College Park, Maryland. John, single, has gone through 3 wives like waste through a tin horn because of his inveterate proclivity for infinite, insulting, loquacity of the nth degree. He is an adamant and ultimate jackass (democrat), a self made philosopher, and a corny raconteur, constantly delivering sermons in strictly monologue fashion. Like my fraternity brother Greeley often said -a diarrhea of words and a constipation of thoughts. John can contribute the height of aggravation, especially while we are - or attempting to - relax and eat our 5 o'clock sustenance. In spite of his one way diatribes on politics and religion, he can be occasionally affable.

Also at Hampton Hall retirees, there are two couples with whom I've become quite fond. One is Faye and Glenn Guaon. Glenn resides beside me at our #4 table and Faye sits diametrically opposite me. Glenn was a WWII rear gunner and bombardier in the South Pacific and Italian invasion theaters, flying twenty plus missions. He recounts a most intriguing and unusual incident while flying to Denmark in the summer of '42. The plane emptied the gas tanks and unfortunately they were forced to make an emergency landing on Iceland. They were rescued by boat and continued their journey while the poor plane became hopelessly imbedded in the ice in a state of eternal preservation. Healthwise, Glenn is literally a miracle man as he has had severe myocarditis for several years and has had insertion of five cardiac stents and probably a scant dozen hospitalizations. In spite of all his flirts with the Grim Reaper, he maintains a happy, devil may care, positive attitude and goes merrily on his way. Wife Faye is positively his Girl Friday and guardian angel. She watches over him like a hawk, and tends to his every whim and need. He is partially blind and hard of hearing, but Faye is quite robust and cuts his meat and butters his bread. Realistically she is a big help to me also as she gets my hot chocolate, water, milk, and cares for my cane. She and I do have a common bond, for we watch a common soap opera on TV at noon and are all wrapped up in the harrowing vicissitudes and plus/minus experiences of the characters. Its fun to project what Machiavellian events will occur to the storied persona in the imagination of the script writers. I'm absolutely certain that Faye, with her energy and passion, missed her definitive calling as a loving nurse. She practically breathes for Glenn.

The other married couple, Steve and Eileen Ostash, is most unusual and imbued with the milk of human kindness. Steve was born in southern Russia and was a fellow comrade in WWII in the army. He is quite intelligent and perceptive. He is besieged with multiple physical infirmities of life threatening status. Eileen Ostash is a lovely, fair lady who keeps us up on the latest nosey news. She likes to massage and tweak my shoulders as she swings by me and engages in family type conversation. She is thin as a rail, eats like a bird.

Another twosome, Kenneth and Jane, occupy our table. Ken is a widower, afflicted with romantic feelings and dwarfism. Jane was unfortunately married to a basket case husband. One of her masculine partners has recently given up the ghost and she has latched on to Ken.

There was a good natured, sharp gentleman who is now deceased who sat opposite me. We had a close relationship and he too was a WWII army service man. He had a peculiar, uncontrollable sleep disturbance and would doze off in the middle of our repast. He told me of the time he was on CQ (charge of quarters) night duty and fell asleep and was revived to consciousness by none other than the commanding officer. Needless to say, he was relieved of that duty permanently.

Our present proctor, Sandy, is the ideal leader of our group. She is loving, doesn't spare the horses, and goes all out to please us and make us happy. Sandy is full of energy, witty, cheerful, and loaded with novel ideas to keep us stimulated. On Halloween, she outdid herself and really let out the shaft with all sorts of tricks and treats.

There was a day of depression when our previous culinary genius retired several months ago. She had been a fixture as chief cook for several years and she was taken for granted until she decided to call it quits. Unbelievably she was the proud mother of nine loving children. One of her progeny was an USA naval officer and when she visited him stationed on La Madelena, she connected socially with my daughter, Susan, who was teaching her grandchildren stationed there. Our present chef, Peggy, is quite substantial but different from her predecessor. A large proportion of the "Happy Hearts" members are overweight as food is our principal means of pleasure. The meals are of good quality and quantity, very simply prepared, and adequate with the basic nutriments.

We're a closely knit bunch of elderly guys and gals with congenial camaraderie. In fact, all of the Hall seniors, except our culinary chef Peggy, are in the same boat, i.e. afflicted with mortal health burdens. In spite of such gloomy infirmities, we are all (except for John Scantlebury), happy, devil may care, humans on the edge. We support each other faithfully.

Chapter 40

Evangelical Seniors

My third senior category is relegated to my spiritual or ecclesiastical connections which I deem of paramount importance. My relationship to God and Mother Nature is actually the bedrock spine and foundation of my existence. My creator has been extremely kind and gracious to me for which I render undying thanks and gratitude. He/She is my enabler, my inspiration, my breath of life, my sustenance, my everything. All religions of mankind worship and bow down to the Supreme Being. I firmly believe we are here on this earth for a definite purpose - to render support and assistance to all our fellow mortals and creatures with all of our God given talents. Also, I do believe we will be rewarded in the after existence, according to our positive contributions to our fellow humans and feral beings.

As I previously mentioned, my boyhood was rooted in the reformed church in Greensburg PA. When I found none in Bay City, my partner, L. Fernald Foster convinced me to join our First Presbyterian Church. Realistically, First Presbyterian is basically comparable to my youth church in Greensburg. I am proud of my 64 years as a member of First Presbyterian. I have served many years as Elder and Deacon, and recently have participated in serving communion to the handicapped and elderly shut-ins. Also I have been a faithful Sunday attendee of church services, most notably since my retirement in1999, and since surrendering my fascination with that little dimpled ball on the golf links. I sit in the pew fourth from the rear with affable Walter and Mary Howland and I am occasionally joined by my dear Terrapin buddy Joan Cummings.

There is a church group of seniors that meets every 3rd Wednesday for a hearty cuisine luncheon and then a very interesting lecture by a prominent Bay City professional. In addition, we have spaghetti dinners and ice cream socials. Our church has a <u>very</u> large program of activities for all ages.

Our pastor, Reverend Doctor Jeffrey Weenink is the busiest church leader I have ever seen, anywhere. He thrives on church activities every day and night of the week. Jeff is a demon of academia and lives the Christian life he preaches. His sermons are forceful, dynamic, practical, and carry a spiritual message of evangelical explosiveness. I'm certain he and his wife and three female progeny practice what they preach. Jeff is from Holland, Michigan, and his father is a minister of the gospel, now retired. God has blessed us heavenly in steering Jeff our way.

Our choir is resplendent and sings like a bunch of angels led by a choirmaster, a college PHD who has a gifted baritone voice and is an accomplished pianist able to sermonize with expert talent. His wife Antoinette has an ultra magnificent operatic voice. She really can hit the rafters on the high notes. They make a wonderful complementing couple and are quite a boon to our church.

Chapter 41

Our Physical Infirmities

Ripening age bestows a multitude of illnesses in the latter third of our existence. They are inevitable because our wonderful organs wear out and give up the ghost, even iron rusts out in time. Death is the only absolute, and therefore the greatest, happening in life. One person's life is but a drop in the bucket of time. Life can aptly be compared to a set of tires. With proper care and strict obedience to the laws of nature, you can make them last to their maximum age with full, fiery enjoyment or, alternatively, you can live it up at a fast pace and wear out all the tread in a short time. My philosophy in a nutshell has always been to stay in the middle of the road and avoid both extremes of living. Don't swim up stream and when possible go down wind and avoid the pot holes and speed bumps.

Another good way to prolong your life is for a person to avoid arguments, for you will never convince your adversary in a million years that you are gospel and he is wrong, even if water doesn't run up hill and gravity does contribute to falls. Time is too precious a commodity to waste, and getting oneself hot under the collar will not win friends or solve any problems. Our physical bodies, in spite of nature's fantastic handiwork, were never constructed to last longer than 15 decades under perfect specifications, and that is a fact. Therefore, it behooves us to maximize our efforts to learn all possible, to devote ourselves to helping other humans and wildlife, to develop ourselves to our greatest potential, to contribute our utmost to improving our fellow beings - especially those less fortunate than we - and to take care of our delicate, fragile bodies with the greatest solicitude. In other words, strongly emphasize the positive and don't mess with mister in-between. One of our greatest attributes is to be relaxed with an inner peace of mind but to take our duties and mission in life passionately and develop our God given talents to a serious degree.

I have been most fortunate, pretty much all of my life, in maintaining good health. I've previously described to you some of the health challenges and issues that have crossed my path. All in all, a Higher Power has decided to let me live on to a ripening age.

As is well known, two factors in achieving longevity are an appropriate diet and the appropriate amount of battery recharging sleep. We've come to realize that we must go easy on the salt, sugar, and saturated fats, while keeping the calories under control to avoid obesity. Low carbohydrates and high protein are the order of the day. A general diet encompassing a little portion of <u>all</u> foods, while abstaining from going overboard on any particular food group, is healthful. As I have said anon and anon simply take care of your body and your body will take care of you. Mostly, it is just common horse sense with no magic or mysterious formula. You would surmise that while working with contagious and infectious diseases constantly day in and day out that I would be a sitting duck for contracting some of these illnesses, but by the grace of God, frequent hand washings, minimal direct contact, and the immunizing effect of small, frequent doses of organisms, I miraculously managed to escape unscathed during my practice.

However, senescent infirmities have caught up with me. The human organs, tissues, muscles, and blood vessels all wear out and deteriorate with father time. Nothing lasts forever and even the sea anemones die after centuries. My first glimpse of the aging process came after my WWII service when I developed diabetes Type II out of the blue. It really was no profound shock, for my paternal grandmother, Anna, died while in our Greensburg home from terminal diabetes. My maternal grandfather, J.T. Haines, contracted diabetes Type II at age 60 years, manifested by mellifluous diabetic dermatitis. He was a stubborn old cuss and refused to take diabetic insulin injections and in his time there were no anti-diabetic sulfonyeurea meds.

Ninety percent of elderly diabetes falls under the Type II classification. In this type there is a tissue glycemic insensitivity to insulin, glucose toxicity, and impaired B cell response to glucose. Fortunately, my diabetes was mild and could mainly be controlled by diet and exercise until my eighties and then by small dosages of a 2 ½ mg pill every day or two. I can't forget the 4 weeks to Europe in the summer of '05 (which I shall recount shortly) when I forgot to take my glucose testing apparatus and was on automatic pilot. In spite of this handicap, I decided to bank on my inherent sense of well being and sense of equilibrium and all was roses.

In 1986, an inexorable, intense, pervasive lumbar backache developed and in spite of several months of physiotherapy my pain magnified. I knew it couldn't be a disc for Dr. Gueramy (bless his wizard way) had rectified my T12 and L1 fractured disc pads by deftly injecting meat tenderizer. A bright idea struck my cerebrum; it must be cancer of the prostate for it metastasizes to the spine and ribs. So, Steve Asherl shot an arrow into my prostate to obtain a biopsy and voila, sure enough the undeniable answer was prostate cancer with metastisis to the spine and ribs. Dr. David Cook said, "Howard you are scheduled for surgery in 2 days with Fugivara for bilateral archidectomy." I was resigned to my fate and acquiesced with fervor. Because of the metastasis spinal and rib lesions, the prostate was not extirpated (removed). A prostate scan a year prior was negative and I'm sure that the cancer was there for at least a couple years before diagnosis. Magically, about 4 hours postoperatively, my ungodly pain in my back began to ameliorate and in a few hours it was practically nil. This proves to me that there is an overwhelming linkage between testosterone and cancer of the prostate. Luckily, I escaped pulmonary cancer spread to date. My treatment post surgery has consisted of oral chemo, positive thinking, proper diet, a strong will to live, and prayer.

It's almost 18 years now postoperatively, and my biggest concern is congestive heart failure. I like to think that there is poignant, purposeful reason for my existence. Maybe I can make a significant contribution to happiness for my fellow men/women and the little creatures. My main cardiac problem revolves around aortic valvular leakage, insufficiency, and anemia. Lack of energy and shortness of breath are rampant, and exercise is limited, but I have no angina and can walk with a cane. I have had a mild, harmless dysrhythmia with extra systoles periodically for several years. (Back in the sixties Hal Shafer (bless his heart) said Howie does not need cardiac cath and there is no serious heart problem for sure.) Although my physical activity and exercise is limited, I navigate fairly well on excellent, sturdy legs in spite of balance and equilibrium problems. Daughter, Susan, insisted vigorously on my employing a cane, so she obtained a hefty German cane and it really is a great support. Thank the Lord that I still am fully in possession of my faculties and senses to pilot my wonderful '96 Crown Victoria. I've driven circa ¾ million miles in 79 years of driving. I forbid myself to drive at night in spite of my great 20/20 vision, due to lessening of reflexes and billions of distracting lights.

My anemia has hovered around 10.5 grams hemoglobin for the past half dozen years, but recently has taken a dip to 9.0 grams and has alarmed David Cook, my oncologist. Therefore, I am getting 60,000 units procrit weekly, and after 4 weeks the Hg has crept up to 10 grams. Procrit is a hormone manufactured by the kidneys and its purpose is to jack up and give a wake-up call to the bone marrow to get off its dead rear and get the hemoglobin into full production. The injections are useful, especially in cancer patients where new blood formation is stagnant. My BUN (nitrogen) and creatinine are slowly creeping the wrong way (up) indicating aging kidneys and interference with procrit formation.

Another problem which confronted me in the year 2000 was discovery of

DVT (deep vein thrombosis) of my right popliteal vessel on ultrasound exam. Fortunately, Tony Vasquez found my carotids to be in mint condition meaning my diet apparently was up to snuff. However, I do have to put the damper on my salt intake in deference to my renal buddies. I have been compelled to take Warfarin or Coumadin for approximately six years to prevent clot formation and dissemination to the lungs and cerebrum. My daily 80mg aspirin tablet (20 years) also aids my nonclotting mechanism immeasurably, as well as helping avoid myocardial infarction and stroke (Apoplexy).

Another goodie that has come to roost in my tree is the inevitable development of vertebral stenosis, cervical as well as thoraco-lumbar. This means an encroachment and squeezing of the spinal cord and that can be disastrous. I've had acute, intermittent, excruciating pain in my neck muscles for these many years. This condition of the walls infinitesimally closing in on vital structures is well nigh insoluble. Pain killers help for a few minutes, Physiotherapy contributes fleeting, partial relief, and exercise and massage are all adjunctive helpful factors in relieving the agony temporarily. A funny, unexpected turn of events is that my cervical aches and pains have surprisingly diminished in the past six months or so. Unexplainable. I have never really taken any pain modifiers, and from the beginning have decided to fight it with a Christian Science mentally, grin and bear it and "change the subject."

The hospital physical therapy department saw a lot of me a couple years ago and they were extremely supportive and helpful, but I realized I must face the music and let nature take its course. Never do I cease to be amazed that the greatest physician of them all truly is God or Mother Nature, take your pick. Always, I have shunned pain medication addiction, especially for chronic pain. When it's all said and done, morphine is the <u>greatest</u> drug of all for acute, agonizing pain. In the great World War II, we had morphine surettes available for overwhelming injury pain and they were a godsend,. We just pulled off the cap and injected it intramuscularly to give instantaneous relief. However, I can understand the reluctance to subject the carriers of morphine surrettes to the intense temptation of self use. But actually, morphine is not really very addictive, like its child, heroin. I found this out when I was taking morphine orally for my backache due to cancer.

One last malady my cross has to bear is a right, indirect inguinal hernia, which could be worse if it were bilateral. This appeared unannounced circa Thanksgiving '05. Apparently my lower inguinal abdominal musculature weakened from wear and tear, although I have always taken great pride in my total absence of "bay window" or "pot belly". Clearly, a pregnant male abdomen is an anathema to the body and bodes no good for longevity of life. A large belly is incongruous to form and shape, proper positioning of the belt and slacks, and denotes a slovenly, obese appearance. In other words - repulsive. I decided against surgery as the hernia is producing no untoward pain or symptoms. Practically any surgery at my age is a light beacon to death, if not actually a death warrant. Surgery here is exceedingly damaging and shocking to the entire body and all the vital organs. In addition, the loss of blood and the major deleterious effects of anesthesia are mortally inescapable. I suppose if an acute appendix infection reared its ugly head, it could be extirpated by local and antipain drugs. I honestly believe that straining at defecation was my waterloo in this instance. My dear mother had excessive, lifelong constipation and I'm afraid congenital passage, plus poor management on my part, plus oodles of enema and catharties in my infancy were contributory. There is a condition of extreme stonewall constipation which affects children rarely, known as Hirshsprung's disease caused by absence of nerves to the large intestine. Maybe my nerve innervation to my descending colon was deficient, but I'm sure the answer to my plight was not a Hirschsprung, just a less degree.

In spite of my multi-factorial infirmities, I am resigned to my fate as the price of aging and I love life and so I bite the bullet. I believe that yours truly is the luckiest guy in the world because my state of health could be affected greatly by the disabling, prodigious pain of arthritis, impaired sight and hearing, inability to walk, loss of memory, or ability to drive a car. Independence is of gigantic importance. I also have DVT (deep vein thrombosis) and spinal stenosis, but they come with age.

Chapter 42

July 2005 Safari to Europe

After ruminating and agonizing for several months, weighing all the pros and cons with my wife and children, I decided to make the Atlantic leap to the "Old Country". My daughter, Susan, was especially affirmative about my coming to visit her, her husband Val, and her three wonderful children (my grandchildren) Lisa, (recently wedded to Michael Heidan), Jon the architect, and Sara the fourth year medical student. I became convinced, beyond all doubt, that being in my mid-nineties it was now or never for me. I fully knew that this venture wouldn't be a walk on the beach, but I conned myself into believing these old bones were up to the task -damn the torpedoes and full speed ahead. All my four offspring were 100% in favor of my voyage and said it with ample support, especially Tom with a new set of luggage and Melissa with green backs to finance the trip.

My embarking from my point of origination, MBS Airport locally, was facilitated greatly by my good Terrapin and Ecclesiastical friend, Joan Cummings. She managed my wheelchair (which Susan demanded I bring) as though it were a toy. My wheelchair and passport did come in handy at the multiple immigration stations at the airports. I must have appeared quite innocuous/harmless because I zipped through all the examining posts with gazelle celerity.

Marvin and Patricia Brilinski were my mentors and body guards supreme on the trip. Of course, they knew all my children and grandchildren quite well from their frequent visits to their home. I was very happy to be traveling with Marv and Pat. I was well cared for under their supervision on our flight to Gatwick Airport near London, England from Detroit Metro Airport the night of July 10th, 2005.

We had a tedious, boring eight hour wait at the Detroit airport for our Northwest Airlines Atlantic flight. The Brilinskis and I were separated by a few seats, but luckily my next door neighbor on the plan was a comely, young, congenial lady who was joining her air corps GA army husband prior to his shipping out for service in Iraq. We held intermittent conversation and fitful repose. Pat came to check on me a couple times; and the entire flight was as smooth as glass. The attendants were cordial and offered me the use of their private washroom. Our repast wasn't a cornucopia of nutriments but it was quite adequate to keep the wolf from the door.

London time wise is six hours in advance of our EST and we arrived at Gatwick Airport around 10 a.m. their time. We decided to entrain from the airport, and made it in an hour plus to the center of London. Pat had booked reservations at the Grosvenor Hotel, a stately, antique high class abode directly across the avenue from Hyde Park. We were fascinated with the English pronunciations and enunciations of words. They slurred and combined their syllables to shorten and jazz up their discourse. They pronounced Grosvenor Hotel as "Groaner". Their expressions were undyingly pure British. To us their charges were most exorbitant: -5 pounds ($10.00) for a cup of coffee and 18 pounds ($36.00) for breakfast at the hotel. Our lodging cost 200 pounds ($400.00) per night, so you in no way can call us "cheapies".

I was based in London at the Grosvenor for a week exactly. Marv pushed me in my wheelchair all over London to the innumerable English, French, Italian, and German bistros and eateries within a radius of 2 miles from our Hotel. (We also ran into numerous of our old friend restaurants, like McDonald's, scattered throughout Great Britain and Germany.) Marvin is a 60'ish, mighty muscular, he-man, in good health. But he may have sacrificed a few years of life with his love for food, tobacco (until July '05), and alcohol (until midlife). Recently he has come to grips with diabetes Type II and had a cardiac stent inserted to combat arteriosclerotic vascular obstruction. In any event, with his Tarzan like physical build, Marvin handled me like a baby - with ease.

I had only one wheelchair accident which happened in Bath on July 13th while navigating a curb. I fell forward landing full weight on my left knee at the tibial plateau. I was quite concerned that I might have a fracture - like one of my teen female patients who fractured her right tibial plateau playing kickball, developed deep popliteal vein thrombosis, and kicked the bucket with rare pulmonary embolism. My pain was excruciating and hung on for a lengthy period; but I was able to walk on the knee without too much difficulty. An X-ray was number one priority but they talked me out of getting one. I got my X-ray after I got back to Bay City in August. It was negative. Icepacks helped the tumor and dolor, and antiseptic ointment prevented infection. It healed in about a month. Guess my bones are pretty dense.

In another incident while on the trip, I slipped and fell while climbing in the bath tub and sustained a glancing blow to my frontal cranium. It was an old concrete tub necessitating dexterous agility and a ladder to enter the tub. Getting out of the tub was an effort in futility and showers were extinct.

There was just a little knob on my forehead from the fall and I didn't even contract a headache, so it all came out in the wash.

The tour of London was a complete failure for me because I was glued to the 2-tiered bus and could only glimpse the highlight buildings and prominent spectacles while rooted in my seat. Westminster Abby and the Tower of London would have been my choices for exploration. However Pat, Marvin and I did negotiate two unforgettable excursions to Bath, Stonehenge, and York. We traveled by bus westward, about 100+ miles to Bath, where the invading Romans established the famous Roman Baths. There were two more historical invasions of Britain by the Vikings and Normans which left their telltale landmarks as well.

We reached Stonehenge early in the evening and spent about two hours touring the environs. It is ultimately amazing how our ingenious ancestors of about 4000 years ago conceived a scheme for transporting those humongous megaliths from the Irish Sea to the Stonehenge destination. They must have employed some type of barges or wooden ships to cross the water; and then pulled them on terra firma many miles by sleds. The piece de resistance was arranging the prodigious granite stones dug and excised from a quarry into a huge circle, erecting them, and hoisting some of them to rest on the tops about 25 feet high. It must have taken hundreds of thousands of people, decades to produce such a prodigious and stupendous a project. It was accomplished without tools, ropes, or mathematics and ranks almost on a par with the pyramids. Apparently the pillars represented the moon, sun, stars, and heavenly firmaments. My hat is off to our brawny, prehistoric ancestors.

Our journey to York, about a three hour train ride, was the following day. It was smooth as glass and the countryside of rolling hills on a sunny day was revealing and joyful. When we reached York, we learned that this was the day of the annual horse races and that Queen Elizabeth was in attendance. The Brits were dressed in all their finery, fit to kill. The ladies all had gorgeous, large garden hats, beautiful evening gowns, and sculpted makeup. The men all wore fancy tuxedos, top hats, spats, and immaculate facial shrubbery. We cavorted around York and had a great day. The fireworks occurred when we toured back to London on the train. The British race patrons, now train passengers, unabashedly let down their hair and threw their proprieties to the wind with alcoholic revelry, swearing, and loud boisterous arguments. It was quite a show and stark entertainment to say the least.

The Brilinskis left me on Friday, July 15th, by plane for the Isle of Man. Their destination was a world famous resort in the Irish Sea about forty miles off the north eastern Irish coast and approximately thirty miles off the mid western coast of England. Susan and Val came in on Saturday, the 16th of July and we enjoyed catching up on the news since our hiatus of a year's separation.

On Sunday, we toured Hyde Park from stem to stern, and enjoyed watching the crowds of motley people, a vivid cross section of diverse humanities. On the following Monday, we left London and planed to Frankfurt, Germany on a smooth uneventful flight. We were met at the airport by Lisa, Michael, Jon and Sara and my buddy Ekki Prengel, Susan's first husband.

We toured to Lisa and Michael's abode in Wiesbaden, where we all congenially and joyously celebrated my 94th birthday. I was the recipient of lavish, unique gifts including the "Guttenberg Bible" and a large, handsome stein. My birthday cake, fortunately, did not embody the full quota of candles, so we didn't start a 5 alarm fire. Lisa is a sales representative for Thompson. She is a very energetic, prudent, and par excellent sales lady with all out passion for her job. Her husband Michael is an expert engineer who runs a manufacturing facility making sun roofs for cars.

My erstwhile, loyal, good friend and former son in law, Ekki, hosted a family welcoming party in my honor at a famous riverside bistro overlooking the Main River. The German wines and beers are as good as they come and, unlike the American beer counterparts, are not carbonated.

One day later, Susan, Val, Ekki and I visited my grandson, Jon Prengel at his architectural office in Frankfurt. He shares an office with two young architects there. Jon is a very vigorous, proficient, and knowledgeable architect. He is totally devoted to his profession. He has accomplished amazing designs for several unique buildings erected in the city of Frankfurt.

My three grandchildren speak impeccable English, as well as the German language and are both American and German citizens. I'm afraid the die is cast and they will prefer residence in Germany, although granddaughter Sara may give the USA preferential consideration. I'm nourishing a glimmer of hope that she may choose my country. Maybe she will marry an American.

After five days of royal red carpet treatment at Lisa and Michael's home, Susan, Val and I moved from Wiesbaden to their home in Wurzburg, Germany. Wurzburg is a quaint, thriving, 1300 year old city offering historical and cultural amenities, museums, artist work, shops, castles, and a glorious fortress. It is renowned for its magnificent architectural edifices, works of art, architects, artists, and world famous university.

Susan is a teacher and counselor par excellante at Wurzburg High School for the US army personnel children. Husband number two, Val Valenzuela, is totally the maestro in charge of the household appurtenances. Val served over 20 years in the US Army as an English teacher to the enlisted personnel, as well as numerous other pedantic duties, and is now retired. Due to Susan's position, they are the benefactors of full remuneration for their bailiwick which is rented. Their house is a spacious three story residence with a large basement for dairy and frozen victuals. The first floor consists of kitchen, dining room, huge parlor, large outdoor patio overlooking fifty miles of lush countryside, bathroom, and an ample bedroom. The second floor contains three bedrooms and one bath. One of the upstairs bedrooms was my abode. The sharp winding staircase to the second floor was a bit of a hazard for me. But I really navigated it easily with assistance. In addition, they have a two car garage and a large garden plot. They are really living in a palace, in the lap of luxury.

On our first night, Susan and Val took me to a quaint, fortified village and we indulged in a luscious dinner. Three days later, the Brilinskis arrived from their week's visit to the Isle of Man via London to the Stuttgart Airport about 30 miles south of Wurzburg. Pat and Marvin Brilinski described in minute detail their wonderful vacation experience at the Isle of Man. They got a huge jolt out of driving on the left side of the road and engineering those right turns. Pat regretted not paying a smidgeon of a visit to Ireland, but apparently the trip charges to this island were rather exorbitant, even making the steep British fare look like a piker.

The meteorology in Germany was beastly hot, +100F degrees in the shade, and I was veritably rendered lifeless on a trip to the U.S. Army Post installation about 25 miles south (not in the shade). My body core temperature must have risen immeasurably; but I escaped heat illness thanks to the good Lord.

Susan and Val veritably laid out the red carpet for us Bay Cityians. They wined and dined us royally and their Mediterranean diet is mighty heart healthy. We took numerous excursions to the surrounding countryside and had fabulous dinners at all the gourmet restaurants within a radius of 20 miles. The crowning jewel of our marvelous three week Wurzburg sojourn was a three day trip to the Austrian Alps near the end of our stay. Susan has a Mercedes auto with smaller European dimensions. There were only five persons in the car, but it was a smallish car and three were large, with Val and I being the skinnies. Val is a wonderful driver, par excellence. Pat sat in front with Val. Susan, Marvin and yours truly occupied the rear seating. Poor Marvin was literally sitting on the edge of his seat in the middle, and Susan and I were squished in like sardines beside him. We traveled about 200+ miles to our elegant hotel in Austria, in the heart of the mountains. We made numerous tours in the surrounding environs. Those alpine mountains are gorgeous beyond description and rival the Alaskan elevations.

One very special excursion took us up a steep mountain in a horse drawn carriage to a famous castle near the peak. It was a humongous stress and strain for the poor, six laboring horses to pull a dozen people on a 30 degree upward trail. This magnificently indescribable royal castle named, Konigschloss Neuschwanstein was erected during 1869 to 1886 by Koenig Ludwig II von Boyern, King of Bavaria from 1845 to 1886. He built this castle several miles away and further upward on the mountains from the castle of his father, which was much more modest. Susan and I, toured the castle grounds and the panoramic views were literally breathtaking. Susan is no spring chicken and vigorously pushing me in my trusty royal chariot, especially on elevated cobble stones, taxed her athletic ability to the nth degree. Susan and Val took the journey to the upper castle. Ludwig's riotous and dissipated life was terminated in its prime by a suspected drowning.

Susan, Lisa, and I engaged in a rather heated controversy about my stay in Germany while we were residing at Lisa's dwelling. Lisa and Sue were downright adamant in forcefully arguing that I should reside in Germany with them for at least several months and pointed out the huge list of advantages. I countered with convincing arguments about living stateside. In the end, as usual, we each stubbornly maintained our stands and the entire fiasco concluded in a veritable stalemate. On another occasion, Susan and I had a slight disagreement at a delightful high class bistro in Wurzburg, just after we had placed our orders. I can't remember now, for the life of me, what our differences were all about, but I know that I calmly remarked, "Well, that's a two way street.". Upon saying this my daughter got a bit warm under the collar and she arose and bolted for the doorway in spite of pleadings to come back. I was left speechless. Apparently, I had innocently hit a nerve bulls eye; and I felt terribly sorry and embarrassed. In spite of this, Pat, Marvin, and I continued with our meal and maintained a peaceful attitude and conversation. About ¾ of the way home we caught up with Susan who was gingerly walking. She smiled and motioned for us to continue homeward and refused a ride. Later Susan and I kissed and passed the peace pipe. I'm sure she had a legitimate right for her behavior and her side of the story and it was an infinitesimal misunderstanding. Susan and I are cut out of the same cloth genetically. We're both determined and obstinate, liking to exert our control over any situation. We both are used to giving orders to our scholars and patients. My dear daughter is an exact replica of my mother who was quite headstrong and had a strong backbone. My mother inherited tenacity from her father, J.T. Haines, and passed it on to me, and then I on to Susan. It is an admirable characteristic, but there is sometimes a downside and a more mature solution would undoubtedly be compromise.

There was one weekend when Sara, Jon, Ekki, Lisa, and Michael all came together with us at the homestead in Wurzburg. We had a most wonderful and joyful celebration both Saturday and Sunday. I have to be exceedingly nice to my Susan for she has also put forth a gallant effort to type part of my book manuscript on the computer in spite of grueling, vigorous teaching duties as a person of eminence in the high school.

My very own gorgeous granddaughter, Sara, now a 4th year medical student at Mainz University Medical School, escorted me on a complete tour of all the buildings there. She gave me the grand, detailed tour painting verbal pictures of all her studies. I am exceedingly happy and proud to state that Sara is progressing with lofty grades in all her subjects and is delighted to be entering the clinical phase of medicine whereby she interviews and does real workups face-to-face with real patients. She is actually quite passionate about her medical endeavors and lights up like a Christmas tree when she describes her professors, fellow students, and studying all hours of the day and night. I empathize deeply with her arduous schedule because I've been there. It is an arduous mess of blood, sweat, and tears but the rewards and final designation of M.D. degree is super well worth it. Sara is tough and rugged, full of perseverance, and I'm positive she will attain her goal with guns blazing. She has also been dealt a full deck cerebrally.

On the day Brilinski's and I left for the airport in Frankfurt to plane homeward, there was literally a cloud burst of rainstorms. I am sure the driving was mighty tedious and difficult, but Val is most experienced, reliable, and indefatigable as a driver. He was up to it. We all convened at the airport, all of Susan's family plus Ekki. Parting is such sweet sorrow; and we all expressed our heartfelt gratitude for such a great lifetime experience. They all expressed a sincere desire for me to return next year, if able, which put a song in my heart. I am hoping fervently for a <u>great</u> grandchild. This would make a great occasion for a return trip. However, there is one male newborn, yet unseen looming on the dim horizon. My former son-in-law Ekki became a proud father in 2005 with his brand new Chinese wife. He met her on a safari to China a couple of years ago and they have been lawfully wedded. Although Ekki is much superior in age to his lovely bride, from all appearances, they appear to be melding famously.

Our flight back to the good old U.S.A. from Frankfort was uneventful. We had about a dozen exhausting immigration and inspection interviews before we finally escaped at our destination, the MBS Airport. Marvin's son Matt met us at the airport and I felt like kissing the good earth but could only find cement. Upon reaching home I barely made it to my bedstead and promptly collapsed, diving beneath the covers. I was never, ever so glad to see a bed. I slept almost continuously for 48 hours, in deep anesthesia. It was just about the most wonderful adventure of my life but I don't believe I could/would ever live in Europe. The people there are the salt of the earth, the countries are beautiful, and their histories are fabulous, but there is no place like home.

I don't believe I have been so deenergized in my existence. My tank was veritably on empty. My battery voltage probably wouldn't even have shocked a robust flea. The old gray mare was ticking on one cylinder, but miraculously by the grace of God my spark was nurtured and revivified again over a period of a couple months after the trip back to full throttle. Susan urged me to return the following summer. The spirit is high, but the flesh is weak, which negated a physical return.

Chapter 43

Our Beloved Feline Brood

Cats are wonderful and glorious animals, especially kittens. The kittens become somewhat disenchanted as they grow older. Cats also pose serious, unremitting drawbacks and hazards to humans. Transmission of toxoplasmosis to newborns from infected mothers via poorly cooked meats is 1 in 10,000. Mothers in gestation can also contract toxoplasmosis gondii from feline infected stools in the cats litter, so they should always use gloves to scoop stools. Pregnant mothers become infected from oocysts excreted in the infected animals waste; and the organisms are transmitted to the fetus in utero. These furry beasts can also become infected by toxacara cati and canis (dogs) roundworms causing ocular lara migraines. Humans acquire this infection from eggs ingested from soil in gardening. Children are susceptible to this disease. As I previously mentioned, one particularly hazardous disease kittens can provoke in children is cat scratch fever caused by scratching of dirt and bacteria intravenously, usually into hands and arms. It causes large adenopathies and high fever and there is no treatment. It just has to wear out over several months. Allergy to fur and saliva is also a serious concern.

We are blessed/cursed with a gathering group of magnificent feline creatures which are a reasonable facsimile and substitute for a childless family. We have inherited them over the years by our inveterate love of animals from previous owners who were negligent and unloving. Most of these chats (French for cats) showed up in our garage or backyard, enticed by our offerings of delectable victuals and water holes which are perennially available to all outside thirsty critters. They all need tender loving care (TLC) and are amenable to kind hearted, loving humankind.

Preceding our role as cat lovers, we were hung up on Pekingese (Peeks) canines for a few years. However, after several adverse painful experiences, we decided to change to tougher, hardier, healthier Genus Felis. One incident that really fractured our hearts happened when our dog Jetty (Chet the Jet Hanulak) was crushed by an oncoming car when he was chasing another hound in front of our home on busy Henry Street. Several times the Peeks had eye orbit problems for their eye sockets are shallow and the eyeballs are easily extruded.

We have managed to accrue a motley conglomeration of all breeds of cats under the sun. We originally let them out of the house, but the consequences were disastrous. Two of our most prized kitties (Hercules and Lady Pink), were sent to animal heaven by auto accidents for Borton Avenue is a perennial busy highway for east / west Essexville traffic. We, therefore, decided to build a cat cage (house), 10x10x10 feet, in our backyard for them to cavort about in fresh ambient air. After several months, the task of carrying them in and out of the cage became over burdensome and time consuming, so we decided to just keep them in house.

Each chat has its very own, special habitat and beware anyone who dares to confiscate that sacred perch. They are definitely night animals, rabid carnivores, and independent. But they are also very loving animals under their veneer of stoicism. My wife is exceedingly caring and affectionate with our 21 furry critters. They certainly thrive and reach maximum growth under her skillful tutelage. Having been a most excellent pediatric charge nurse for many years at Samaritan and Bay Medical Center, she is a great caretaker. Actually, the cats are like human infants in their moods, desires, habits, and reactions. Their responses and emotions are predictable; and they possess a distinct language of their own. Their intelligence and curiosity are top notch with each chat having a singular personality. Some are feisty and others are felicitous; but generally they respect each other's territory and rights. At one time, we had around 30 of these beasts, but we have lost a slew over time. Our eldest cat is circa 25 years young and most are nearing the magic year of two decades. At present, their names are as follows: Minnie, Sinbad, March, April, May, Lydia, Myself, Sammy, Jewels, Vincent, Angel, Sunny, Sweet Boo, Comfort, Precious, Jennifer, Caesar, Sage, Miss mew, Charles, and Mumbles. Those who have a big affinity for me are Minnie, March, Myself, Lydia, Caesar, Charles, and Sammy. Sinbad haunts me as my shadow, following me constantly. Minnie is one of my prime favorites and miraculously escaped the jaws of Mister Brink after we found her. Caesar loves cottage cheese and glues to me every breakfast to lick my knife, for I love bagels. Sinbad, March, and Vincent like to snuggle up to me at night on the bed. I'm certain Steffie (wife) has her favorites with her at night. I don't permit any to sleep with me for I have an allergic nose and lungs. But they are mighty stealthy and crafty. They often pilfer a spot above my pillow when I am in the arms of morpheus.

There is one chat, Bud lite, who will always be emburnished in my memory because we were constant comrades. He has departed this life but his ashes remain on my desk. It's amazing how the intensity and duration of profound true affection can develop between man and beast; akin to filial intensity. Steffie devotes unbridled attention to our felines and keeps all our household floors immaculately clean even though it is a Herculean job. An air purifier surely would be a mighty helpful right arm. As they vamoose, there will be no replacements.

Cats have inherent instinctive inborn catanysms. Daytime is their Rip Van Winkle time and night time is prime activity time. Chats are always underfoot and it takes extreme athleticism to avoid trampling on their mammoth tails. They are forever slowly strolling in front of you and by divine mental telepathy, they always know your exact destination. Feline animals are skittish and at the same time quite phlegmatic. Too bad they can't play basketball, as they can jump and leap amazingly. They exhibit remarkably unexpected behavior, such as running 100 yard dashes out of a clear blue sky. They are quite independent like a hog on ice; and nimbly float through the air like Casey. All in all they are vastly distinctive, intelligent, and gifted in their kittish way. They are as independent as a hog on ice. Ours are all neutered and licensed. Trichobezours (hairballs) in the stomach, vomiting, and diarrhea are the downside.

Chapter 44

Keyboard Maestro Kevin Cole

My original meeting with Kevin Cole was in a physician - patient relationship. Kevin was desperately sick with a third degree gastric ulcer. He was writhing with acute, unbearable epigastric pain and had lost tons of weight from nausea, vomiting, and anorexia intermittently, over a period of several months. He was athreptic and a pitiful presentation. His mother was deeply distraught and at her wits end. In spite of extensive expert medical care employing all the tricks in the medical arms bag, he had grown progressively worse. My challenge with Kevin was centered in the etiology or the whys and wherefores of his condition. These were the crux to solving his deep seated problem. After chiseling off the superficial layers of causes, which could be a host of physical or medication reasons, I discovered the bulls eye of his problem. It was rooted in his class room and his profound proclivity for a musical instrument. Kevin had an unwavering love for his piano and practiced playing it day and night with undying fervor. This penchant did not allow him recreational playtime with his fellow classmates. Therefore his comrades couldn't condone this unusual behavior for no one else of age six years was devoted so relentlessly to such adult behavioral activity. His school buddies teased and taunted Kevin relentlessly and unmercifully. As a result, he was immersed in worry, guilt, and anxiety being entirely on the defensive. He was alone and had no buffers or supports to counterattack these vicious peer attacks, like rain dropping on your head with no letup. I could understand, very easily, how he developed his stomach ulcer, and how his condition worsened gradually from the chronic onslaught of razing and mental torture.

My psychotherapy then consisted mainly in fortifying Kevin's gut and spinal counterattack to these raw insults by his peers. He was encouraged to fight fire with fire. He had done nothing wrong, and should be exceedingly proud of his accomplishments on the piano. They were just jealous. They really desired his friendship and company. I logically explained the mental situation to his mother and father, Betty and Mendell. They agreed with my sensible explanation and would pass on the solution to Kevin giving him unflagging support. We also decided to face his teacher and delineate his problem in detail to her. In turn, she could give his classmates a convincing harangue on the seriousness of Kevin's life and death battle, and the deleterious part they were playing - in other words call off the wolves. Comfort and love from everyone was of the essence in his recovery. Medication, except mild sedation, was powerless. A healthful culinary diet of all foods, especially his favorites, was the order of the day with a "go easy" on fibrous nutrients to avoid diarrhea. On this regime his Mom and yours truly slowly stemmed the tide. Over a period of a few years, we gradually succeeded in restoring Kevin's basic health and an attitude of peace with the world. Kevin continued to develop his musical, God given, prodigious abilities.

Everyone has inherent, genius qualities lying dormant but ready to be exploited if only that individual can discover his/her hidden talents. It's never too late to harvest this singular skill or the power to perform, as witness Johannes Brahms who was in his forties when his first symphony emanated. Kevin Cole has had a vast penchant and proclivity for Ira Gershwin's musical creations. He has become just about the number one interpreter and player of Ira's hallowed piano productions. He comes home to Bay City every few months to see his parents and siblings. On these occasions, he produces and performs a concert at The Players, St. Stanislaus Church, or the State Theater.

I have attended several of Kevin's magnificent concerts and always come away with a wonderful feeling, a glow of enchanting fulfillment. Joan Cummings, my Terrapin and Evangelical buddy, is hooked on Kevin's renditions. We have attended several of his concerts together. Joan missed one in December '05, at the State Theater in Saginaw so Diane Oberlies, a church acquaintance, accompanied me. Diane is a very lovely person in all attributes, who has a stately home all to herself on the country club environs. She teaches at Western High in Auburn. After this concert, I introduced Diane to Kevin and related my connection with him. Kevin was overjoyed, giving us a royal welcome. He signed his CD's for us.

Then, two days later, Joan escorted me to Kevin's identical Christmas concert in Bay City at The Players habitat on Columbus Avenue. It was a perfect day in my brief life, chock full of unique surprises. After church services, we went to Jim and Betsy Stoddard's home to bestow Christmas greetings. Lo and behold, the Stoddards gave me an unexpected present. Then we proceeded to the country club where we ate a sumptuous cornucopia of all food categories. I was tempted to have "Eggs Benedict" for the first time, but settled for my favorite, western omelet. After gorging and surfeiting by the fireplace at the country club, we killed an hour's time checking out the Christmas lights until Kevin's 3 p.m. concert at The Players. The Players was jam packed, standing room only. We had rabbit's foot luck and got seats down front with Kevin's family. As always, Cole's piano and voice rendition were elegant and superb. Towards the end of his repertoire, Kevin pulled a rabbit out of his hat and gave me a real shocker out of the clear blue. He stated, "I have composed and dedicated a song to Dr. Knobloch. He has enabled me to be alive here by his medical care; and I render my eternal thanks to him." I had a sudden tingling feeling all over of jubilation and ecstasy - and disbelief. I had to pinch myself to confirm reality, but Joan squeezed my arm for me. After the concert, I thanked him but shared the credit for his survival with his mother. On the way home, my feet hardly touched the ground for I felt like I was in the Aurora Borealis. I said to myself, be humble for God really deserves the lions share of the credit for Kevin's recovery.

Chapter 45

A Milestone - 70th Medical Reunion May, 2006

I was all a twitter and flying high in orbit while anticipating with bated breath my 70th (1936) medical school class reunion, May 5th/6th, 2006, at Davidge (John Beale) Hall, at the University of Maryland. It gave me soaring pride to know my children, #4 Melissa and #2 Tom, would be escorting me to the blessed reunion. I had been dreaming for several years of possibly attending this hallowed event, hoping I would be alive and physically fit to bring this occurrence to fruition. The alumni association at U of Md. has informed me there are 7 of us out of 98 graduates surviving, albeit with the baggage of old age infirmities. I telephoned four remaining members and they signified that they were unable to make the reunion. So, I was to be the one and only attendee from my class apparently! It saddened me immensely to ascertain that my beloved roommate for three years in medical school, Harry Clay Bowie had gone to his final reward. As I mentioned before, we were inseparable partners. We walked to classes every day, shared all our study hours, dissected the same three cadavers, and ate all our meals together. Harry was one of my <u>best</u> friends ever and we were 100% loyal and truthful to each other. We each were no nonsense, devoted 100% to medicine, and reaped the rewards of becoming honor students being in the first five in our graduating class. We had rare dates with the sweeter sex. I had a couple dates with a gorgeous blond with alabaster, peaches and cream skin, Peggy Doubleday (General Abner Doubleday's great great granddaughter). But my studies were paramount, above all, until I succumbed to fall madly in love with my wife (Doris Mathilde) in the spring of 1935. Harry had a couple dates with a comely lass, Helen Phillips, but it proceeded nowhere. Harry and I were like twin brothers, sharing our study successes, hunger pangs, sweat, blood and tears, exams, and poverty in the midst of a horrible countrywide depression. Ours was a true Damon-Pythias relationship.

Davidge Hall, where my medical classes were given, was constructed in 1807 and dedicated by the one and only Marquis De Lafayette of Revolutionary

War fame. It is the oldest teaching medical school building in the U.S.A. and Maryland is about the 5th oldest medical school in our country. The U of Md. Alumni Association planned to give a special luncheon for the 70th reunion class of '36 and the fifty year class of '56. Noteworthy events planned were a special post mortem analysis of a famous person, a crab feast, a trip to Washington DC (50 miles) to see the WWII Memorial, and an amphibious tour of historic sites in Baltimore and the Chesapeake Bay including Fort McHenry, famed for Francis Scott Key's writing of The Star Spangled Banner.

To get to the reunion, my faithful nurse, Joan, was to motor me to Flint. I was to travel to Atlanta, where Melissa would meet me at the airport. We were then on to Baltimore, where Tom's plane arrived from Vancouver B.C. within 10 minutes of ours. We were planning to stay at the Marriott Hotel in Baltimore, which is located 3 blocks from the medical school.

After all this fervent anticipation of attending my 70th medical school reunion, I was stymied by a serious, vital organ collapse resulting from probable food poisoning, a week before my planned departure. I was hospitalized by my oncologist and internal medicine physicians because of heart failure, diabetic relapse, and kidney failure. In spite of the hospitalization, it never occurred to me that I would be unable to fulfill my desire to reunite with my Maryland brothers and sisters and make the vaunted trip. My two wonderful children, Melissa and Tom, Tarzan muscle man, did almost surrender their role of escorting and wheeling me to the exalted reunion in light of my health collapse. But I knew, that as usual, being elastic I would bounce back like a rubber ball. I had always dodged my health bullets previously with celerity. And in fact, I did it again with God's help!

I traveled to Atlanta, from Flint, MI, thanks to my benevolent Terrapin friend, Joan, and picked up Melissa. We flew with ease to Baltimore, where we met Tom who planed in from Vancouver. We had a fantastic get together and great, positive relations throughout our three days of wonderful events in Lord Baltimore's own city.

Two events to remember did turn out to be the honoring of my class of '36 and the fifty year class of '56, at the Westminster Hall (burial place of noted Edgar Allen Poe); and the treatise and tribute to Booker T. Washington, preeminent African American, analyzing his life and the pre and post mortem circumstances of his death at Davidge Hall. It was a distinct pleasure for me to attend as the lone representative of my class of '36. We also had a most interesting trip to see the WWII Memorial in Washington D.C., 40 miles from Baltimore, followed by an elegant picnic lunch, and a jolly land and sea tour of the city's points of interest and the Chesapeake harbor.

On the fourth day, we toured by vehicle from Baltimore to College Park,

MD, to be treated by Alumni Director Brian Shook to a grand tour of the brand spanking new Alumni Center Building (Samuel Riggs IV). It is an indescribably well planned, practical, and organized structure of immense proportions. To my sheer delight, we were pleasantly surprised with the company of two friends and fine supporters of the University of Maryland, Ed and Marian Fry, from Chestertown MD. I had previously spent time with Ed and Marian on my visit to Chestertown in 2004. We planed from Baltimore back to Atlanta, where we arrived at Melissa and Martin's super delightful abode on Lake Arrowhead, fifty miles northeast of Atlanta, in the Smokey Mountain foothills. The setting is idyllic and heavenly; but the weather was cool and windy, as in Bay City. Indubitably, we had a most cordial stay there with our hostess with the mostest, Melissa. Melissa, pacifist, superb organizer, focuser, and chef extraordinaire served up several delicious culinary dinners. Poor Martin, a renowned nuclear physicist, had a most traumatic occurrence just before we returned to Atlanta when he slipped and jammed his right forefinger and fractured his hand necessitating a horrid cast. Tom returned to Vancouver, BC, after a four day sojourn and I returned to Bay City, MI, after a seven day visit. This excursion actually was my lifetime adventure, along with my travel to Maryland for the homecoming football game in October '04 and my trip to Europe in '05. Every event went off perfectly, like timed clockwork. Dare I plan for my 75th medical school reunion in 2011??

Like Joshua who blew down the walls of Jericho and saw the Hebrew promised land, I have in my 63 years in medicine had a glimpse of the promised land of medicine, courtesy of the Good Lord. The daily, improving medical discoveries have given me a spectacular historical ride of immense proportions. Technology in medicine is now the humongous, developing mode. I thank God profusely and now bequeath my baton to my wonderful granddaughter Sara.

Chapter 46

Conclusion

The famous classical pianist Brahms wrote his first symphony in his 50's. It seems that I have now composed my first book in my 90's. A modest analogy between Brahms and myself can be made. It is certainly true that one can start something very new and different at any age.

I feel I have thoroughly covered my life and adventures of 95+ years so far. (And still counting!) But it's now time to wrap up my autobiography and get it off to the printers. At the end of the book, I have included a collection of adages, tenets, aphorisms, and pearls of wisdom gathered from my life odyssey which may, hopefully, be somewhat enlightening for my readers. I wish good health, Godspeed, and an interesting life to all.

When I'm laid to eternal rest, I hope my epitaph will say "He was one of the good guys and a champion of children."

Adages, Tenents, Aphorisms, and Pearls of Wisdom

1. Control stress with a healthy brain.
2. Cerebral power governs physical power.
3. Church adds two years to your life.
4. Family life is numero uno.
5. Choose your parents and genes wisely.
6. Add 10 years by diet - go heavy on vegetables, fruits, grains, nuts and beans.
7. Emphasize acetyl 1, carnitine, and alpha 3 fatty acids (pecorino cheese).
8. Always forward and upward, never look back.
9. Avoid caffeine. Drink red wines in moderation.
10. Get daily quota of vitamin C.
11. Eat mono and polysaturated fats; avoid trans fats like the plague.
12. Use salt sparingly and avoid sugar. Go for pastas.
13. Good music is a tonic for the soul.
14. Be kind to your heart and liver.
15. Hard work never injured anyone.
16. Nourish the child in you for life.
17. The diabetic diet is your model.

18. Choose friends wisely in the extreme.

19. Cultivate a love spark for all time.

20. Avoid the protuberant abdomen at all costs.

21. Don't swim upstream.

22. Always be positive and don't argue.

23. Keep a song in your heart.

24. Say daily prayers and thanks for your blessings.

25. Welch's grape juice, grapefruit, and blueberries are great oxidizers.

26. Work relaxed.

27. Hit the road running.

28. To err is human; to forgive is Divine.

29. Love yourself, love your parents, love your family, and love your neighbors.

30. Get loads of sleep.

31. The best medicine is laughter.

32. Time and tide wait for no one.

33. Position in life, being in the right place at the right time, is a great positive force.

34. Take <u>special</u> care of your heart, you only have one.

35. Be kind to animals, they lead a tough life.

Photographs from the Life of

Howard T. Knobloch, M.D.

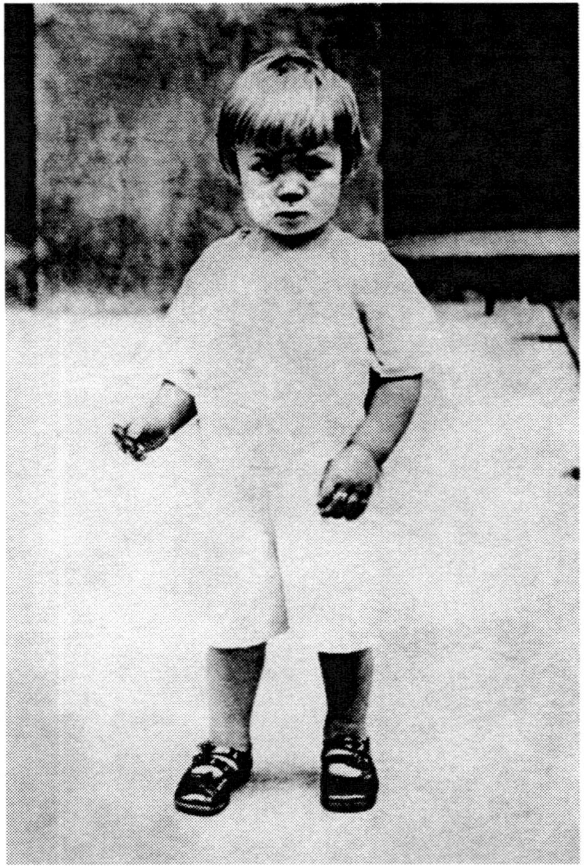

The stubborn toddler

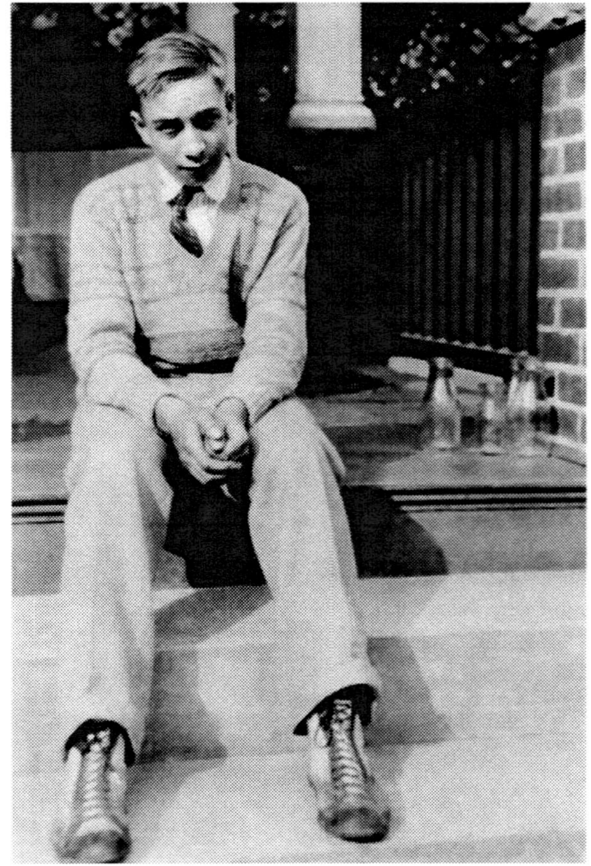

The confused teenager at home in Greensburg

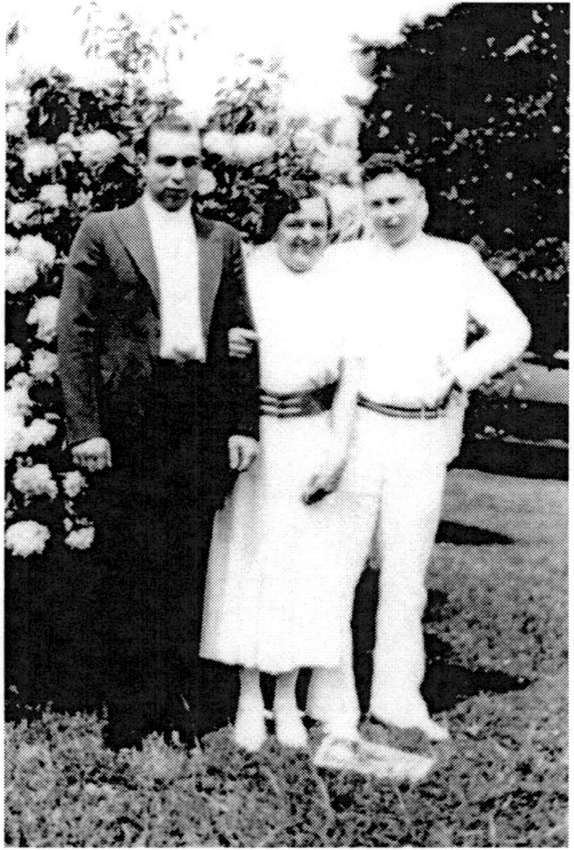

At home with mother and uncle Arthur

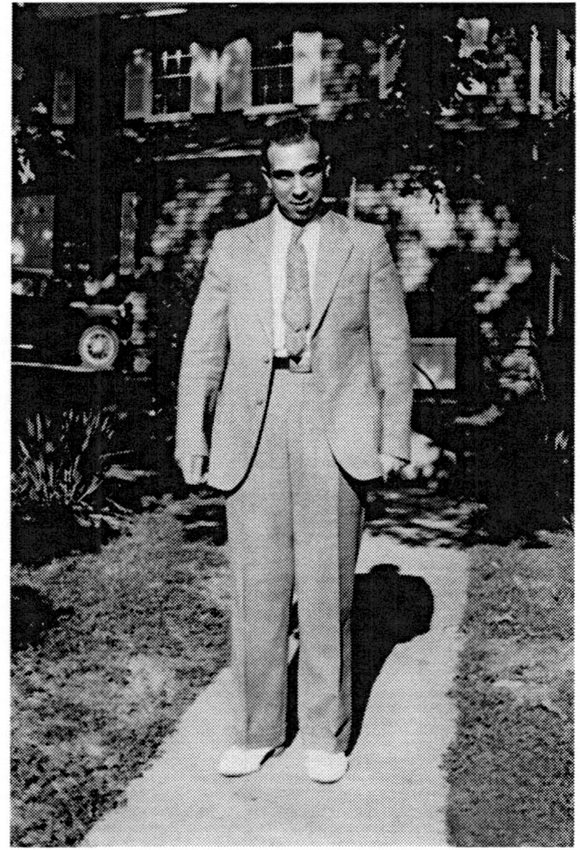

Ready for medical school

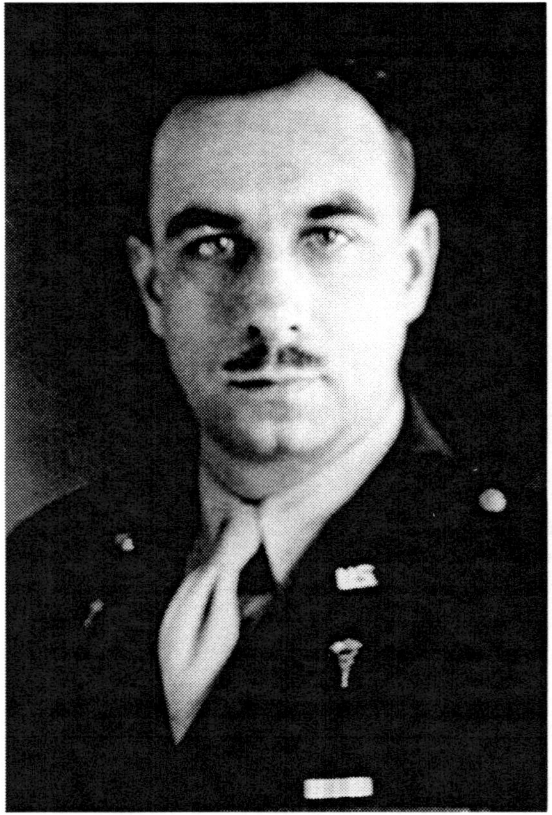

Captain Knobloch, US Army, WW II

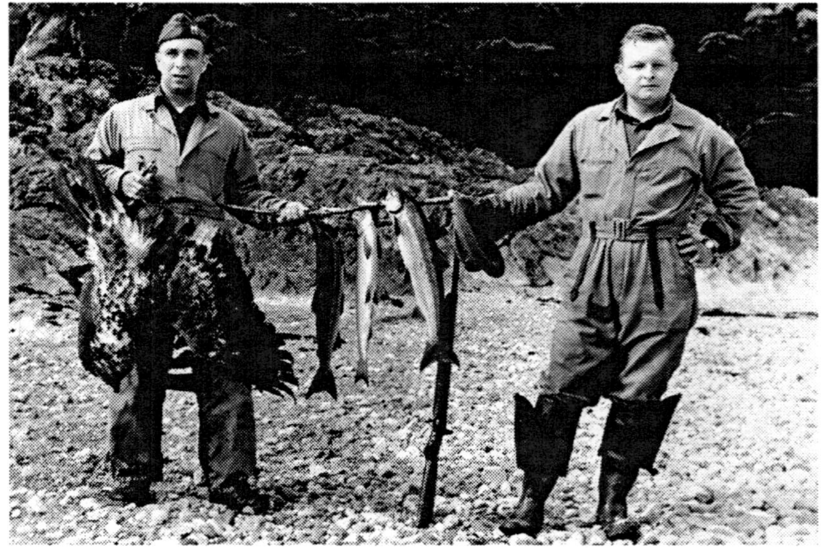

Salmon fishing on Annette Island in Alaska during Army duty

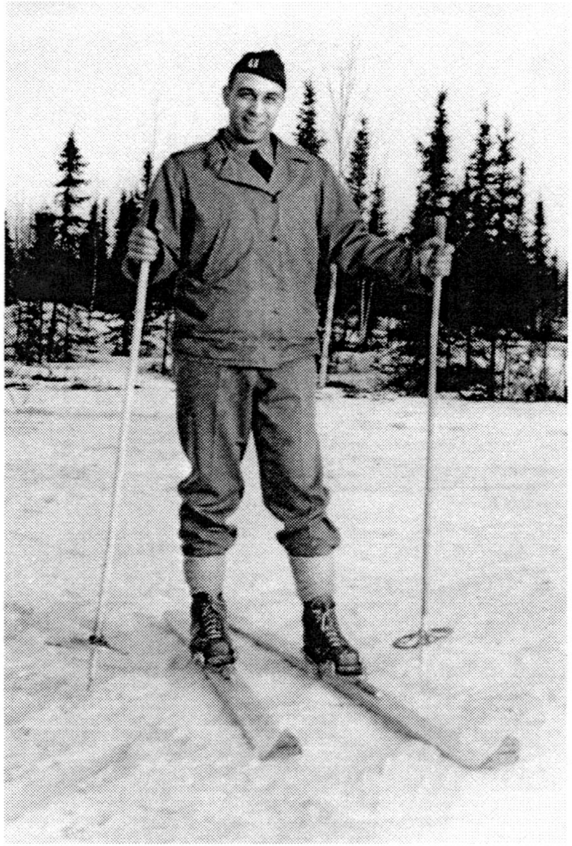

Sking at Fort Richardson in Alaska during Army duty

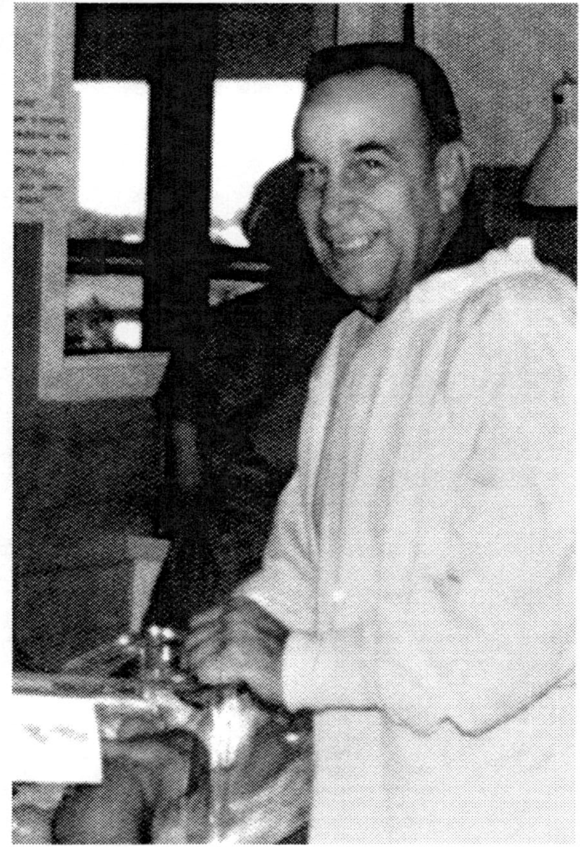

Early days of medical practice

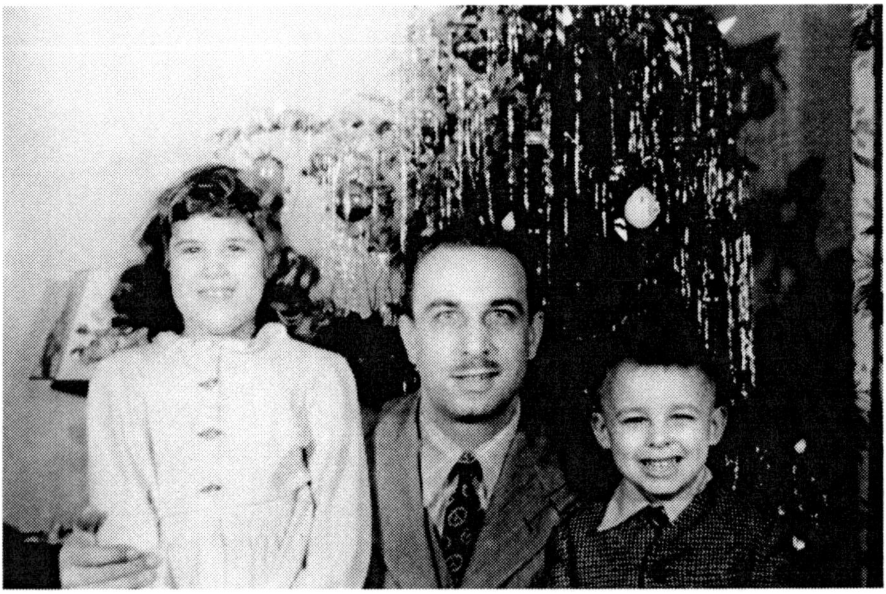

Christmas with Susan and Tom at 1911 Center Ave.

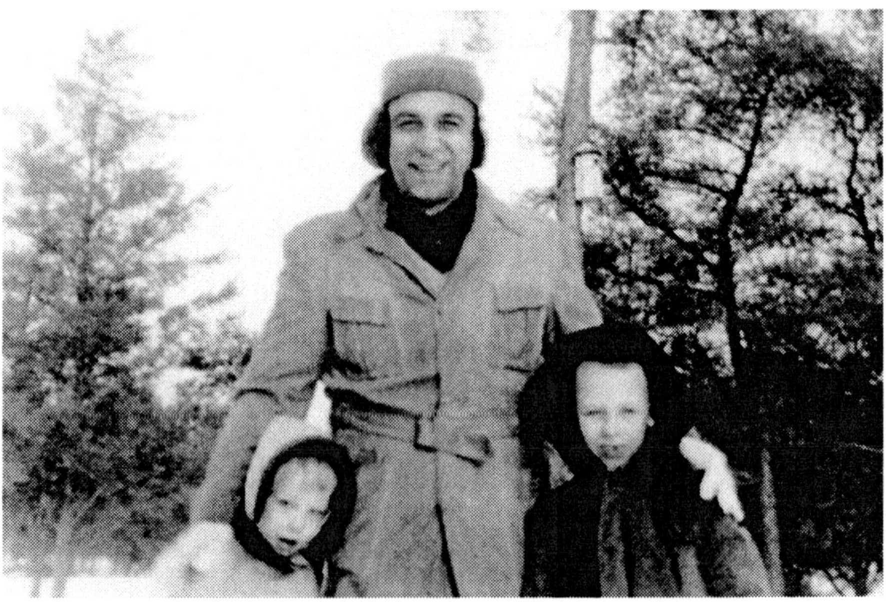

An outing with Greg and Melissa

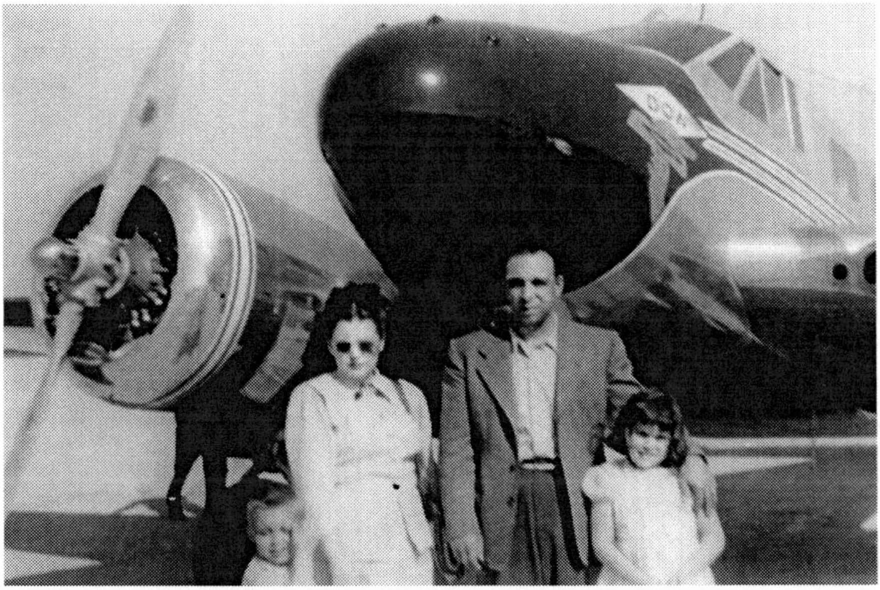

Traveling with Tom, Doris, and Susan

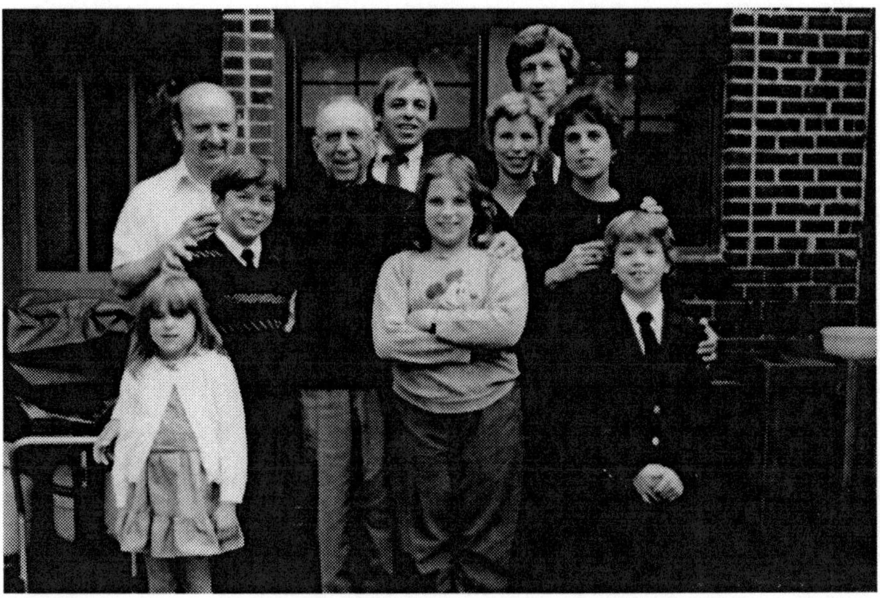

Family get-together 1984

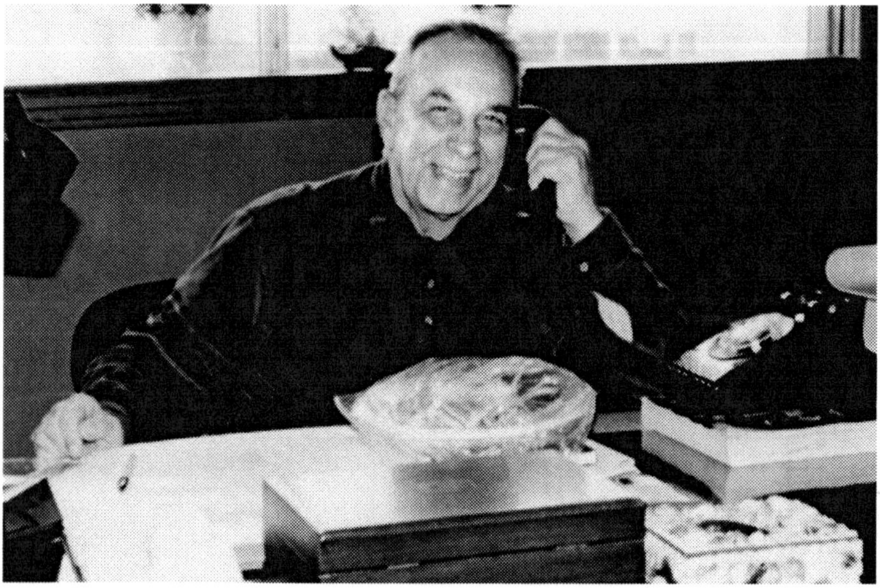

Returning patient calls from the office

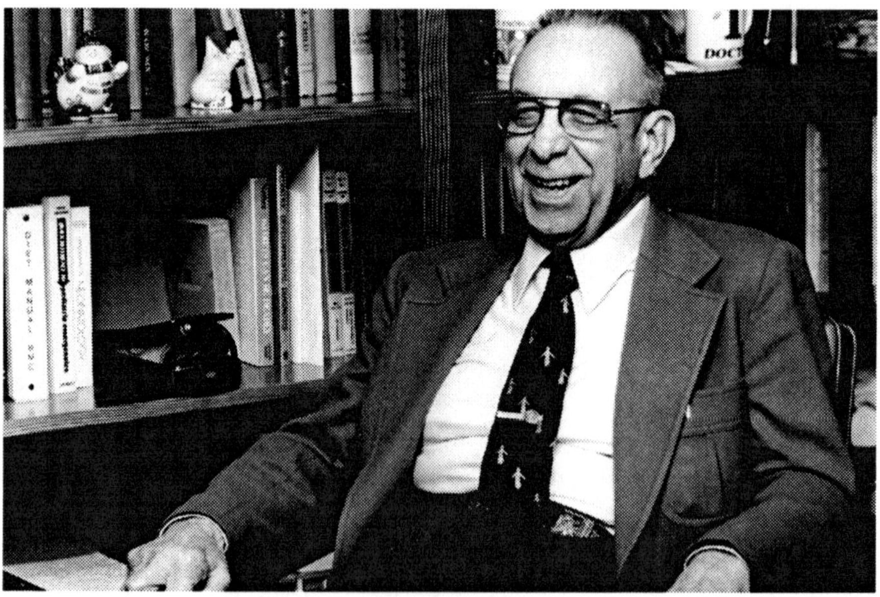

A free moment during office hours

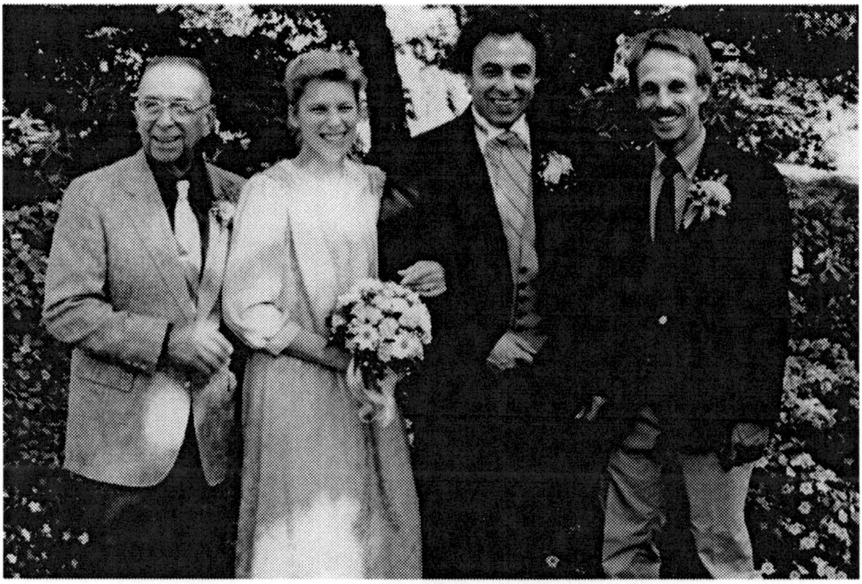

Tom's wedding 1987 in Vancouver, British Columbia

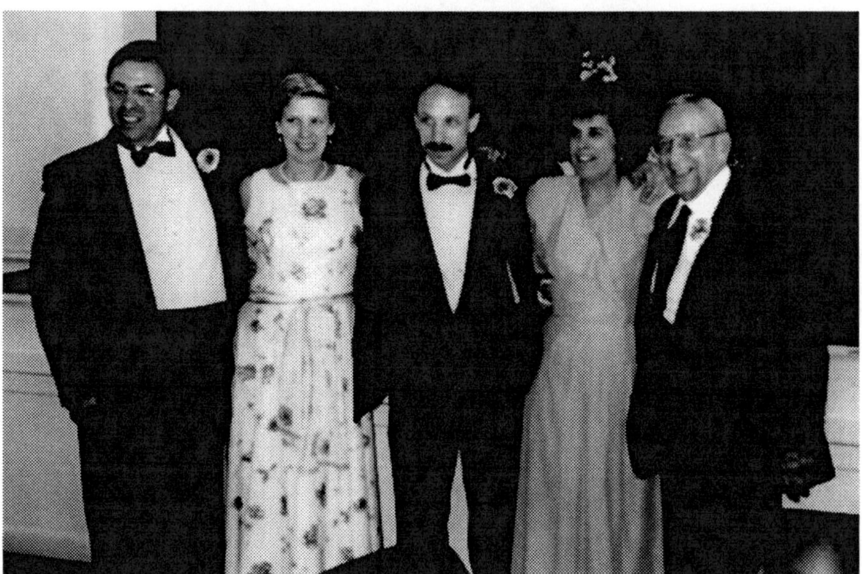

Greg's wedding 1996 in Atlanta, Georgia

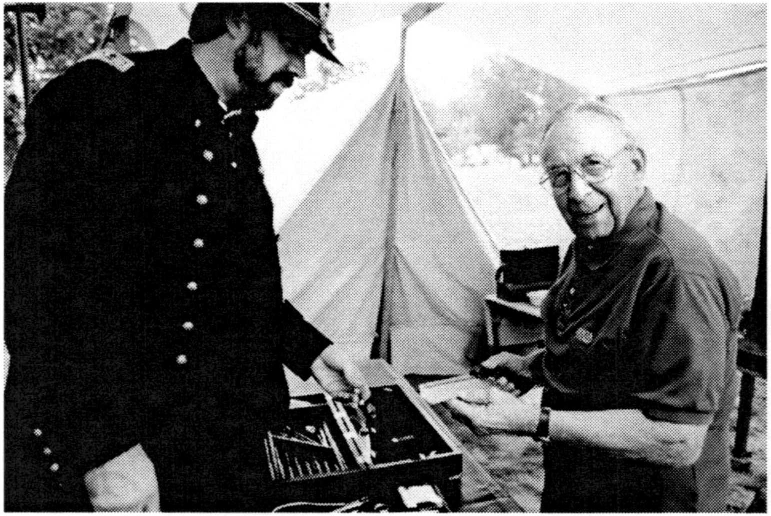

Surgeon's insturments at Civil War
Renactment In Atlanta 1993

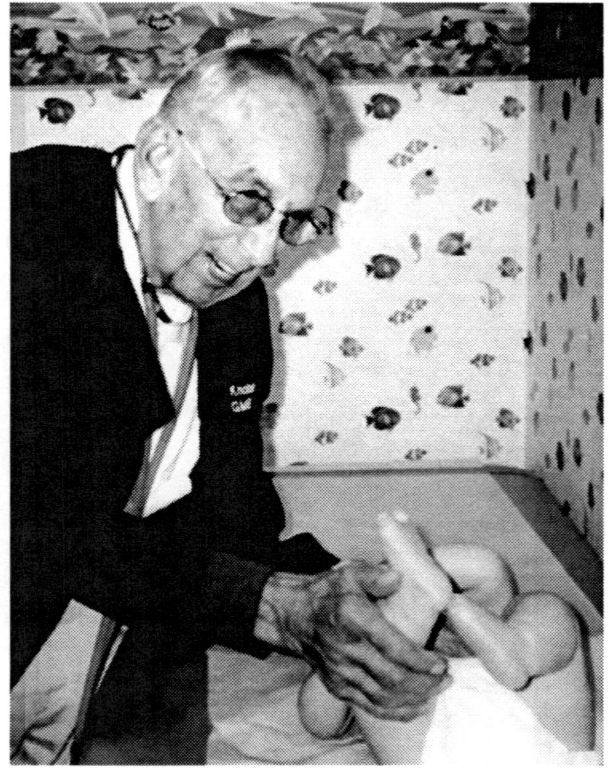

Baby examination in later years

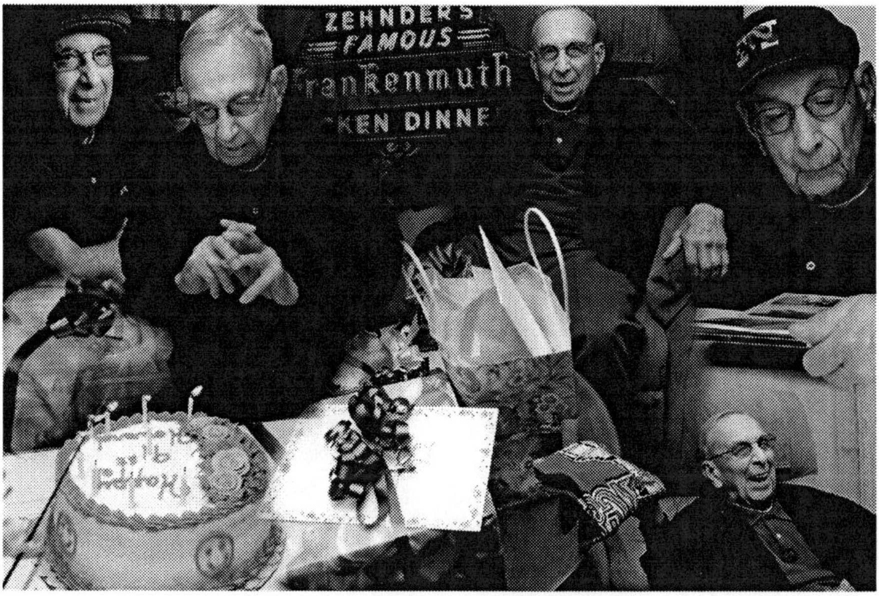

Ninetyith birthday celebration 1996

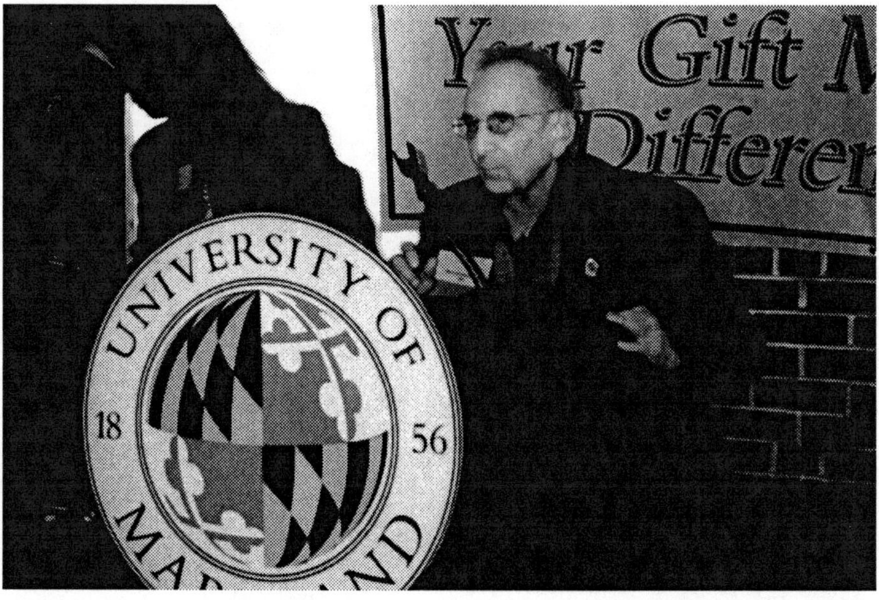

Speaking to Colenade Society at the University of Maryland 2005

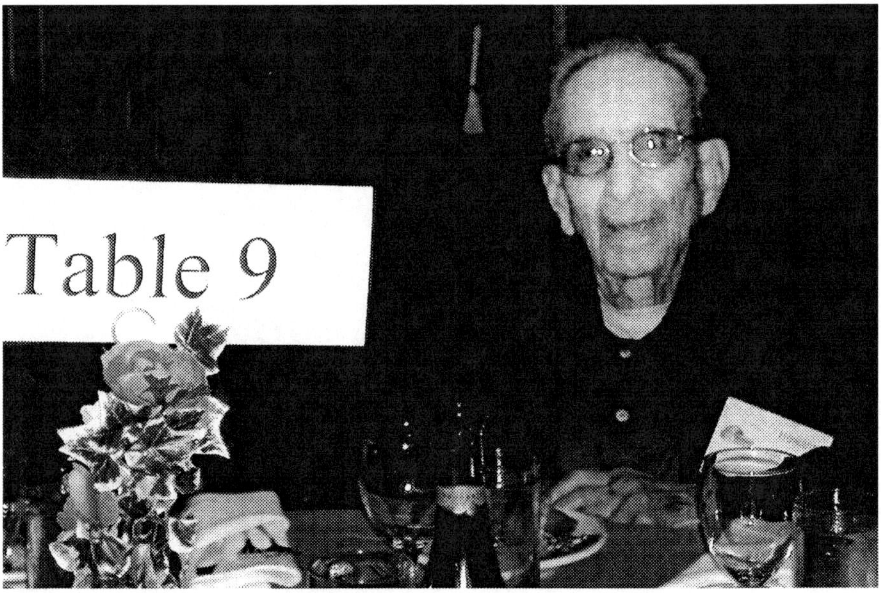

70th class reunion U of MD Medical School - Honoring Luncheon 2006 (sole delegate from class of 1936)

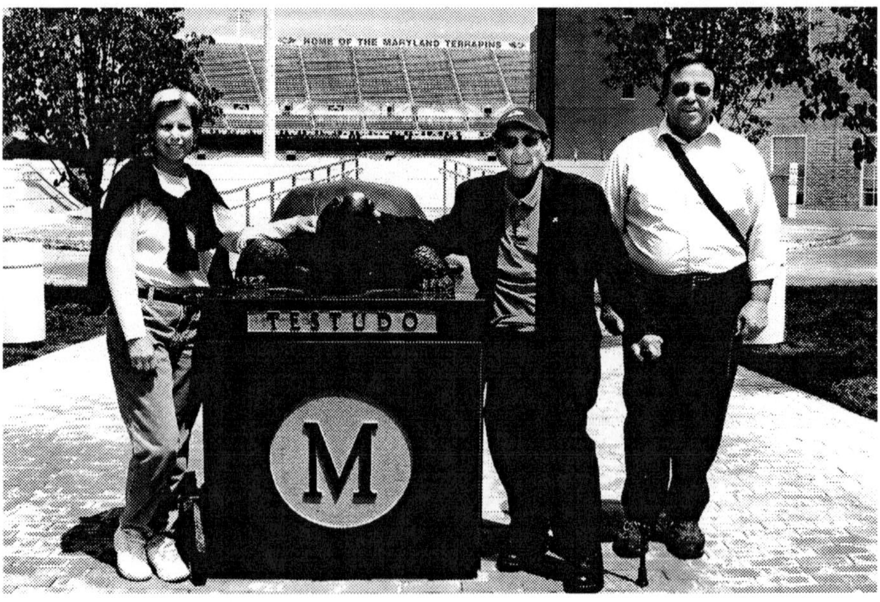

U of MD College Park Campus - Testudo 2006

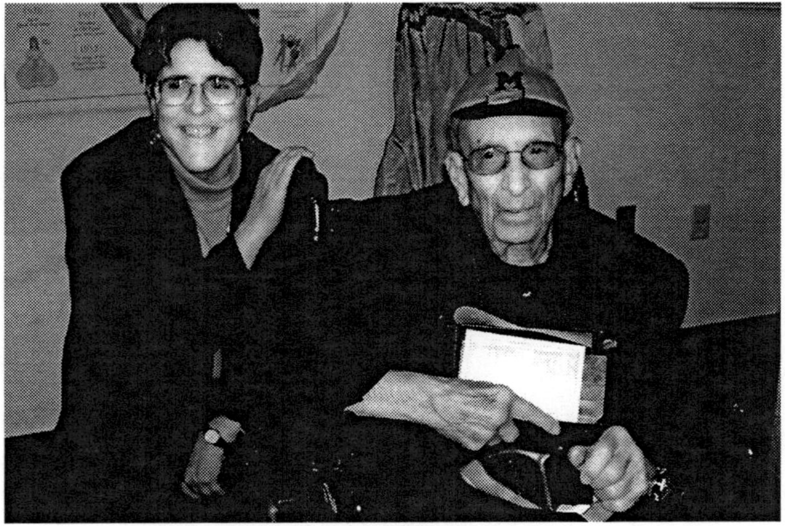

"Rat Cap" freshman year circq 1929,
U of MD Historical Exhibit 2006

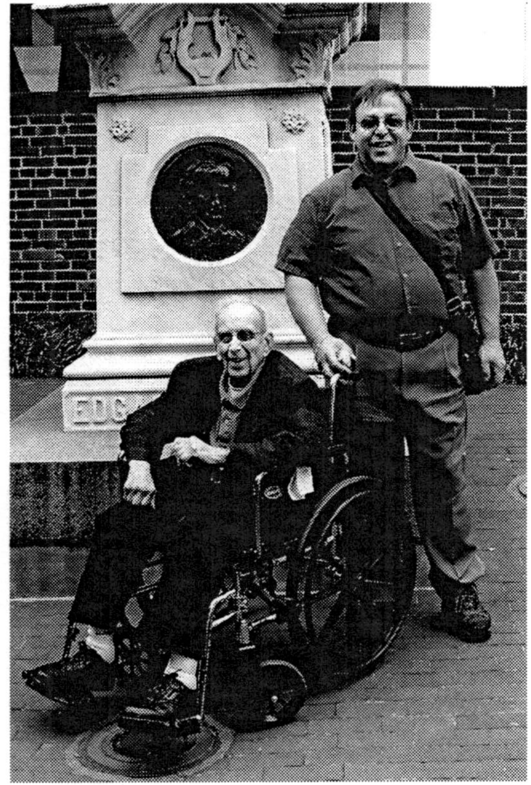

E.A. Poe's grave on Green St. in Baltimore 2006

Printed in the United States
84080LV00002B/88-189/A